Abdominal and Gastrointestinal Emergencies

Editors

AUTUMN C. GRAHAM
JOSEPH P. MARTINEZ

EMERGENCY MEDICINE CLINICS OF NORTH AMERICA

www.emed.theclinics.com

Consulting Editor
AMAL MATTU

May 2016 • Volume 34 • Number 2

ELSEVIER

1600 John F. Kennedy Boulevard • Suite 1800 • Philadelphia, Pennsylvania, 19103-2899
http://www.theclinics.com

EMERGENCY MEDICINE CLINICS OF NORTH AMERICA Volume 34, Number 2
May 2016 ISSN 0733-8627, ISBN-13: 978-0-323-44461-3

Editor: Patrick Manley
Developmental Editor: Casey Jackson

Emergency Medicine Clinics of North America (ISSN 0733-8627) is published quarterly by Elsevier Inc., 360 Park Avenue South, New York, NY, 10010-1710. Months of issue are February, May, August, and November. Business and Editorial Offices: 1600 John F. Kennedy Boulevard, Suite 1800, Philadelphia, PA 19103-2899. Customer Service Office: 6277 Sea Harbor Drive, Orlando, FL 32887-4800. Periodicals postage paid at New York, NY, and additional mailing offices. Subscription prices are $100.00 per year (US students), $320.00 per year (US individuals), $579.00 per year (US institutions), $220.00 per year (international students), $450.00 per year (international individuals), $711.00 per year (international institutions), $220.00 per year (Canadian students), $385.00 per year (Canadian individuals), and $711.00 per year (Canadian institutions). International air speed delivery is included in all *Clinics'* subscription prices. All prices are subject to change without notice. **POSTMASTER:** Send address changes to *Emergency Medicine Clinics of North America*, Elsevier Periodicals Customer Service, 11830 Westline Industrial Drive, St. Louis, MO 63146. Customer Service (orders, claims, online, change of address): Elsevier Periodicals **Customer Service, 11830 Westline Industrial Drive, St. Louis, MO 63146. Tel: 1-800-654-2452 (U.S. and Canada); 314-453-7041 (outside U.S. and Canada). Fax: 314-453-5170. E-mail: journalscustomerservice-usa@elsevier.com (for print support); journalsonlinesupport-usa@elsevier.com (for online support).**

Reprints. For copies of 100 or more of articles in this publication, please contact the Commercial Reprints Department, Elsevier Inc., 360 Park Avenue South, New York, NY 10010-1710. Tel.: 212-633-3874; Fax: 212-633-3820; E-mail: reprints@elsevier.com.

Emergency Medicine Clinics of North America is covered in *MEDLINE/PubMed (Index Medicus), Current Contents/Clinical Medicine, EMBASE/Excerpta Medica, BIOSIS, SciSearch, CINAHL, ISI/BIOMED,* and *Research Alert.*

Contributors

CONSULTING EDITOR

AMAL MATTU, MD, FAAEM, FACEP
Professor and Vice Chair, Department of Emergency Medicine, University of Maryland School of Medicine, Baltimore, Maryland

EDITORS

AUTUMN C. GRAHAM, MD
Associate Residency Program Director, Department of Emergency Medicine, MedStar Georgetown University Hospital, MedStar Washington Hospital Center Emergency Medicine Residency, Washington, DC

JOSEPH P. MARTINEZ, MD
Associate Professor, Departments of Emergency Medicine and Medicine, University of Maryland School of Medicine, Baltimore, Maryland

AUTHORS

JENNIFER AVEGNO, MD
Assistant Professor, Section of Emergency Medicine, University Medical Center, Louisiana State University Health Sciences Center, New Orleans, Louisiana

DAVID J. CARLBERG, MD
Assistant Professor of Emergency Medicine, Georgetown University School of Medicine, Washington, DC

MATTHEW CARLISLE, MD, MAS
Assistant Professor, Section of Emergency Medicine, University Medical Center, Louisiana State University Health Sciences Center, New Orleans, Louisiana

SHARMISTHA DEV, MD, MPH
Departments of Emergency Medicine and Internal Medicine, University of Michigan, Ann Arbor, Michigan

JEFFREY S. DUBIN, MD, MBA
Chair, Department of Emergency Medicine, MedStar Washington Hospital Center; Associate Professor of Clinical Emergency Medicine, Georgetown University School of Medicine, Washington, DC

SEAN M. FOX, MD, FACEP, FAAP
Associate Professor, Assistant Program Director, Emergency Medicine Residency Program, Department of Emergency Medicine, Carolinas Medical Center, Charlotte, North Carolina

ALEXA R. GALE, MD
Attending Physician, Department of Emergency Medicine, MedStar Washington Hospital Center, Washington, DC

AUTUMN C. GRAHAM, MD
Associate Residency Program Director, Department of Emergency Medicine, MedStar Georgetown University Hospital, MedStar Washington Hospital Center Emergency Medicine Residency, Washington, DC

ALEX KOYFMAN, MD
Clinical Assistant Professor of Emergency Medicine, UT Southwestern Medical Center, Parkland Memorial Hospital, Dallas, Texas

JERRY LEE, MD
Emergency Medicine Resident, Division of Emergency Medicine, Duke University Medical Center, Durham, North Carolina

STEPHEN D. LEE, MD
Assistant Professor of Emergency Medicine, University of Maryland School of Medicine, Baltimore, Maryland

AMY LEUTHAUSER, MD, MS, FACEP
Consultant, Department of Emergency Medicine, Bay of Plenty District Health Board, Tauranga Hospital, Tauranga, New Zealand

KYLE D. LEWIS, MD
Department of Emergency Medicine, University of Texas Medical School at Houston, Houston, Texas

SAMUEL D. LUBER, MD, MPH
Associate Professor, Department of Emergency Medicine, University of Texas Medical School at Houston, Houston, Texas

ABRAHAM MARKIN, MD
Departments of Emergency Medicine and Internal Medicine, Henry Ford Hospital, Detroit, Michigan

JOSEPH P. MARTINEZ, MD
Associate Professor, Departments of Emergency Medicine and Medicine, University of Maryland School of Medicine, Baltimore, Maryland

JONATHAN McKEAN, MD
Clinical Instructor, Department of Emergency Medicine, University of Cincinnati College of Medicine, Cincinnati, Ohio

BENJAMIN McVANE, MD
Resident, Department of Emergency Medicine, Icahn School of Medicine, Mount Sinai Hospital, New York, New York

JOSE V. NABLE, MD, MS, NRP
Department of Emergency Medicine, MedStar Georgetown University Hospital, Assistant Professor of Emergency Medicine, Georgetown University School of Medicine, Washington, DC

JUMANA NAGARWALA, MD
Assistant Residency Director, Department of Emergency Medicine, Henry Ford Hospital; Assistant Clinical Professor, Department of Emergency Medicine, Wayne State University School of Medicine, Detroit, Michigan

SREEJA NATESAN, MD
Assistant Professor, Division of Emergency Medicine, Duke University Medical Center, Durham, North Carolina

JESSICA PALMER, MD
Department of Emergency Medicine, MedStar Washington Hospital Center, Washington, DC

JOHN C. PERKINS Jr, MD
Assistant Program Director, Virginia Tech Carilion Emergency Medicine Residency, Department of Emergency Medicine, Assistant Professor of Emergency and Internal Medicine, Virginia Tech Carilion School of Medicine, Roanoke, Virginia

THUY VAN PHAM, MD
Assistant Professor, Department of Emergency Medicine, University of Maryland School of Medicine, Baltimore, Maryland

ELIZABETH PONTIUS, MD, RDMS
Assistant Professor of Emergency Medicine, Georgetown University School of Medicine; Department of Emergency Medicine, MedStar Washington Hospital Center, Washington, DC

PATRICK ROBINSON, MD
Emergency Medicine Resident, Virginia Tech Carilion Emergency Medicine Residency, Department of Emergency Medicine, Roanoke, Virginia

SARAH RONAN-BENTLE, MD, MS
Assistant Professor, Department of Emergency Medicine, University of Cincinnati College of Medicine, Cincinnati, Ohio

MANPREET SINGH, MD
Health Sciences Clinical Instructor and Ultrasound Fellow, Department of Emergency Medicine, Harbor-UCLA Medical Center, Torrance, California

JEREMIAH SMITH, MD, FAAP
Pediatric Emergency Medicine Fellow, Department of Emergency Medicine, Carolinas Medical Center, Charlotte, North Carolina

KATRIN Y. TAKENAKA, MD, MEd
Associate Professor, Department of Emergency Medicine, University of Texas Medical School at Houston, Houston, Texas

TRACI THOUREEN, MD
Assistant Professor and Director of Simulation, Division of Emergency Medicine, Duke University Medical Center, Durham, North Carolina

CHRISTINA LYNN TUPE, MD
Assistant Professor, Department of Emergency Medicine, University of Maryland School of Medicine, Baltimore, Maryland

HEATHER VOLKAMER, MD
Emergency Medicine Resident, Division of Emergency Medicine, Duke University Medical Center, Durham, North Carolina

MATTHEW WILSON, MD
Attending Physician, Department of Emergency Medicine, MedStar Washington Hospital Center, Washington, DC

Contents

can cause peritoneal and retroperitoneal symptoms. Evaluation and management of lower intestinal disease requires a nuanced approach by the emergency physician, sometimes requiring computed tomography, ultrasonography, MRI, layered imaging, shared decision making, serial examination, and/or close follow-up. Once a presumed or confirmed diagnosis is made, appropriate treatment is initiated, and may include surgery, antibiotics, and/or steroids. Appendicitis patients should be admitted. Diverticulitis and inflammatory bowel disease can frequently be managed on an outpatient basis, but may require admission and surgical consultation.

Patients commonly present to the emergency department with anorectal complaints. Most of these complaints are benign and can be managed conservatively; however, there are a few anorectal emergencies that clinicians must be aware of in order to prevent further complications. The history and physical examination are especially important so that critical disorders can be recognized and specific treatment plans can be determined. It is important to maintain a broad differential diagnosis of anorectal disease and to distinguish benign from serious processes.

Vomiting and abdominal pain are common in patients in the emergency department. This article focuses on small bowel obstruction (SBO), cyclic vomiting, and gastroparesis. Through early diagnosis and appropriate management, the morbidity and mortality associated with SBOs can be significantly reduced. Management of SBOs involves correction of physiologic and electrolyte disturbances, bowel rest and removing the source of the obstruction. Treatment of acute cyclic vomiting is primarily directed at symptom control, volume and electrolyte repletion, and appropriate specialist follow-up. The mainstay of therapy for gastroparesis is metoclopramide.

Diarrhea generates a wide range of diagnostic considerations and has profound individual and public health significance. The setting and circumstances under which a patient presents with diarrhea drastically influences the concern brought to the encounter. Nausea, vomiting, and diarrhea are often provisionally labeled "gastroenteritis" with appropriate expectant management. In resource-poor countries, the significance of diarrhea is even greater. This review focuses on diarrhea and its initial evaluation and management in the emergency department.

Acute gastrointestinal bleeding is a commonly encountered chief complaint with a high morbidity and mortality. The emergency physician is challenged with prompt diagnosis, accurate risk assessment, and appropriate resuscitation of patients with gastrointestinal bleeding. Goals of care aim to prevent end-organ injury, manage comorbid illnesses, identify the source of bleeding, stop continued bleeding, support oxygen carrying capacity, and prevent rebleeding. This article reviews current strategies for risk stratification, diagnostic modalities, localization of bleeding, transfusion strategies, adjunct therapies, and reversal of anticoagulation.

Abdominal vascular catastrophes are among the most challenging and time sensitive for emergency practitioners to recognize. Mesenteric ischemia remains a highly lethal entity for which the history and physical examination can be misleading. Laboratory tests are often unhelpful, and appropriate imaging must be quickly obtained. A multidisciplinary approach is required to have a positive impact on mortality rates. Ruptured abdominal aortic aneurysm likewise may present in a cryptic fashion. A specific type of ruptured aneurysm, the aortoenteric fistula, often masquerades as the more common routine gastrointestinal bleed. The astute clinician recognizes that this is a more lethal variant of gastrointestinal hemorrhage.

Abdominal pain is a common complaint that leads to pediatric patients seeking emergency care. The emergency care provider has the arduous task of determining which child likely has a benign cause and not missing the devastating condition that needs emergent attention. This article reviews common benign causes of abdominal pain as well as some of the cannot-miss emergent causes.

Abdominal pain in the elderly can be a challenging and difficult condition to diagnose and treat. The geriatric population has significant comorbidities and often takes polypharmacy that can mask symptoms. The presentation of common conditions can be different than that in the younger population, often lacking the traditional indicators of disease, making it of pivotal importance for the clinician to consider a wide differential during their workup. It is also important to consider extra-abdominal abnormality that may manifest as abdominal pain.

Patients with human immunodeficiency virus, those who are posttransplant, and those undergoing chemotherapy are populations who are immunocompromised and present to the emergency department with abdominal pain related to their disease processes, opportunistic infections, and complications of treatment. Emergency department practitioners must maintain vigilance, as the physical examination is often unreliable in these patients. Cross-sectional imaging and early treatment of symptoms with aggressive resuscitation is often required.

EMERGENCY MEDICINE
CLINICS OF NORTH AMERICA

THE CLINICS ARE NOW AVAILABLE ONLINE!
Access your subscription at:
www.theclinics.com

PROGRAM OBJECTIVE

The goal of *Emergency Medicine Clinics of North America* is to keep practicing emergency medicine physicians and emergency medicine residents up to date with current clinical practice in emergency medicine by providing timely articles reviewing the state of the art in patient care.

LEARNING OBJECTIVES

Upon completion of this activity, participants will be able to:
1. Review the relationship between the opioid epidemic in the United States and related gastrointestinal issues.
2. Recognize different causes of acute gastrointestinal pain.
3. Discuss the evaluation of gastrointestinal pain by abdominal quadrant.

ACCREDITATION

The Elsevier Office of Continuing Medical Education (EOCME) is accredited by the Accreditation Council for Continuing Medical Education (ACCME) to provide continuing medical education for physicians.

The EOCME designates this enduring material for a maximum of 15 *AMA PRA Category 1 Credit*(s)™. Physicians should claim only the credit commensurate with the extent of their participation in the activity.

All other health care professionals requesting continuing education credit for this enduring material will be issued a certificate of participation.

DISCLOSURE OF CONFLICTS OF INTEREST

The EOCME assesses conflict of interest with its instructors, faculty, planners, and other individuals who are in a position to control the content of CME activities. All relevant conflicts of interest that are identified are thoroughly vetted by EOCME for fair balance, scientific objectivity, and patient care recommendations. EOCME is committed to providing its learners with CME activities that promote improvements or quality in healthcare and not a specific proprietary business or a commercial interest.

The planning committee, staff, authors and editors listed below have identified no financial relationships or relationships to products or devices they or their spouse/life partner have with commercial interest related to the content of this CME activity:

Jennifer Avegno, MD; David J. Carlberg, MD; Matthew Carlisle, MD, MAS; Sharmistha Dev, MD, MPH; Jeffrey S. Dubin, MD, MBA; Anjali Fortna; Sean M. Fox, MD, FACEP, FAAP; Alexa R. Gale, MD; Autumn C. Graham, MD; Hong K. Kim, MD, MPH; Alex Koyfman, MD; Indu Kumari; Stephen D. Lee, MD; Jerry Lee, MD; Amy Leuthauser, MD, MS, FACEP; Kyle D. Lewis, MD; Samuel D. Luber, MD, MPH; Patrick Manley; Darren P. Mareiniss, MD, JD; Abraham Markin, MD; Joseph P. Martinez, MD; Amal Mattu, MD, FAAEM, FACEP; Jonathan McKean, MD; Benjamin Mcvane, MD; Jose V. Nable, MD, MS, NRP; Jumana Nagarwala, MD; Sreeja Natesan, MD; Jessica Palmer, MD; John C. Perkins, Jr, MD; Thuy Van Pham, MD; Elizabeth Pontius, MD, RDMS; Patrick Robinson, MD; Sarah Ronan-Bentle, MD, MS; Erin Scheckenbach; Manpreet Singh, MD; Jeremiah Smith, MD, FAAP; Katrin Y. Takenaka, MD, MEd; Traci Thoureen, MD; Christina Lynn Tupe, MD; Heather Volkamer, MD; Richard Gentry Wilkerson, MD; Matthew Wilson, MD; Thomas Andrew Windsor, MD, RDMS.

UNAPPROVED/OFF-LABEL USE DISCLOSURE

The EOCME requires CME faculty to disclose to the participants:
1. When products or procedures being discussed are off-label, unlabelled, experimental, and/or investigational (not US Food and Drug Administration [FDA] approved); and
2. Any limitations on the information presented, such as data that are preliminary or that represent ongoing research, interim analyses, and/or unsupported opinions. Faculty may discuss information about pharmaceutical agents that is outside of FDA-approved labelling. This information is intended solely for CME and is not intended to promote off-label use of these medications. If you have any questions, contact the medical affairs department of the manufacturer for the most recent prescribing information.

TO ENROLL

To enroll in the *Emergency Medicine Clinics* Continuing Medical Education program, call customer service at 1-800-654-2452 or sign up online at http://www.theclinics.com/home/cme. The CME program is available to subscribers for an additional annual fee of $235 USD.

METHOD OF PARTICIPATION

In order to claim credit, participants must complete the following:

1. Complete enrolment as indicated above.
2. Read the activity.
3. Complete the CME Test and Evaluation. Participants must achieve a score of 70% on the test. All CME Tests and Evaluations must be completed online.

CME INQUIRIES/SPECIAL NEEDS

For all CME inquiries or special needs, please contact elsevierCME@elsevier.com.

Foreword

"Oh, My Aching Belly!"

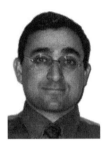

Amal Mattu, MD, FAAEM, FACEP
Consulting Editor

Anyone who works in acute care medicine knows that abdominal pain is one of the most common complaints among patients. If one looks at the differential diagnosis for abdominal pain, it becomes obvious why so many patients experience this complaint: there are numerous conditions that produce abdominal pain, including many nonspecific conditions (eg, stress, dehydration), many common conditions (eg, pharyngitis, viral illness), and many extra-abdominal conditions (eg, pneumonia, urinary tract infection). It almost seems that the abdomen is a final common pathway for almost all medical conditions, mild to severe!

A further challenge to this chief complaint is that many entities in the differential diagnosis are rapidly fatal if not diagnosed and treated quickly. The classic emergency mantra of "rule out worst first" is critical when caring for patients with abdominal pain. The astute clinician must consider vascular causes both inside (eg, aortic disasters, mesenteric ischemia) and outside (eg, acute myocardial infarction) the abdomen first and then gradually work backward toward the benign diagnoses. Unfortunately, this process can be time-consuming, and dangerous diagnoses can be easily overlooked. I often refer to the abdomen as the true "black box" of the human body, where danger often lurks unseen, hidden among a multitude of organs that conspire to fool you! My own paranoia, I'll admit, is based on the two most memorable cases of my career in which intra-abdominal disasters were initially missed by us all and resulted in poor outcomes.

A thorough read of this issue of *Emergency Medicine Clinics of North America* is sure to help you avoid such unfortunate outcomes. In this issue, Guest Editors Drs Autumn Graham and Joseph Martinez have assembled an outstanding group of authors who address all of the major acute concerns of the abdomen. The chief complaint of abdominal pain itself is addressed in not one but *eight* articles. These articles address special populations, such as pediatric patients, immunocompromised patients, post-bariatric surgery patients, and elderly patients. Nonspecific common complaints, such as vomiting and diarrhea, are addressed, and less common but deadly

Emerg Med Clin N Am 34 (2016) xv–xvi
http://dx.doi.org/10.1016/j.emc.2016.02.002
0733-8627/16/$ – see front matter © 2016 Published by Elsevier Inc.

conditions, such as vascular emergencies, also receive their due attention. The article on gastrointestinal bleeding discusses advances in therapies and also potential discharge of low-risk patients. A final article addressing anorectal complaints finishes off the "top-to-bottom" approach that this group of authors has taken.

This issue is an invaluable addition to the *Emergency Medicine Clinics of North America* series. It represents a fairly comprehensive curriculum in abdominal and gastrointestinal emergencies. The guest editors and authors are to be commended for shedding some additional light on the true black box of the human body. I have no doubt that the reader will gain confidence in his or her approach to these challenging conditions, and lives will be saved!

Amal Mattu, MD, FAAEM, FACEP
Department of Emergency Medicine
University of Maryland School of Medicine
Baltimore, MD 21201, USA

E-mail address:
amalmattu@comcast.net

Preface

Abdominal and Gastrointestinal Emergencies

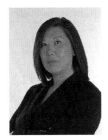 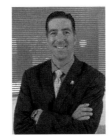

Autumn C. Graham, MD   Joseph P. Martinez, MD
Editors

Abdominal pain remains one of the most common reasons for an acute visit to a health care professional. While many patients will not receive a specific diagnosis as the cause of their symptoms, a systematic approach to each patient is imperative as life-threatening processes present with gastrointestinal complaints. In this issue of *Emergency Medicine Clinics of North America*, we have brought together a group of articles that provides such a systematic approach. Many of us approach the abdomen in an anatomic fashion, considering the abdomen as a series of interconnected boxes that house unique disease pathology with localizing symptoms. This issue has articles divided in just such a manner. In addition, we have dedicated articles to common symptom presentations, such as vomiting, diarrhea, or gastrointestinal hemorrhage. As previously mentioned, the abdomen houses a number of life-threatening conditions. One article delves into the vascular catastrophes, those conditions that require action that is measured in minutes rather than hours or days. Special populations are discussed as well, including pediatric patients, geriatric patients, immunocompromised patients, and those patients that have undergone bariatric surgery. Today's expert clinicians are expected to practice medicine in an evidence-based fashion. With this thought in mind, we have added an article on the evidence-based approach to a patient with abdominal pain. Keeping in mind the age-old adage that "the diaphragm is not a brick wall," we have also included an article on nonabdominal causes of abdominal pain. It has been our privilege assembling this talented group of authors. We have learned a tremendous amount through their efforts, and it is our hope that you will as well.

Emerg Med Clin N Am 34 (2016) xvii–xviii
http://dx.doi.org/10.1016/j.emc.2016.02.001
0733-8627/16/$ – see front matter © 2016 Published by Elsevier Inc.

emed.theclinics.com

Autumn C. Graham, MD
Georgetown University Hospital/
Medstar Washington Hospital Center
Emergency Medicine Residency
Department of Emergency Medicine
3800 Reservoir Road NW
Washington, DC 20007, USA

Joseph P. Martinez, MD
Departments of Emergency Medicine and Medicine
University of Maryland School of Medicine
685 West Baltimore Street, HSF-1
Room 150
Baltimore, MD 21201, USA

E-mail addresses:
autumn.graham@medstar.net (A.C. Graham)
jmartinez@som.umaryland.edu (J.P. Martinez)

Evidence-Based Medicine Approach to Abdominal Pain

Sreeja Natesan, MD*, Jerry Lee, MD, Heather Volkamer, MD,
Traci Thoureen, MD

KEYWORDS

- Evidence-based medicine • Abdominal pain • Approach to abdominal pain
- Abdomen • EBM approach

KEY POINTS

- A systematic approach to evaluating abdominal pain can provide patients with efficient and accurate care.
- A thorough history to localize the abdominal pain and associated symptoms can help to create a differential diagnosis.
- The cough test, inspiration test, and peritonitis test can help to determine if a patient has a concerning abdominal examination.
- Bedside ultrasound and upright plain radiograph are of utility in an unstable patient to determine the cause of the abdominal pain.
- Pain medication should not be withheld in a patient presenting with abdominal pain.

INTRODUCTION

The chief complaint of abdominal pain accounts for 5% to 10% of all presentations in the emergency department (ED).[1] With such broad differential and diagnostic modalities available, a systematic approach to evaluating abdominal pain is essential to provide patients with efficient and accurate care. Using evidence-based principles, the approach to abdominal pain can be simplified.

HISTORY OF PRESENTING ILLNESS

The history of presenting illness is arguably the single most important part in the evaluation of a patient with abdominal pain. History and physical examination alone were able to determine between organic and nonorganic causes of abdominal pain in 79%

Disclosure statement: none.
Division of Emergency Medicine, Duke University Medical Center, 2301 Erwin Road Duke North, Suite 2600, Durham, NC 27710, USA
* Corresponding author.
E-mail address: Sreeja.natesan@dm.duke.edu

Emerg Med Clin N Am 34 (2016) 165–190
http://dx.doi.org/10.1016/j.emc.2015.12.008
0733-8627/16/$ – see front matter Published by Elsevier Inc.

emed.theclinics.com

of patients.[2] Another study demonstrated that a careful history alone can lead to the correct diagnosis in up to 76% of cases.[3] Several key characteristics of a patient's history can help guide the differential diagnosis.

Onset

The timing of patients' pain can help determine acuity, progression of symptoms, and likelihood of emergent cause. Acute severe pain is more likely to be associated with serious, emergent cause, such as ruptured abdominal aortic aneurysm (AAA), mesenteric ischemia, and bowel perforation.[4] A large retrospective and prospective study demonstrated this when most of the patients with a perforated peptic ulcer presented within 12 hours of symptom onset.[5] More insidious pain correlates with a developing inflammatory or infectious pathologic conditions, such as cholecystitis, appendicitis, or small bowel obstruction (SBO).[6] An example was found in one study demonstrated most patients with appendicitis presenting at 12 to 23 hours of symptoms onset and most patients with diverticulitis presenting after 48 hours.[5]

Location

Location of pain is a key part in determining the affected organs. Understanding the embryologic derivation of the gastrointestinal organs can help the examiner narrow down a differential. Localized pain in the epigastrium is highly specific for diseases of the foregut structures, including the stomach, pancreas, liver, and proximal duodenum.[7] Periumbilical pain is 99% specific for diseases of the midgut region or intestine,[7] including the remaining small bowel, proximal third of the colon, and the appendix. Finally, localized suprapubic pain is associated with the hindgut organs or the remaining two-thirds of the colon, the bladder, and the genitourinary organs.[6] **Table 1** demonstrates potential differential diagnosis based on the information obtained from the history of presenting illness.[8]

Table 1
Differential diagnosis based on location of abdominal pain

Location	Differential Diagnosis
RUQ	*Biliary:* cholecystitis, cholelithiasis, cholangitis *Hepatic:* hepatitis, hepatic abscess *Others:* pneumonia, pulmonary embolism, pancreatitis, peptic ulcer disease, retrocecal appendicitis
LUQ	*Splenic:* splenic infarct, splenic laceration *Cardiac:* myocardial infarction, pericarditis *Others:* pneumonia, pulmonary embolism, pancreatitis, peptic ulcer disease, diaphragmatic hernia
Epigastric	*Gastric:* peptic ulcer disease, gastritis *Pancreatic:* pancreatitis *Biliary:* cholecystitis, cholelithiasis, cholangitis
RLQ	*Colonic:* appendicitis, cecal diverticulitis, cecal volvulus *Genitourinary:* nephrolithiasis, ovarian torsion, PID, ectopic pregnancy, testicular torsion, inguinal hernia *Others:* mesenteric adenitis
LLQ	*Colonic:* sigmoid diverticulitis *Genitourinary:* nephrolithiasis, ovarian torsion, PID, ectopic pregnancy, testicular torsion, inguinal hernia *Others:* abdominal aortic aneurysm

Abbreviations: LLQ, left lower quadrant; LUQ, left upper quadrant; PID, pelvic inflammatory disease; RLQ, right lower quadrant; RUQ, right upper quadrant.

Furthermore, many abdominal pain diagnoses are associated with a typical location of pain. For example, right lower quadrant pain has proven to be highly sensitive for appendicitis,[9] whereas right upper quadrant pain is highly sensitive for cholecystitis.[10] Both right lower quadrant pain and right upper quadrant pain are only moderately specific for appendicitis and cholecystitis, respectively, as there are other processes that can manifest in these areas. Left lower quadrant pain is highly associated with diverticulitis.[11] Finally, a study on bowel obstructions demonstrated that generalized abdominal pain is 93.1% specific for this disease process.[12]

Character

The character of pain can help determine the pathophysiologic process causing patients pain. Visceral nerve fibers, or the fibers that innervate organs, are typically poorly localized. These fibers, when activated, cause an aching or dull pain. Activation of these fibers may occur from stretching, increased peristalsis, or ischemia. The high specificity of colicky abdominal pain for a SBO, for example, demonstrates activation of visceral nerve fibers.[12]

Somatic fibers innervate the peritoneum. When activated or irritated by blood or inflammation, these nerve fibers cause a sharp, well-localized pain. One study designed to identify factors of the history and physical associated with ectopic pregnancies found that when compared with an intrauterine pregnancy, ectopic pregnancies are much more likely to present with sharp abdominal pain.[13]

Radiation

Inquiring about radiation of pain can further help the clinician deduce the pathophysiologic process causing patients' abdominal pain. In disease processes, such as those involving the liver, biliary tract, or appendix, radiation or migration of pain can be very pertinent. Gallstone pain, for example, is highly associated with radiation from the right upper quadrant to the upper back.[14] Right subcostal pain is also highly specific for diseases of the liver and biliary tract.[7] Migration of pain from the periumbilical region to the right lower quadrant has proven to be both highly sensitive and specific for appendicitis.[15]

Palliative, Provoking, or Associated Factors

Association of pain with outside factors can provide insight into the differential diagnoses. For example, relief of pain by vomiting and also increased pain with eating is highly specific for SBO.[12] Associated vomiting is a less specific symptom but is seen in 100% of cases of gastroenteritis and 77% of cases of cholecystitis. Furthermore, anorexia is associated with most cases of SBO, appendicitis, and cholecystitis.[16]

Table 2 demonstrates a summary of the clinical features that are associated with each disease process with the associated sensitivity and specificity.

Past Medical, Surgical, and Social History

Patients' past medical, surgical, and social history can provide crucial information to further aid in constructing the appropriate differential diagnosis. Recurrence of a similar pain can often be seen in cases of nephrolithiasis, diverticulosis, or gallstone disease, as seen in a study that showed that most patients with cholecystitis reported previous episodes of abdominal pain.[5] This finding is in contrast to new onset of abdominal pain, which is highly sensitive for appendicitis.[9]

Comorbid conditions can help point to a specific diagnosis. For example, patients with type II diabetes have almost a 1.5 times higher risk of acute pancreatitis than nondiabetic patients.[19] Acute abdominal pain in patients with a history of atrial fibrillation has been shown in some studies to be highly sensitive for mesenteric

Table 2
Clinical features with sensitivities/specificities based on diagnosis

Diagnosis	Clinical Features	Sensitivity (%)	Specificity (%)
Appendicitis[9,17]	RLQ pain	81	53
	Pain before vomiting	100	64
	Anorexia	68	36
	No pain previously	81	41
	Migration of pain	69	84
	Nausea and emesis	74	36
Cholecystitis[10]	RUQ pain	81	67
	Nausea	77	36
	Emesis	71	53
	Anorexia	65	50
	Fever	35	80
Mesenteric ischemia[18]	History of atrial fibrillation	7.7–79.0	—
	Hypercoagulable state	2.4–29.0	—
	Acute abdominal pain	60–100	—
	Nausea/vomiting	39–93	—
	Diarrhea	18–48	—
	Rectal bleeding	12–48	—
SBO[12]	Generalized pain at onset	22.9	93.1
	Colicky pain	31.2	89.4
	Relief of pain by vomiting	27.1	93.7
	Increased pain with eating	16.7	94
	Previous abdominal surgeries	68.8	74
	Vomiting	75.0	65.3
	History of constipation	43.8	95

Abbreviations: RLQ, right lower quadrant; RUQ, right upper quadrant.

ischemia.[18] Another study showed that half of patients diagnosed with mesenteric ischemia have a history of prior deep vein thrombosis.[20]

Medication use can provide insight into the cause of patients' pain as well. Nonsteroidal antiinflammatory drug (NSAID) use in elderly patients was associated with a 4-fold increased risk of upper gastrointestinal (GI) bleeding or death from a peptic ulcer from that of nonusers.[21]

A history of multiple abdominal surgeries may raise the diagnostician's concern for SBO. One study showed that more than three-quarters of patients with a SBO had previous abdominal surgery.[5]

Additionally, a comprehensive social history can shed light on potential leading diagnoses. A smoking history puts patients at a 7.6 times higher risk of developing an AAA when compared with nonsmokers.[22] Illicit drug use is also an important risk factor, as multiple case reports have documented cocaine abuse and its association with acute mesenteric ischemia.[23,24]

Not to be ignored is the gynecologic history in female patients. History of vaginal bleeding, discharge, prior ectopic pregnancies, and exposure to sexually transmitted infections (STIs) are just a few of the components that can lead to an alternate diagnosis. Ectopic pregnancies have proven to be associated with a prior history of intrauterine device (IUD), history of infertility, and tubal ligation.[13]

PHYSICAL EXAMINATION

Once a thorough history of presenting illness is obtained, the physical examination helps further narrow the differential diagnosis and better localize patients' abdominal pain to specific areas and/or organ systems. A complete physical examination includes a review of patients' vital signs and an inspection of other body areas outside of the GI system, particularly the genitourinary system, cardiopulmonary system, and skin.

General Appearance

Patients' general appearance can be very useful in assessing severity/acuity of their abdominal pain.[1,25] Patients who are pale, confused, or in severe distress tend to have a higher-acuity illness. However, atypical presentations of abdominal pain can be seen in certain patient populations, such as elderly patients who might not mount an adequate response.[26] The physical examination may demonstrate this, as the slightest movement of abdomen will elicit pain, raising concerns for the presence of peritonitis.[6,27,28] Another observation from the general examination can be seen in patients who cannot seem to find a comfortable position while lying on the bed. This pain is suggestive of renal colic. These simple observations on initial evaluation of patients can demonstrate acuity, severity, and characteristics of the abdominal pain.

Vital Signs

Vital sign abnormalities can signify a more serious cause of abdominal pain, but normal vital signs do not exclude emergent diagnoses.[26] **Box 1** demonstrates clinical considerations regarding analysis of vital signs.

Approach to Unstable Patients with Abdominal Pain

If patients appear ill with unstable vital signs, such as hypotension, volume resuscitation should be started immediately in conjunction with assessing for life-threatening pathologies requiring immediate surgical intervention. **Box 2** reviews differential diagnosis considerations in unstable patients with abdominal pain.

Physical Examination Findings

Table 3 demonstrates the classic presentation and considerations for various diagnoses considered in patients with abdominal pain.[7]

Inspection

Inspection of the abdomen is a fast and easy way to collect useful information. The presence of a surgical scar indicates a history of abdominal surgery, which is a risk factor for certain pathologies, such as bowel obstruction or viscus perforation in the right clinical context. The presence of abdominal distention has a high likelihood ratio (LR) for bowel obstruction (LR+ = 5.6–16.8), though ascites or even intraperitoneal bleed can also present this way.[30] **Table 4** demonstrates clinical clues from inspection and differential diagnosis associated with symptoms.

Box 1
Vital signs clinical considerations

1. Fever: It is suggestive of infection or inflammation and may be absent in elderly and immunocompromised patients.[26]

2. Blood pressure: Hypotension may indicate sepsis, hemorrhage, and severe dehydration.

3. Heart rate: Tachycardia is suggestive of pain, sepsis, hemorrhage, and volume depletion from third spacing and may be absent in patients on beta-blockers.

4. Respiratory rate: Tachypnea can indicate metabolic acidosis with respiratory compensation or increased pain. Nonspecific findings are seen in cardiac/pulmonary diseases.

Box 2
Differential diagnosis for the unstable patient

GI bleed

Ruptured AAA

Massive pulmonary embolism

Perforated viscus

Ruptured ectopic pregnancy

Auscultation

Auscultation is often done but might be of limited use.[33] Nevertheless, the presence of high-pitched bowel sounds could indicate early SBO, whereas hypoactive bowel sounds could indicate late bowel obstruction, ileus, or many other pathologies, as it is a nonspecific finding.

Table 3
Classic presentation and clinical consideration based on diagnosis

Differential Diagnosis	Classic Presentation	Considerations
Appendicitis[9,29]	Periumbilical abdominal pain localizing to RLQ, anorexia, nausea, fever	RLQ tenderness is LR+ = 8.0. Psoas sign is LR+ = 2.38.
Bowel obstruction[30]	Abdominal distention, nausea, anorexia, constipation	Distention is LR+ = 5.6–16.8.
Cholecystitis[10]	Periumbilical abdominal pain localizing to RUQ, anorexia, nausea, fever	Murphy sign is a strong positive predictor of cholecystitis: LR+ = 2.8.
Diverticulitis[11]	LLQ, fever	Localizing tenderness in LLQ is LR+ = 10.4.
EP[13]	Abdominal pain, amenorrhea, vaginal bleed	Presence of cervical motion tenderness, peritonitis, and lateralizing symptoms all increase the likelihood of EP.
Mesenteric ischemia[18]	Abdominal pain out of proportion with examination finding, nausea, anorexia	Presence of peritonitis, abdominal distention, or diffuse pain can be suggestive of diagnosis.
Pancreatitis	Abdominal pain radiating to back, nausea, vomiting	Grey-Turner or Cullen sign can suggest necrotizing pancreatitis.
Perforated viscus	Severe generalized abdominal pain, peritoneal sign	—
Peptic ulcer disease	Epigastric pain that is associated with food intake	—
Ovarian torsion[31]	Sudden onset of severe, unilateral lower abdominal pain, nausea	A known history of ovarian cyst/mass increases the likelihood of torsion.
Ruptured AAA[32]	Abdominal pain and/or back pain + pulsatile abdominal mass	Pulsatile abdominal mass LR+ for presence of AAA = 12.0–15.6
Ureterolithiasis	Acute onset flank pain radiating to groin, nausea	It can mimic ruptured AAA.

Abbreviations: EP, ectopic pregnancy; LLQ, left lower quadrant; LR, likelihood ratio; RLQ, right lower quadrant.
Data from Refs.[11,13,18,31]

Table 4
Differential diagnosis based on inspection clues

Inspection Clues	Diagnosis to Consider
Surgical scar	Obstruction Perforated viscus
Ecchymosis	Retroperitoneal bleed

Grey-Turner:
  bilateral
  flanks
	Acute pancreatitis, retroperitoneal hematoma, ruptured ectopic
	  pregnancy

Cullen: umbilicus	Ectopic pregnancy, acute Pancreatitis, retroperitoneal hematoma
Fox: inguinal canal	Traumatic injury to pancreas, kidneys, aorta, ascending/descending colon
Bryant: scrotal	Ruptured AAA
Abdominal distension	Obstruction, ascites

Vesicular rash in
  dermatome
  distribution
	Herpes zoster

Palpation

Percussion can be used to distinguish between distention caused by air (tympanic) and fluid (dull + fluid wave). If in doubt, bedside ultrasound can be used.

Detecting the presence of peritoneal irritation should be the primary goal of any proper abdominal examination as peritonitis is often a sign of more emergent pathologies. Unfortunately, physical examination is not error proof in confirming peritonitis. Rebound tenderness and involuntary guarding are traditionally used, but they are not perfect. Several other examination techniques in our arsenal can help in evaluating peritonitis more reliably. **Box 3** demonstrates a differential diagnosis for patients with concerns of peritonitis on bedside physical examination.

Box 3
Differential diagnosis for the acute surgical abdomen

Cholecystitis

Perforated appendicitis

Boerhaave syndrome

Perforated peptic ulcer

Perforated viscus

Peritonitis

Malignancy

Mesenteric ischemia

Strangulated hernia

Spontaneous bacterial peritonitis

Tubo-ovarian abscess

Volvulus

Guarding

Involuntary guarding (or rigidity) indicates reflex spasm of abdominal muscle due to peritoneal irritation. This guarding is unlike voluntary guarding, which can be due to fear, anxiety, ticklishness, and so forth, and is distractible. True guarding is best exemplified by rigidity and can be characterized by continuous increase in muscle tone throughout respiratory cycle, whereas patients with voluntary guarding would generally show decreased tone during inspiration. Beware relying on involuntary guarding to diagnose elderly patients, as they might not exhibit any guarding or rigidity.[34]

Rebound Tenderness and Alternative Techniques

The rebound tenderness maneuver is done by slow, deep palpation followed by abrupt removal of the examiner's finger. The test is positive if pain increases with release of the finger as opposed to during compression. However, this test can be falsely positive in one-quarter of patients.[35] Thus, alternative ways have been devised, including cough test,[36] jump test, and heel-strike test.[29] In general, the more tests that are positive in patients, the likelier that the diagnosis is true peritonitis. The cough test has similar sensitivity as traditional rebound testing but with a higher specificity (79% vs 40%–50%).[36] Together with clinical correlation, these techniques can help us in detecting patients with peritoneal irritation and, thus, possible abdominal catastrophe. **Box 4** shows a summary of the techniques to elicit if patients have rebound tenderness.

Localized Tenderness

Localized tenderness has a broad differential, but we can narrow this differential based on which quadrant is maximally tender.

Special Examination Techniques to Help with Specific Diagnoses

There are special examination techniques that have been associated with specific diagnosis to help determine the likelihood of this entity. For example, the Murphy sign has an LR of 2.8 for acute cholecystitis with a specificity of 87%. Out of all examination findings studied, the Murphy sign is the strongest positive predictor for acute cholecystitis.[10]

Psoas, obturator, and the Rovsing signs are associated with appendicitis. Although these maneuvers have not been studied extensively, they have been demonstrated to have low sensitivity plus high specificity in several studies, meaning they are more useful if present but do not rule out appendicitis if absent.[9,29,37] The psoas sign has an LR of 2.4 for appendicitis. However, various other conditions that cause retroperitoneal inflammation can also elicit this sign, including psoas abscess, pancreatitis, and pyelonephritis. The obturator sign has a similar LR as the psoas sign. It suggests

---

Box 4
Evaluation techniques for peritonitis

Maneuvers to elicit signs of peritonitis

- *Cough test*: positive when pain is elicited with coughing

- *Inspiration test*: positive when pain is exhibited when exhaling and puffing the stomach out

- *Peritoneal irritation*: positive when asking patients to jump (especially in children), tapping the heel, or bumping the bed

Data from Bundy DG, Byerley JS, Liles EA, et al. Does this child have appendicitis? JAMA 2007;298(4):438–51; and Bennett DH, Tambeur LJ, Campbell WB. Use of coughing test to diagnosis peritonitis. BMJ 1994;308(6940):1336.

an inflammatory process adjacent to the pelvic wall musculature, including appendicitis. The Rovsing sign is an indirect test for rebound tenderness. **Box 5** demonstrates special maneuvers used in diagnosing appendicitis.

Examination for pulsatile mass is an examination maneuver specific for diagnosis of AAA. This examination finding has a high LR+ of 12.0 to 15.6, depending on AAA size. Palpation of AAA is safe and has not been reported to precipitate rupture. It is the only examination maneuver that has been found to be of any value in detecting AAA, especially ones large enough to warrant intervention.[32,38]

Rectal Examination

Digital rectal examination has a limited role in the evaluation of undifferentiated abdominal pain or acute appendicitis, and its routine performance in patients with undifferentiated abdominal pain has not been supported by literature.[39,40] However, in select cases it can yield useful information, as in the case of constipation, anorectal complaints, or GI bleed. **Box 6** demonstrates when a rectal examination may be useful.

Extra-abdominal Examination

A thorough cardiopulmonary examination should be done, as any intrathoracic disease process can present as abdominal pain.

Pelvic examination should be done to assess for pelvic peritoneal through testing for cervical motion tenderness and to directly visualize cervix for signs of vaginal discharge or bleeding. Although some evidence suggests empiric pelvic examinations performed in the ED on all female patients with abdominal pain might not yield useful data, guidelines still recommend performing a pelvic examination on almost all female patients with lower abdominal pain.[41–43]

Similarly, male genitourinary examination is important in male patients with abdominal pain to assess for signs of testicular torsions, trauma, strangulated hernias, or infections, including Fournier gangrene and STIs. The flank/back should be tested for the presence of costovertebral angle (CVA) tenderness, which can reflect the presence of pyelonephritis or obstructive uropathy. **Box 7** discusses extra-abdominal diagnosis considerations.

LABORATORY TESTING IN ABDOMINAL PAIN

Multiple studies over the years have tried to distinguish laboratory findings to point us to the definitive diagnosis of acute abdominal pain. The following will review several tests that have been investigated.

Box 5
Special maneuvers based on suspected diagnosis

Special examination maneuvers

- *Murphy sign:* positive if patients exhibit inspiratory arrest during deep RUQ palpation

- *Psoas sign:* positive if pain is elicited with passive hip extension

- *Obturator sign:* positive if pain is elicited with passive internal/external rotation of the right hip

- *Rovsing sign:* positive if pain is elicited in RLQ when the examiner exerts pressure on the LLQ

Abbreviations: LLQ, left lower quadrant; RLQ, right lower quadrant; RUQ, right upper quadrant.
   Data from Refs.[9,10,29,37]

Box 6
Diagnoses whereby rectal examination may have utility

Rectal examination may be useful in

Acute GI bleed

Colon cancer

Intussusception

Ischemic colitis

Perirectal disorder (abscess)

Rectal foreign body

Stool impaction

White Blood Cell Count

Leukocytosis has been looked at for the evaluation of multiple causes of abdominal pain. Commonly, a complete blood cell count will be ordered in the workup of acute abdominal pain. An elevated white blood cell (WBC) count is often seen with appendicitis, mesenteric ischemia, SBO,[44] and pancreatitis. It is highly sensitive but not specific.[44] Leukocytosis may be helpful in distinguishing illness from a normal variant, especially when the neutrophil count is greater than 80%.[45] However, elevation of WBC count can be misleading or less helpful in certain populations, such as pregnant patients who have a physiologic elevation.[45] Diagnostic significance of leukocytosis in elderly patients may also be a challenge if they are on medications, such as steroids that cause demargination.[25] The elderly may not develop a leukocytosis, even when they have surgical pathology in the abdomen. In combination with other objective variables, such as hypotension and abnormal abdominal radiographs, leukocytosis may be predictive of adverse outcomes[25] but alone has not shown to have significance. It is also important to note that with a high pretest probability, a normal WBC count cannot rule out diagnoses, such as appendicitis or cholecystitis.[46] It also has not been shown to be a good discriminator between urgent and nonurgent causes of abdominal pain.[47]

C-Reactive Protein

Primarily an inflammatory marker, C-reactive protein (CRP) has been shown to increase rapidly in response to infectious and inflammatory conditions.[48,49] CRP has

---

Box 7
Differential diagnosis for extra-abdominal pathology

Cardiopulmonary disease

Ectopic pregnancy

Fournier gangrene

Inguinal hernia

Pelvic inflammatory disease

Pyelonephritis

Spontaneous abortion

Testicular torsion

Tubo-ovarian abscess

been noted to have the highest diagnostic accuracy for perforated appendix in one study[50] and correlates with the CT severity of appendicitis.[51] In other studies it has been looked at in conjunction with other laboratory values, such as WBC count, and has not been shown to be able to discriminate between urgent and nonurgent causes of abdominal pain.[48] A low CRP level (0–5 mg/L) does not rule out positive findings on CT in the clinical setting of the acute abdomen. CRP is more specific than WBC count but is less sensitive in early appendicitis.[52,53] However, increasing levels of CRP predict, with increasing likelihood, positive findings on CT.[54] It has also been shown that the combined use of WBC count and CRP may increase the negative predictive value in appendicitis.[55]

Procalcitonin

Procalcitonin is a precursor for calcitonin and is secreted primarily by cells in the thyroid and lung. In normal, healthy individuals, it is undetectable. If an endotoxin or inflammatory cytokine stimulates these cells, then procalcitonin is produced. It is different from CRP because it is not stimulated by sterile inflammation or viral infections.[56,57] Procalcitonin has been investigated in the diagnostic workup of appendicitis and intestinal ischemia.[58,59] Procalcitonin was found to be more accurate in diagnosing complicated appendicitis, as opposed to early, acute appendicitis, with a pooled sensitivity of 62% (33%–84%) and specificity of 94% (90%–96%).[59] In multiple studies, procalcitonin has been shown to have relatively high sensitivity (72%–100%) and a high negative predictive value (81%–100%) for the diagnosis of ischemia and necrosis.[60–63]

D Dimer

D dimer is a fibrin degradation product. It is increased in many conditions, including trauma, malignancies, venous thromboembolism, and aortic dissection.[64–66] More recently, it has been looked at in relation to acute abdominal conditions.[67–69] D dimer showed promise with relatively high sensitivity in mesenteric ischemia[67] but ultimately was judged to not have sufficient sensitivity to rule out the disease. Its role with appendicitis is even less clear. It has shown low sensitivity and diagnostic value[64,69] in a few studies and high sensitivity in others,[68] thus rendering it an unreliable study thus far in the workup of appendicitis.

Intestinal Fatty Acid Binding Protein

Intestinal fatty acid binding protein (I-FABP) is a low molecular mass cytoplasmic protein. It is found specifically in the epithelial cells of the small intestine. When there is intestinal injury and/or mucosal barrier disruptions due to poor mesenteric blood flow and necrosis, I-FABP is rapidly released into the circulatory system. I-FABP is present in both the small and large bowel; but it has much higher concentrations of cells in the duodenum, jejunum, and ileum. Studies have looked at I-FABP levels in ischemic models and have shown good correlation between the protein level and amount of ischemia. This research supports the concept that I-FABP may be a good marker for detecting small bowel ischemia[70–75] in the future should human trials confirm these findings.

Lactate

Lactate is the end product of anaerobic glycolysis. It is then processed in the liver and metabolized to pyruvate. Elevations of lactate can be seen when the conversion capacity in the liver is overloaded from release of lactate from the tissues. Vascular causes of abdominal emergencies have often been thought to have a higher value for lactate secondary to decreased tissue perfusion/hypoxia, thus making it a good test for early diagnosis. This idea has not been shown to be true, as normal values are often found early in the disease process.[76–79]

Lipase/Amylase/Liver Function Tests

Serum amylase and lipase are often sent to evaluate causes of epigastric pain and, more specifically, pancreatitis. Studies have shown that the tests are somewhat redundant, and both tend to increase with pancreatitis. It is important to note that serum lipase will increase later than serum amylase and will remain elevated longer and that both tests can also have false elevations in renal insufficiency secondary to their partial renal clearance.[80] Several studies have shown that lipase is a more specific test with pancreatitis, especially pancreatitis secondary to alcohol.[81,82] In cases of suspected gallstone pancreatitis, several studies have looked at the accuracy of noted abnormalities in aspartate transferase (AST), alanine transferase (ALT), alkaline phosphatase, and bilirubin.[83,84] An ALT level of greater than 150 IU/L had a positive predictive value of greater than 95%[84] for gallstone pancreatitis. However, only one-half of all patients with gallstone pancreatitis have elevations in ALT, giving it a low sensitivity. AST has been found to be almost as predictive as ALT in gallstone pancreatitis, but alkaline phosphatase and bilirubin have not been found useful in diagnosis.[80]

DIAGNOSTIC IMAGING MODALITIES

Table 5 reviews the most used diagnostic modalities and their sensitivities and specificities for the specific causes.[7,85] Having a clear understanding of the best imaging modality can help ED workers expedite care.

Table 5	
Diagnostic imaging consideration based on diagnosis	
Diagnostic Imaging Modality	**Considerations**
Appendicitis	CT 93%–95% sensitive if appendix seen
Bowel obstruction	Plain radiograph 71%–77% sensitive; CT 93% sensitive
Cholecystitis	US 91% sensitive, hepatobiliary iminodiacetic acid scan 97% sensitive
Diverticulitis	CT 93%–100% sensitive
Ectopic pregnancy	Transvaginal ultrasound
Mesenteric ischemia	CT angiography 96% sensitive
Pancreatitis	CT 78% sensitive, 86% specific
Perforated viscus	Upright chest radiograph 80% sensitive; CT 87%–98% sensitive
Tubo-ovarian abscess	Transvaginal US preferred imaging
Ovarian torsion	Pelvic US with Doppler flow
Renal/ureteral colic	Noncontrast spiral CT preferred
Ruptured AAA	Bedside US 100% sensitive for enlarged aorta

Abbreviation: US, ultrasound.

Data from Cline D, Maisel J, Sokolosky M, et al. Gastrointestinal emergencies. In: Cline D, Ma O, Cydulka R, et al, editors. Tintinalli's emergency medicine just the facts. Kansas city (KS): McGraw-Hill Companies, Inc; 2012. p. 140–81; and Broder J. Diagnostic imaging for the emergency physician. Philadelphia: Elsevier Saunders; 2011.

Plain Radiographs

The utility of plain radiographs during the initial stages of evaluation of abdominal pain can serve as a value adjunct to the physical examination. Plain radiographs can be obtained far more quickly than typical ultrasound or CT images in many EDs. This promptness is especially important in time-critical diagnoses whereby physical examination findings are concerning. **Box 8** demonstrates clinical considerations when potentially using a plain radiograph for evaluation of abdominal pain. In patients who have peritoneal signs, an upright radiograph that reveals air under the diaphragm allows the clinician to expedite a surgical consult rather than waiting for CT imaging. **Fig. 1** shows a picture of free air under the diaphragm, which is concerning for perforation.[85]

One caveat to the use of plain radiograph is being cognizant of the limitations of the study, especially with regard to the sensitivity. If imaging with plain radiographs lacks sensitivity for a condition, the clinician may be misguided and falsely reassured by a normal plain radiograph when in fact further modalities of images are warranted for the patients' presentation. SBO is a perfect example of this. The search for the pathognomonic air fluid levels on abdominal plain radiograph many times makes this the first imaging modality used to evaluate abdominal pain. However, the sensitivity of plain radiographs in detecting SBO is only 71% to 77%,[7,85] with the plain radiograph shown to be the least useful imaging modality for the diagnosis of SBO. **Fig. 2** shows the classic findings associated with SBO.[82] Normal or nonobstructive gas pattern can occur in the presence of an SBO, and multiple studies show that the insensitivity of plain radiograph limits its utility as a screening choice for SBO.[86] In fact, plain radiographs for SBO has a pooled positive LR of 1.64 in comparison with CT and MRI, which were both accurate in diagnosing SBO with +LRs of 3.6.[85] **Table 6** summarizes findings seen with each specific diagnosis.

Research has found that for those patients who will likely have a CT of the abdomen/pelvis, the use of a plain abdominal radiograph adds very little additional value and can often be misleading.[30]

Computed Tomography Scan

CT scan of the abdomen/pelvis has become the diagnostic modality test of choice for evaluation of abdominal pain. Large changes in technology have led to clearer images and the ability to evaluate a multitude of complaints when trying to deduce the cause of abdominal pain. Despite the increased cost and longer length of stay, recent data show a shift toward the utility of CT scans in the diagnosis of atraumatic abdominal pain in the ED.[87]

CT scan has transformed the diagnostic evaluation of abdominal pain. It is superior to other modalities for specific diagnoses. Possessing both a high sensitivity and specificity, CT scan with contrast has become the study of choice for entities, such as diverticulitis.[88] **Fig. 3** demonstrates findings consistent with diverticulitis.[82] A misleading nonobstructive gas pattern in patients who clinically cause concern for SBO can be diagnosed by CT imaging, which carries a higher sensitivity and specificity than plain radiograph imaging for this disease process.[85]

Box 8
Plain radiograph clinical considerations

Pros: quick, inexpensive

Cons: sensitivity varies, may delay definitive test

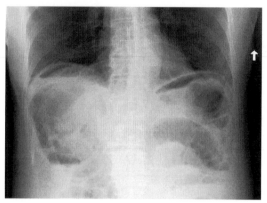

Fig. 1. Free air under the diaphragm. (*Courtesy of* Joshua Broder, MD.)

In order to optimize the diagnostic modality being used, the clinician must consider the clinical differential diagnosis in order to choose which type of CT scan protocol would best answer the clinical question being asked. The use of the wrong protocol could result in false reassurance from the results. For example, obtaining the wrong protocol for a CT scan in evaluation for mesenteric ischemia could provide falsely reassuring results causing the clinician to miss this catastrophic vascular disease that yields with it a mortality rate of 30% to 90%. CT angiography (CTA) should be considered the first line in cases of acute or chronic mesenteric ischemia because of its high sensitivity and specificity. A specificity of greater than 94% and sensitivity of greater than 96% can be found regarding the appearance of the bowel wall in addition to the vascular findings in patients with mesenteric ischemia. Ordering the wrong protocol, such as a noncontrast CT, in acute mesenteric ischemia has lower sensitivity and specificity.[89]

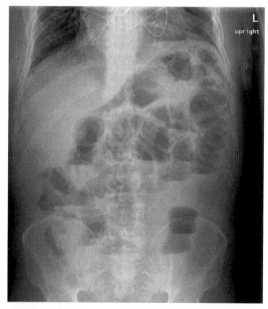

Fig. 2. SBO with air fluid levels. (*Courtesy of* Joshua Broder, MD.)

Table 6
Plain radiograph findings with differential diagnosis

Radiograph Finding	Differential Diagnosis Consideration
Air under the diaphragm	Perforated viscus
	Recent laparoscopic surgery
Air fluid levels (often described as string of pearls or stack of coins)	SBO
Appendicolith, gas in appendix	Appendicitis
Double bubble	Malrotation with midgut volvulus
Sentinel loop sign	Acute pancreatitis (L hypochondrium)
	Acute appendicitis (R iliac fossa)
	Acute cholecystitis (R hypochondrium)
	Diverticulitis (L iliac fossa)
Target or crescent lucency	Intussusception
Bent inner tube	Sigmoid volvulus
Coffee bean	Cecal or sigmoid volvulus

Abbreviations: L, left; R, right.

To further complicate matters, contrast can be provided orally, rectally, or intravenously. Although it does carry the risk of nephrotoxicity and contrast allergy, the use of intravenous contrast can be beneficial to enhance imaging, especially in the context of inflammation or infection.[90] **Fig. 4** demonstrates the appearance of appendicitis with the use of both oral and intravenous contrast.[85]

Much research has been dedicated regarding the utility of oral and rectal contrast because of conflicting thoughts regarding its addition to increase diagnostic accuracy. Although institution dependent, in most cases of patients with abdominal pain requiring CT imaging, there has been a trend away from the use of oral and rectal contrast. These studies report that the use of oral contrast has been found to increase the length of stay in the ED and to increase radiology turnaround time without offering much additional information in imaging interpretation. This finding resulted in a movement toward eliminating routing oral contrast use for CT abdomen/pelvis in the ED with multiple studies finding success in decreasing the length of stay by almost

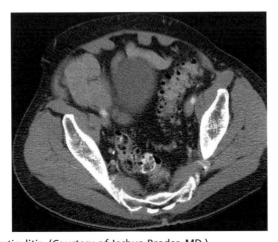

Fig. 3. CT of diverticulitis. (*Courtesy of* Joshua Broder, MD.)

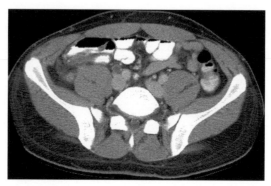

Fig. 4. CT with intravenous/oral contrast of appendicitis. (*Courtesy of* Joshua Broder, MD.)

100 minutes as well as decreasing time from order to CT by more than 60 minutes while not compromising the diagnosis of patients with abdominal pain.[91] A CT abdomen/pelvis *without oral contrast* in the ED setting has been found to be both safe and positively impacts both and emergency medicine and radiology workflow.[92]

As the role of CT has become more dominant in the realm of diagnosis for patients with acute emergent abdominal pain, clinicians must be stewards in determining who truly requires this type of imaging. Many studies have been conducted to try to decipher who requires CT imaging. Unfortunately, laboratory testing does not offer additional information in risk stratifying those patients who require CT imaging.[93] CT scans are not without their risks. The concern for radiation exposure must be considered, especially in younger patients. Sadly, as CT scan becomes more predominant, time-efficient, and available, experts are predicting an increase in radiation-induced cancers.[94–96] Despite the high sensitivity and specificity of CT scan, the exposure to radiation should not be discounted; providers should be cautious of using this modality for diagnostic investigation. This point holds especially true when treating the pediatric and young female population. Ultrasound, in the experienced hand of the sonographer, is the preferred modality in children despite CT being more accurate for appendicitis because of ultrasound's lack of ionizing radiation. However, if the results are equivocal, a follow-up CT will often be required. The approach of CT after ultrasound has been determined to have excellent accuracy, with reported sensitivity and specificity of 94%.[97]

Ultrasound

The increasing availability of ultrasound makes it a valuable tool in the workup of patients with abdominal pain. Lacking radiation, ultrasound is an alternative to CT imaging in specific clinical situations. Transforming the way abdominal pain is evaluated, bedside ultrasound has become an efficient adjunct to the physical examination.[98] Ultrasound can be helpful in identifying many structures, such as the gallbladder, liver, spleen, pancreas, kidney, urinary bladder, and aorta.

Moreover, ultrasound serves as an indispensable tool in unstable patients with undifferentiated abdominal pain in which a focused abdominal ultrasound can give much useful information. For example, ultrasound can help determine if free fluid is present, expediting the emergent surgical consultation. Free fluid on ultrasound on its own may be suggestive of either ascites or blood. Additionally, a focused bedside aortic ultrasound can be used in unstable patients with concerning findings to rule out AAA. The pooled operating characteristics of ED ultrasound for the detection of AAA were a sensitivity of 99% and a specificity of 98%.[99] An example of an AAA can be seen in **Fig. 5**.[85]

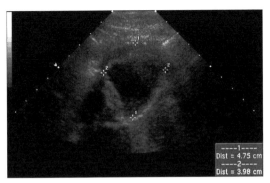

Fig. 5. Ultrasound of AAA with mural thrombus. (*Courtesy of* Joshua Broder, MD.)

Bedside ultrasound can also reveal large fluid shift/leakage into the peritoneal cavity from perforation or other intra-abdominal catastrophe. Combined with a high index of suspicion, a positive, concerning bedside ultrasound finding should prompt an expedited transport of patients to the operating room for exploration.

Ultrasonography has, in some cases, been found superior to CT imaging. An ultrasound rather than a plain radiograph or CT scan would more appropriately image patients who present with right upper quadrant pain suggestive of cholecystitis because of its higher sensitivity and specificity.[85] In cholecystitis, emergency physicians detected stones at a sensitivity of 94% with a positive predictive value 99%, specificity of 96%, and negative predictive value of 73%, making it a highly sensitive and reliable indicator of the presence of gallstones.[100] Some research suggests that, in the hand of a highly experienced emergency physician skilled in sonography, the detection rate of acute cholecystitis is similar to that of radiology sonography.[101] This is, however, limited, based on technical skills and experience. An example of a positive gallbladder for cholecystitis can be seen from **Fig. 6**.[85]

Ultrasound is the first diagnostic test of choice in patients presenting with concerning findings of gallbladder, hepatic, or biliary disease.[102] Likewise, for suspected ovarian torsion, a Doppler ultrasound would offer the most valuable information. Arterial flow can be reduced in ovarian torsion, but typically this occurs only with a concomitant venous flow abnormality.[103] The most frequent finding is either decrease or absence of venous flow (93%), which may reflect the early collapse of the compliant

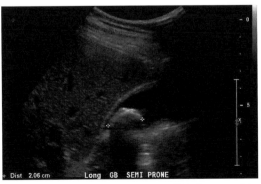

Fig. 6. Ultrasound of cholecystitis with stone in gallbladder, pericholecystic fluid, and increased gallbladder wall thickness. (*Courtesy of* Joshua Broder, MD.)

venous walls. Abnormal ovarian venous flow[104] may be the only abnormal ultrasound sign observed during the early stage of adnexal torsion, although the effectiveness of ultrasound in diagnosing ovarian torsion yielded a positive predictive value of 87.5% and specificity of 93.3%,[105] corroborating the potential for expeditiously making this diagnosis. Equipped with this knowledge, if patients who clinically appear to have ovarian torsion still have a significant amount of pain on reevaluation despite a normal Doppler ultrasound of the ovaries, gynecology consultation may be indicated.

THERAPEUTIC MANAGEMENT AND DISPOSITION
Gastrointestinal Cocktail

Treating patients' associated symptoms can be just as important as treating patients' abdominal pain. Aside from common analgesics, the GI cocktail is often used in the treatment of dyspepsia or epigastric pain. A GI cocktail consists of viscous lidocaine, an antacid, and an anticholinergic. The exact contents and combination of this cocktail are often studied. A comparison between the different combinations of antacids; antacid and a belladonna alkaloid combination medication that includes atropine, hyoscyamine, phenobarbital, and scopolamine; and antacid, viscous lidocaine, and a belladonna alkaloid combination medication that includes atropine, hyoscyamine, phenobarbital, and scopolamine demonstrated no statistically significant difference in pain improvement between the treatment groups.[106] This finding is in contrast to another study demonstrating a significant improvement in pain in patients receiving an antacid with viscous lidocaine as compared with those receiving an antacid alone.[107] Treatment with a viscous analgesic, whether it is benzocaine or lidocaine, is associated with a statistically significant improvement in pain.[108] Thirty-four percent of patients with abdominal and chest pain got relief from GI cocktail alone,[109] making this medication a useful adjunct in the treatment of epigastric pain. GI cocktail, however, has not been shown to be an accurate test to exclude cardiac disease as a cause of chest or epigastric pain.[110]

Antiemetics

Antiemetic agents can be useful in treating associated nausea and vomiting. Many commonly used antiemetics include ondansetron, metoclopramide, prochlorperazine, and promethazine. Ondansetron is a common, safe, first-line antiemetic in the ED.[111] It results in less sedation than promethazine[112] and is not associated with akathisia like metoclopramide or prochlorperazine.[111] However, ondansetron has not proven to be superior to promethazine[112,113] or metoclopramide in reducing patients' nausea or vomiting. Furthermore, a large, prospective, randomized trial comparing ondansetron, metoclopramide, and placebo favored treatment with the antiemetics, although the results did not show a statistically significant difference in their efficacy.[114] Finally, prochlorperazine, when compared with promethazine, has proven to be more effective and immediate in the treatment of nausea and vomiting.[115] When choosing an antiemetic, it is important to weigh the potential adverse effects of the medication with potential benefits and efficacy.

Use of Pain Medication with Abdominal Pain

Patients with abdominal pain, including those concerning for a surgical abdomen, should be treated adequately with analgesics in the ED as soon as possible. Historically, clinicians have practiced the strategy of withholding pain medications until a diagnosis has been made in fear of masking symptoms/signs and ultimately leading to diagnostic error. However, literature has largely debunked this practice; multiple studies have suggested that analgesics administration does not significantly increase the risk of diagnostic or management error during initial evaluation of acute abdominal pain.[116] Based on the available data, that study's investigators concluded that a practice of early administration of analgesics to patients with undifferentiated abdominal pain is both humane and would have no negative impact on the eventual diagnostic accuracy.[117]

Disposition

Serial abdominal examinations

Delays in intervention and potential for deterioration concern many physicians in the evaluation of acute abdominal pain. Close observation and serial examinations make this outcome less likely. When compared with delays in patients' hospital stay, as seen in a period of observation, it was prehospital delays, or delays in patients seeking care, that led to statistically significant advanced pathology.[118] A systematic review demonstrated no statistical significance between the rates of complications, rates of readmission, or length of hospital stay in patients who were observed for abdominal pain versus those who underwent early laparoscopic intervention.[119] In patients whose diagnosis is uncertain but concerning, a period of observation and serial examinations can help the examiner determine the appropriate course of action. In patients with an intermediate probability for appendicitis, a period of observation of 10 hours improved the capacity to determine whether or not patients actually had appendicitis.[120]

Watching patients over time gives the examiner an opportunity to evaluate patients for development of signs or symptoms that point to a specific pathology. One study of women with nonspecific abdominal pain demonstrated that of the 51% of women randomized to observation, 39.2% of them eventually underwent surgical intervention for worsened symptoms or development of peritonitis. This study also demonstrated that patients randomized to observation had statistically significant shorter stays in the hospital without differences in mortality or morbidity. At 12 months, there was no statistical significance in the recurrence of abdominal pain in either the group that underwent early laparoscopy[121] or that was observed This finding supports the argument for serial examinations and a period of observation in patients with intermediate or nonspecific abdominal pain.

Additionally, a period of observation with repeat examinations can lead to decreased rates of inappropriate interventions. In a classic surgical study of more than 1000 patients, unnecessary appendectomies were done in 16% of patients presenting with nonspecific abdominal pain and suspected appendicitis.[122] One study demonstrated a decrease from a 33% to a 5%[123] rate of negative findings on laparotomy after a period of observation.[124]

Disposition from the ED depends on the final diagnosis at the time of discharge. However, it can be difficult to appropriately manage patients without any specific diagnosis for their abdominal pain (more than 40% of patients according to one large study). There are several disposition options: patients can be admitted for surgical management, admitted for medical management, placed in observation, or discharged to home with appropriate return precautions and follow-up evaluation. The decision to discharge or to observe depends on several factors:

- Likelihood for patients' condition to evolve into life-threatening/organ-harming processes despite current negative workup
- Their ability to follow-up in a timely manner
- Their ability to return if condition worsens

For patients well enough to be discharged home, it is important to make sure they have normal (or near normal) vital signs, are able to tolerate oral intake, and do not exhibit any concerning findings, such as peritonitis, on discharge physical examination. Discharge instructions should be specific and include worsening pain, persistent pain beyond 8 to 12 hours, and development of fever/vomiting, as these symptoms can suggest evolving appendicitis, SBO, or cholecystitis, which are some of the most common serious diagnoses ultimately given to discharged patients at follow-up reevaluation.[125]

REFERENCES

1. ACEP Board of Directors. Clinical policy for the initial approach to patients presenting with a chief complaint of nontraumatic acute abdominal pain. Ann Emerg Med 1994;23:906–22.
2. Martina B, Bucheli B, Stotz M, et al. First clinical judgment by primary care physicians distinguishes well between nonorganic and organic causes of abdominal or chest pain. J Gen Intern Med 1997;12(8):459–65.
3. Peterson MC, Holbrook JH, Von Hales D, et al. Contributions of the history, physical examination, and laboratory investigation in making medical diagnoses. West J Med 1992;156(2):163–5.
4. Townsend C, Beauchamp D, Evers BM, et al. Sabiston textbook of surgery [electronic resource]: the biological basis of modern surgical practice. Philadelphia: Elsevier Saunders; 2012.
5. Staniland JR, Ditchburn J, De Dombal FT. Clinical presentation of acute abdomen: study of 600 patients. Br Med J 1972;3(5823):393–8.
6. Macaluso CR, McNamara RM. Evaluation and management of acute abdominal pain in the emergency department. Int J Gen Med 2012;5:789–97.
7. Cline D, Maisel J, Sokolosky M, et al. Gatrointestinal emergencies. In: Cline D, Ma O, Cydulka R, editors. Tintinalli's emergency medicine just the facts. Kansas city (KS): McGraw-Hill Companies, Inc; 2012. p. 140–81.
8. Yamamoto W, Kono H, Maekawa M, et al. The relationship between abdominal pain regions and specific diseases: an epidemiologic approach to clinical practice. J Epidemiol 1997;7(1):27–32.
9. Wagner JM, McKinney WP, Carpenter JL. Does this patient have appendicitis? JAMA 1996;276(19):1589–94.
10. Trowbridge RL, Rutkowski NK, Shojania KG. Does this patient have acute cholecystitis? JAMA 2003;289(1):80–6.
11. Wilkins T, Embry K, George R. Diagnosis and management of acute diverticulitis. Am Fam Physician 2013;87(9):612–20.
12. Bohner H, Yang Q, Franke C, et al. Simple data from history and physical examination help to exclude bowel obstruction and to avoid radiographic studies in patients with acute abdominal pain. Eur J Surg 1998;164(10):777–84.
13. Dart RG, Kaplan B, Varaklis K. Predictive value of history and physical examination in patients with suspected ectopic pregnancy. Ann Emerg Med 1999;33(3):283–90.
14. Diehl AK, Sugarek NJ, Todd KH. Clinical evaluation for gallstone disease: usefulness of symptoms and signs in diagnosis. Am J Med 1990;89(1):29–33.
15. John H, Neff U, Kelemen M. Appendicitis diagnosis today: clinical and ultrasonic deductions. World J Surg 1993;17(2):243–9.
16. Brewer BJ, Golden GT, Hitch DC, et al. Abdominal pain. An analysis of 1,000 consecutive cases in a University Hospital emergency room. Am J Surg 1976;131(2):219–23.

17. Alvarado A. A practical score for the early diagnosis of acute appendicitis. Ann Emerg Med 1986;15(5):557–64.
18. Cudnik MT, Darbha S, Jones J, et al. The diagnosis of acute mesenteric ischemia: a systematic review and meta-analysis. Acad Emerg Med 2013; 20(11):1087–100.
19. Girman CJ, Kou TD, Cai B, et al. Patients with type 2 diabetes mellitus have higher risk for acute pancreatitis compared with those without diabetes. Diabetes Obes Metab 2010;12(9):766–71.
20. Harward TR, Green D, Bergan JJ, et al. Mesenteric venous thrombosis. J Vasc Surg 1989;9(2):328–33.
21. Griffin MR, Ray WA, Schaffner W. Nonsteroidal anti-inflammatory drug use and death from peptic ulcer in elderly persons. Ann Intern Med 1988;109(5):359–63.
22. Wilmink TB, Quick CR, Day NE. The association between cigarette smoking and abdominal aortic aneurysms. J Vasc Surg 1999;30(6):1099–105.
23. Osorio J, Farreras N, Ortiz De Zarate L, et al. Cocaine-induced mesenteric ischaemia. Dig Surg 2000;17(6):648–51.
24. Rittenhouse DW, Chojnacki KA. Massive portal venous air and pneumatosis intestinalis associated with cocaine-induced mesenteric ischemia. J Gastrointest Surg 2012;16(1):223–5.
25. Kamin R, Nowicki T, Courtney D, et al. Pearls and pitfalls in the emergency department evaluation of abdominal pain. Emerg Med Clin North Am 2003; 21(1):61–72.
26. Crossley KB, Peterson PK. Infections in the elderly. Clin Infect Dis 1996;22(2): 209–14.
27. Worcester EM, Coe FL. Nephrolithiasis. Prim Care 2008;35(2):369–91, vii.
28. Cartwright SL. Evaluation of acute abdominal pain in adults. Am Fam Physician 2008;77(7):971–8.
29. Bundy DG, Byerley JS, Liles EA, et al. Does this child have appendicitis? JAMA 2007;298(4):438–51.
30. Taylor MR, Lalani N. Adult small bowel obstruction. Acad Emerg Med 2013; 20(6):528–44.
31. Houry D, Abbott JT. Ovarian torsion: a fifteen-year review. Ann Emerg Med 2001; 38(2):156–9.
32. Lederle F, Simel D. Does this patient have AAA? JAMA 1999;281:77–82.
33. Felder S, Margel D, Murrell Z, et al. Usefulness of bowel sound auscultation: a prospective evaluation. J Surg Educ 2014;71(5):768–73.
34. Fenyo G. Acute abdominal disease in the elderly: experience from two series in Stockholm. Am J Surg 1982;143(6):751–4.
35. Taylor S, Watt M. Emergency department assessment of abdominal pain: clinical indicator tests for detecting peritonism. Eur J Emerg Med 2005;12(6):275–7.
36. Bennett DH, Tambeur LJ, Campbell WB. Use of coughing test to diagnosis peritonitis. BMJ 1994;308(6940):1336.
37. Kharbanda AB, Taylor GA, Fishman SJ, et al. A clinical decision rule to identify children at low risk for appendicitis. Pediatrics 2005;116(3):709–16.
38. Fink HA, Lederle FA, Roth CS, et al. The accuracy of physical examination to detect abdominal aortic aneurysm. Arch Intern Med 2000;160(6):833–6.
39. Quaas J, Lanigan M, Newman D, et al. Utility of the digital rectal examination in the evaluation of undifferentiated abdominal pain. Am J Emerg Med 2009;27(9): 1125–9.
40. Manimaran N, Galland RB. Significance of routine digital rectal examination in adults presenting with abdominal pain. Ann R Coll Surg Engl 2004;86(4):292–5.

41. Padilla LA, Radosevich DM, Milad MP. Accuracy of the pelvic examination in detecting adnexal masses. Obstet Gynecol 2000;96(4):593–8.
42. Brown J, Fleming R, Aristzabel J, et al. Does pelvic exam in the emergency department add useful information? West J Emerg Med 2011;12(2):208–12.
43. Close R, Sachs CJ, Dyne PL. Reliability of bimanual pelvic examinations performed in emergency departments. West J Med 2001;175(4):240–4.
44. Flasar MH, Goldberg E. Acute abdominal pain. Med Clin North Am 2006;90(3): 481–503.
45. Babaknia A, Parsa H, Woodruff JD. Appendicitis during pregnancy. Obstet Gynecol 1977;50(1):40–4.
46. McNamara R, Dean AJ. Approach to acute abdominal pain. Emerg Med Clin North Am 2011;29(2):159–73, vii.
47. Gans SL, Atema JJ, Stoker J, et al. C-reactive protein and white blood cell count as triage test between urgent and nonurgent conditions in 2961 patients with acute abdominal pain. Medicine (Baltimore) 2015;94(9):e569.
48. Ballou SP, Kushner I. C-reactive protein and the acute phase response. Adv Intern Med 1992;37:313–36.
49. Gewurz H, Mold C, Siegel J, et al. C-reactive protein and the acute phase response. Adv Intern Med 1982;27:345–72.
50. Panagiotopoulou IG, Parashar D, Lin R, et al. The diagnostic value of white cell count, C-reactive protein and bilirubin in acute appendicitis and its complications. Ann R Coll Surg Engl 2013;95(3):215–21.
51. Laxmisan A, Hakimzada F, Sayan OR, et al. The multitasking clinician: decision-making and cognitive demand during and after team handoffs in emergency care. Int J Med Inform 2007;76(11–12):801–11.
52. Andersson RE. Meta-analysis of the clinical and laboratory diagnosis of appendicitis. Br J Surg 2004;91(1):28–37.
53. Wen SW, Naylor CD. Diagnostic accuracy and short-term surgical outcomes in cases of suspected acute appendicitis. CMAJ 1995;152:1617–26.
54. Coyle JP, Brennan CR, Parfrey SF, et al. Is serum C-reactive protein a reliable predictor of abdomino-pelvic CT findings in the clinical setting of the non-traumatic acute abdomen? Emerg Radiol 2012;19(5):455–62.
55. Stefanutti G, Ghirardo V, Gamba P. Inflammatory markers for acute appendicitis in children: are they helpful? J Pediatr Surg 2007;42(5):773–6.
56. Becker KL, Nylen ES, White JC, et al. Clinical review 167: procalcitonin and the calcitonin gene family of peptides in inflammation, infection, and sepsis: a journey from calcitonin back to its precursors. J Clin Endocrinol Metab 2004; 89(4):1512–25.
57. Assicot M, Gendrel D, Carsin H, et al. High serum procalcitonin concentrations in patients with sepsis and infection. Lancet 1993;341(8844):515–8.
58. Cosse C, Sabbagh C, Kamel S, et al. Procalcitonin and intestinal ishchemia: a review of the literature. West J Gastroenterol 2014;20(47):17773–8.
59. Yu CW, Juan LI, Wu MH, et al. Systematic review and meta-analysis of the diagnostic accuracy of procalcitonin, C-reactive protein and white blood cell count for suspected acute appendicitis. Br J Surg 2013;100(3):322–9.
60. Markogiannakis H, Memos N, Messaris E, et al. Predictive value of procalcitonin for bowel ischemia and necrosis in bowel obstruction. Surgery 2011;149(3): 394–403.
61. Cosse C, Regimbeau JM, Fuks D, et al. Serum procalcitonin for predicting the failure of conservative management and the need for bowel resection in patients with small bowel obstruction. J Am Coll Surg 2013;216:997–1004.

62. Cosse C, Sabbagh C, Browet F, et al. Serum value of procalcitonin as a marker of intestinal damages: type, extension, and prognosis. Surg Endosc 2015; 29(11):3132–9.
63. Nagata J, Kobayashi M, Nishikimi N, et al. Serum procalcitonin (PCT) as a negative screening test for colonic ischemia after open abdominal aortic surgery. Eur J Vasc Endovasc Surg 2008;35(6):694–7.
64. Kaya B, Sana B, Eris C, et al. The diagnostic value of D-dimer, procalcitonin and CRP in acute appendicitis. Int J Med Sci 2012;9(10):909–15.
65. Frost SA, Alexandrou E, Bogdanovski T, et al. Unplanned admission to intensive care after emergency hospitalisation: risk factors and development of a nomogram for individualising risk. Resuscitation 2009;80(2):224–30.
66. Shimony A, Filion KB, Mottillo S, et al. Meta-analysis of usefulness of d-dimer to diagnose acute aortic dissection. Am J Cardiol 2011;107(8):1227–34.
67. Kurt Y, Akin ML, Demirbas S, et al. D-dimer in the early diagnosis of acute mesenteric ischemia secondary to arterial occlusion in rats. Eur Surg Res 2005;37(4):216–9.
68. Akyildiz H, Akcan A, Ozturk A, et al. D-dimer as a predictor of the need for laparotomy in patients with unclear non-traumatic acute abdomen. A preliminary study. Scand J Clin Lab Invest 2008;68(7):612–7.
69. Mentes O, Eryilmaz M, Harlak A, et al. Can D-dimer become a new diagnostic parameter for acute appendicitis? Am J Emerg Med 2009;27(7):765–9.
70. Kittaka H, Akimoto H, Takeshita H, et al. Usefulness of intestinal fatty acid-binding protein in predicting strangulated small bowel obstruction. PLoS One 2014;9(6):e99915.
71. Kanda T, Tsukahara A, Ueki K, et al. Diagnosis of ischemic small bowel disease by measurement of serum intestinal fatty acid-binding protein in patients with acute abdomen: a multicenter, observer-blinded validation study. J Gastroenterol 2011; 46(4):492–500.
72. Kanda T, Fujii H, Tani T, et al. Intestinal fatty acid-binding protein is a useful diagnostic marker for mesenteric infarction in humans. Gastroenterology 1996;110(2):339–43.
73. Kanda T, Nakatomi Y, Ishikawa H, et al. Intestinal fatty acid-binding protein as a sensitive marker of intestinal ischemia. Dig Dis Sci 1992;37(9):1362–7.
74. Gollin G, Marks C, Marks WH. Intestinal fatty acid binding protein in serum and urine reflects early ischemic injury to the small bowel. Surgery 1993;113(5): 545–51.
75. Thuijls G, van Wijck K, Grootjans J, et al. Early diagnosis of intestinal ischemia using urinary and plasma fatty acid binding proteins. Ann Surg 2011;253(2): 303–8.
76. Spangler R, Van Pham T, Khoujah D, et al. Abdominal emergencies in the geriatric patient. Int J Emerg Med 2014;7:43.
77. Demir IE, Ceyhan GO, Friess H. Beyond lactate: is there a role for serum lactate measurement in diagnosing acute mesenteric ischemia? Dig Surg 2012;29(3): 226–35.
78. Cronk DR, Houseworth TP, Cuadrado DG, et al. Intestinal fatty acid binding protein (I-FABP) for the detection of strangulated mechanical small bowel obstruction. Curr Surg 2006;63(5):322–5.
79. Acosta S, Nilsson T. Current status on plasma biomarkers for acute mesenteric ischemia. J Thromb Thrombolysis 2012;33(4):355–61.
80. Smotkin J, Tenner S. Laboratory diagnostic tests in acute pancreatitis. J Clin Gastroenterol 2002;34(4):459–62.

81. Steinberg WM, Goldstein SS, Davis ND, et al. Diagnostic assays in acute pancreatitis. A study of sensitivity and specificity. Ann Intern Med 1985;102(5):576–80.
82. Frank B, Gottlieb K. Amylase normal, lipase elevated: is it pancreatitis? A case series and review of the literature. Am J Gastroenterol 1999;94(2):463–9.
83. Scholmerich J, Gross V, Johannesson T, et al. Detection of biliary origin of acute pancreatitis. Comparison of laboratory tests, ultrasound, computed tomography, and ERCP. Dig Dis Sci 1989;34(6):830–3.
84. Tenner S, Dubner H, Steinberg W. Predicting gallstone pancreatitis with laboratory parameters: a meta-analysis. Am J Gastroenterol 1994;89(10):1863–6.
85. Broder J. Diagnostic imaging for the emergency physician. Philadelphia: Elsevier Saunders; 2011.
86. Hastings R, Powers R. Abdominal pain in the ED: a 35 year retrospective. Am J Emerg Med 2011;29(7):711–6.
87. Scheinfeld M, Mahadevia S, Stein E, et al. Can lab data be used to reduce abdominal computed tomography (CT) usage in young adults presenting to the emergency department with nontraumatic abdominal pain? Emerg Radiol 2010;17(5):353–60.
88. Oliva IB, Davarpanah AH, Rybicki FJ, et al. Expert panel on vascular imaging. ACR Appropriateness Criteria® imaging of mesenteric ischemia. National Guideline Clearinghouse; 2012. Available at: http://www.guideline.gov/content.aspx?id=37910&search=%22abdominal+pain%22+and+emergency. Accessed July 31, 2015.
89. Anderson S, Soto J. Multi-detector row CT of acute non-traumatic abdominal pain: contrast and protocol considerations. Radiol Clin North Am 2012;50(1):137–47.
90. Levenson RB, Camacho MA, Horn E, et al. Eliminating routine oral contrast use for CT in the emergency department: impact on patient throughput and diagnosis. Emerg Radiol 2012;19(6):513–7.
91. Razavi SA, Johnson JO, Kassin MT, et al. The impact of introducing a no oral contrast abdominopelvic CT examination (NOCAPE) pathway on radiology turn around times, emergency department length of stay, and patient safety. Emerg Radiol 2014;21(6):605–13.
92. Smith MP, Katz DS, Rosen MP, et al. Expert panel on gastrointestinal imaging. ACR Appropriateness Criteria® right lower quadrant pain–suspected appendicitis. National Guideline Clearinghouse; 2013. Available at: http://www.guideline.gov/content.aspx?id=47652&search=%22abdominal+pain%22+and+emergency. Accessed August 1, 2015.
93. Brenner DJ, Hall EJ. Computed tomography–an increasing source of radiation exposure. N Engl J Med 2007;357(22):2277–84.
94. Berrington de González A, Mahesh M, Kim KP, et al. Projected cancer risks from computed tomographic scans performed in the United States in 2007. Arch Intern Med 2009;169(22):2071–7.
95. Smith-Bindman R, Lipson J, Marcus R, et al. Radiation dose associated with common computed tomography examinations and the associated lifetime attributable risk of cancer. Arch Intern Med 2009;169(22):2078–86.
96. Balfe DM, Levine MS, Ralls PW, et al. Evaluation of left lower quadrant pain. American College of Radiology: ACR Appropriateness Criteria. Radiology 2000;215(Suppl):167–71.
97. Spence SC, Teichgraeber D, Chandrasekhar C. Emergent right upper quadrant sonography. J Ultrasound Med 2009;28(4):479–96.

98. Miller AH, Pepe PE, Brockman CR, et al. ED ultrasound in hepatobiliary disease. J Emerg Med 2006;30(1):69–74.
99. Rubano E, Mehta N, Caputo W, et al. Systematic review: emergency department bedside ultrasonography for diagnosing suspected abdominal aortic aneurysm. Acad Emerg Med 2013;20(2):128–38.
100. Summer SM, Scruggs W, Menchine MD, et al. A prospective evaluation of emergency department bedside ultrasonography for the detection of acute cholecystitis. Ann Emerg Med 2010;56(2):114–22.
101. Manterola C, Vial M, Moraga J, et al. Analgesia in patients with acute abdominal pain. Cochrane Database Syst Rev 2011;(1):CD005660.
102. Bektas F, Eken C, Soyuncu S, et al. Contribution of goal-directed ultrasonography to clinical decision-making for emergency physicians. Emerg Med J 2009;26: 169–72 (Utility of goal directed ultrasound to guide decisions in the emergency department).
103. Albayram F, Hamper UM. Ovarian and adnexal torsion: spectrum of sonographic findings with pathologic correlation. J Ultrasound Med 2001;20(10):1083–9.
104. Nizar K, Deutsch M, Filmer S, et al. Doppler studies of the ovarian venous blood flow in the diagnosis of adnexal torsion. J Clin Ultrasound 2009;37(8):436–9.
105. Graif M, Itzchak Y. Sonographic evaluation of ovarian torsion in childhood and adolescence. AJR Am J Roentgenol 1988;150(3):647–9.
106. Berman DA, Porter RS, Graber M. The GI cocktail is no more effective than plain liquid antacid: a randomized, double blind clinical trial. J Emerg Med 2003; 25(3):239–44.
107. Welling LR, Watson WA. The emergency department treatment of dyspepsia with antacids and oral lidocaine. Ann Emerg Med 1990;19(7):785–8.
108. Vilke GM, Jin A, Davis DP, et al. Prospective randomized study of viscous lidocaine versus benzocaine in a GI cocktail for dyspepsia. J Emerg Med 2004; 27(1):7–9.
109. Wrenn K, Slovis CM, Gongaware J. Using the "GI cocktail": a descriptive study. Ann Emerg Med 1995;26(6):687–90.
110. Chan S, Maurice AP, Davies SR, et al. The use of gastrointestinal cocktail for differentiating gastro-oesophageal reflux disease and acute coronary syndrome in the emergency setting: a systematic review. Heart Lung Circ 2014;23(10): 913–23.
111. Patanwala AE, Amini R, Hays DP, et al. Antiemetic therapy for nausea and vomiting in the emergency department. J Emerg Med 2010;39(3):330–6.
112. Braude D, Crandall C. Ondansetron versus promethazine to treat acute undifferentiated nausea in the emergency department: a randomized, double-blind, noninferiority trial. Acad Emerg Med 2008;15(3):209–15.
113. Barrett TW, DiPersio DM, Jenkins CA, et al. A randomized, placebo-controlled trial of ondansetron, metoclopramide, and promethazine in adults. Am J Emerg Med 2011;29(3):247–55.
114. Egerton-Warburton D, Meek R, Mee MJ, et al. Antiemetic use for nausea and vomiting in adult emergency department patients: randomized controlled trial comparing ondansetron, metoclopramide, and placebo. Ann Emerg Med 2014;64(5):526–32.e1.
115. Ernst AA, Weiss SJ, Park S, et al. Prochlorperazine versus promethazine for uncomplicated nausea and vomiting in the emergency department: a randomized, double-blind clinical trial. Ann Emerg Med 2000;36(2):89–94.
116. Ranji SR, Goldman LE, Simel DL, et al. Do opiates affect the clinical evaluation of patients with acute abdominal pain? JAMA 2006;296(14):1764–74.

117. Thomas SH, Silen W, Cheema F, et al. Effects of morphine analgesia on diagnostic accuracy in emergency department patients with abdominal pain: a prospective, randomized trial. J Am Coll Surg 2003;196(1):18–31.
118. Ditillo MF, Dziura JD, Rabinovici R. Is it safe to delay appendectomy in adults with acute appendicitis? Ann Surg 2006;244(5):656–60.
119. Maggio AQ, Reece-Smith AM, Tang TY, et al. Early laparoscopy versus active observation in acute abdominal pain: systematic review and meta-analysis. Int J Surg 2008;6(5):400–3.
120. Graff L, Radford MJ, Werne C. Probability of appendicitis before and after observation. Ann Emerg Med 1991;20(5):503–7.
121. Morino M, Pellegrino L, Castagna E, et al. Acute nonspecific abdominal pain: a randomized, controlled trial comparing early laparoscopy versus clinical observation. Ann Surg 2006;244(6):881–6 [discussion: 886–8].
122. Irvin TT. Abdominal pain: a surgical audit of 1190 emergency admissions. Br J Surg 1989;76(11):1121–5.
123. Howie JG. The place of appendicectomy in the treatment of young adult patients with possible appendicitis. Lancet 1968;1(7556):1365–7.
124. Thomson HJ, Jones PF. Active observation in acute abdominal pain. Am J Surg 1986;152(5):522–5.
125. Brewer BJ. "Abdominal pain. An analysis of 1000 consecutive cases in a University Hospital ER" (Laeknabladid "One year follow-up of patients discharged from the ED with non-specific abdominal pain"). Am J Surgery 1976;131(2):219–23.

Approach to Patients with Epigastric Pain

Patrick Robinson, MD[a],*, John C. Perkins Jr, MD[b]

KEYWORDS

- Epigastric pain • Dyspepsia • Esophagitis • Boerhaave syndrome
- Acute pancreatitis • Food bolus impaction

KEY POINTS

- Emergency medicine providers must consider upper-gastrointestinal bleeding in patients presenting with epigastric pain and dyspepsia.
- Empirical trials of proton pump inhibitor therapy in patients with uncomplicated peptic ulcer disease have been shown to improve symptoms and increase the rate of ulcer healing.
- Patients with sudden onset of dysphagia, odynophagia, chest pain, and sialorrhea should be considered to have food bolus impaction and require involvement of gastrointestinal specialists to help determine the most appropriate management.
- Emergency medicine providers should maintain a high index of suspicion for more serious disorders of esophagitis in immunocompromised patients presenting with dyspepsia, odynophagia, and/or dysphagia.
- It is important to consider the broad differential diagnosis of an increased serum lipase level other than acute pancreatitis.
- Acute pancreatitis can have a wide spectrum of mortality and emergency medicine providers should use a Sequential Organ Failure Assessment score or BISAP (blood urea nitrogen, impaired mental status, systemic inflammatory response syndrome criteria, age, pleural effusion) criteria for appropriate disposition.

INTRODUCTION

Abdominal pain is the most frequent presenting complaint in emergency departments (EDs) across the country and the emergency medicine provider (EMP) must be skilled at differentiating and managing this presentation.[1] Approximately 6% of chief complaints involve abdominal pain and, of these, 25% present with epigastric pain.[2]

Disclosure: The authors have nothing to disclose.
[a] Virginia Tech Carilion Emergency Medicine Residency, Department of Emergency Medicine, 1 Riverside Circle, 4th Floor, Roanoke, VA 24016, USA; [b] Virginia Tech Carilion Emergency Medicine Residency, Department of Emergency Medicine, Virginia Tech Carilion School of Medicine, 1 Riverside Circle, 4th Floor, Roanoke, VA 24016, USA
* Corresponding author.
E-mail address: Perobinson@carilionclinic.org

Emerg Med Clin N Am 34 (2016) 191–210
http://dx.doi.org/10.1016/j.emc.2015.12.012   emed.theclinics.com

Abdominal complaints, including epigastric discomfort, can be complicated. A general understanding of visceral pain in the epigastric region with its distinct features can help ED providers understand the appropriate work-up for this complaint type.[1] Abdominal organs communicate stretch, ischemia, and nondescript pain via nociceptors that transmit signals via afferent receptors to the spinal cord.[1] Organs derived from the embryonic foregut, such as the esophagus, stomach, pancreas, biliary system, and proximal duodenum, can all produce pain located in the midline epigastric region.[1] Chest pain as the result of gastroesophageal reflux disease (GERD) and dysphagia are notoriously difficult to distinguish from cardiac disorders because esophageal disease can cause chest pain, but this diagnostic quandary is discussed in further detail elsewhere in this article.[3] This article discusses noncardiac emergency disorders associated with epigastric discomfort. Clinical features and diagnostic and therapeutic options are presented for EMPs trying to appropriately and efficiently evaluate and treat patients with epigastric discomfort, which has a large differential involving both severe and benign disorders.[3]

Peptic Ulcer Disease/Gastritis

Dyspepsia is any symptom of the upper gastrointestinal (GI) tract, including epigastric pain, heartburn, reflux, nausea, vomiting, or discomfort lasting greater than 4 weeks.[4] It is a common presentation thought to afflict 25% to 40% of the population every year.[4,5] This presentation should not be taken lightly, because some studies have shown the incidence of upper-GI bleed secondary to peptic ulcer disease (PUD) to be as high as 41 persons in 100,0000 with an 8.7% risk of mortality.[6] One-quarter of those with dyspepsia are thought to have an underlying organic cause, whereas the other 75% have no identifiable disorder after further evaluation.[5] There has been a common notion that many lifestyle variables, such as smoking, coffee, alcohol, chocolate, obesity, and fat intake, precipitate dyspepsia but evidence does not support this notion.[4] EMPs should recognize that there is a subset of patients presenting with dyspepsia or epigastric pain associated with unique features listed in **Box 1** who should have stool guaiac testing in the ED.[7] A normal hemoglobin test and hematocrit can also be supportive evidence that the dyspepsia is not associated with a GI bleed.

Box 1
Indications for stool guaiac testing

- Symptoms of acute or chronic GI bleeding
- Physical signs of anemia (eg, pallor)
- New anemia on complete blood count
- Report of greater than 2 kg (4.5 lb) of weight loss in past 6 months
- Signs of enteric illness (eg, fever and diarrhea)
- Tenesmus
- History of GI malignancy
- Change in bowel habits
- Use of anticoagulants
- Significant use of nonsteroidal antiinflammatory drugs
- History of esophageal varices

Therapeutic strategies for patients presenting with PUD are focused on relieving symptoms, ulcer healing, and reducing recurrence.[8] Common pharmacotherapy options for the treatment of dyspepsia are listed in **Table 1**.[9–12] EMPs should not interpret the improvement of epigastric discomfort with a GI cocktail (oral viscous lidocaine/antacid plus or minus anticholinergic) as a method to differentiate dyspepsia from cardiac pain.[13] There is evidence that GI cocktails do provide pain relief to patients with cardiac chest pain.[13]

For patients presenting with classic symptoms of PUD, it is appropriate to prescribe a 4-week trial of empiric therapy.[4,12] Historically, it was appropriate to start patients on either a proton pump inhibitor (PPI) or histamine receptor antagonist (H2RA), but a recent Cochrane Review concluded that therapy with PPI was more efficacious than with H2RA.[11] Evidence supports the initiation of an empiric trial of 4 weeks of PPI therapy for patients presenting with dyspepsia instead of the more expensive test-and-treat strategy.[4,12] This strategy is supported by most patients presenting with dyspepsia having symptoms as the result of acid-mediated disorders.[12] Perhaps the most compelling reason to initiate empiric therapy is that PPIs not only reduce symptoms but also increase the rate of ulcer healing if present.[8] However, this therapeutic strategy has not resulted in a reduction of PUD recurrence.[8] An empiric trial of a PPI in patients presenting with dyspepsia should be reserved for patients less than the age of 50 years and without red flags.[12] Red flags listed in **Box 2** are concerning in patients with dyspepsia and should prompt further evaluation with endoscopy because these patients are not appropriate for empiric treatment.[12,14,15] It is important for EMPs to distinguish patients who require urgent/emergent endoscopic procedures from those who can be referred for outpatient evaluation. **Box 3** provides a breakdown of features that can help guide EMPs in determining the appropriate disposition for patients with dyspepsia.[12,14–16]

Table 1 Medical management options for dyspepsia	
PPIs: • Lansoprazole • Omeprazole • Rabeprazole • Pantoprazole	• Most effective therapy supported by literature • IV use should be reserved for patients with acute upper-GI bleeds or emesis because of cost and risk of adverse outcomes in nonulcerative dyspepsia
H2 receptor antagonists: • Ranitidine • Cimetidine • Famotidine • Nizatidine	• Superior to placebo but recent evidence suggests PPI should be first line
Bismuth salts	• Trend towards statistically significant effect compared with placebo
Sucralfate	• No greater symptom relief than placebo, but evidence supports increased rate of ulcer healing

Antacids:
• Magnesium hydroxide
• Aluminum hydroxide
  ○ Maalox
  ○ Mylanta
• Simethicone
	• No greater reduction in symptoms than placebo
	• Must consider decreased absorption of concomitantly ingested medications
	• Prolonged use can cause electrolyte dyscrasias, particularly in patients with chronic renal failure

Abbreviations: IV, intravenous; PPI, proton pump inhibitor.

Box 2
Red flags for patients with dyspepsia

- Unexplained weight loss
- Recurrent vomiting
- Progressive dysphagia
- Odynophagia
- GI blood loss (eg, melena, hematochezia, acute anemia)
- Family history of GI cancer

Helicobacter pylori is associated with most duodenal ulcers. Patients with duodenal ulcers without evidence of *H pylori* infection have a worse prognosis with increased relapse, poor healing, and increased severity of symptoms.[5] The role of EMPs in this setting is to evaluate for red flags associated with the patient's presentation, and, if absent, initiate empiric PPI therapy and arrange for primary care follow-up for evaluation of symptom improvement. It is appropriate for EMPs to make a referral for *H pylori* testing in the outpatient setting. Empiric therapy can be left to the discretion of the provider based on local prevalence and the patient's access to outpatient follow-up.

Complications
Hemorrhage Between 30% and 50% of upper-GI bleeding is the result of peptic ulcers.[17] The specific management of acute GI bleeding is covered elsewhere in this issue (see Jose V. Nable, Autumn Graham: Gastrointestinal bleeding, in this issue.),

---

Box 3
Indications for endoscopy in patients with GERD

Emergent endoscopy: less than 24 hours

- Evidence of acute GI bleed causing unstable vital signs
- Patient with GI bleed and history of esophageal varices or risk factors for variceal bleed

Urgent endoscopy: 1 to 7 days

- Evidence of GI bleeding or anemia but hemodynamically stable
- Dysphagia or odynophagia
- Red flag symptoms or history

Elective endoscopy: greater than 7 days

- Persistent or progressive GERD symptoms despite appropriate medical therapy
- Finding of a mass, stricture, or ulcer on imaging studies
- Evaluation of patients with suspected extraesophageal manifestations of GERD
- Screening for Barrett esophagus (BE) in selected patients (as clinically indicated) or high risk for BE (reflux symptoms, age >50 years, white, male, obese)
- Persistent vomiting
- Patients with recurrent symptoms after endoscopic or surgical antireflux procedures
- Involuntary weight loss greater than 5%

---

but it should be reemphasized that the primary goal of EMPs is aggressive resuscitation with crystalloids and blood products in preparation for therapeutic interventions performed by a gastroenterologist, surgeon, or interventional radiologist. Patients with significant upper-GI bleeding require intensive care monitoring because of their high risk of becoming hemodynamically unstable and associated mortalities as high as 10%.[18] This information further underscores the importance of empiric PPI therapy in appropriate patients and referral to gastroenterology for further diagnostics in patients with concerning features as discussed earlier in this article.

Perforation A rare, but feared, complication of PUD is perforation. Most frequently seen in male patients in their fourth or fifth decade of life, perforation has been noted to occur at rates as high as 7% per year in those with PUD.[19] This presentation is characterized by the abrupt onset of abdominal pain and peritonitis as gastric contents enter the abdominal cavity. Physical examination features such as pain requiring multiple doses of pain medication, tachycardia, diffuse abdominal tenderness, or tenderness in multiple quadrants should increase the provider's suspicion of perforation.[20–22] EMPs cannot rely on radiographic imaging to exclude gastric perforation. Free air under the diaphragm is not always present, and up to 66% of patients have only free peritoneal fluid as their radiographic or ultrasonography abnormality.[23] Plain radiographs have a sensitivity for detecting pneumoperitoneum as low as 15%.[24] Computed tomography (CT) imaging, the preferred imaging method for suspected perforation, has a sensitivity of roughly 85% with the added benefit of being able to identify the source.[24] If high suspicion exists for perforation despite negative imaging, EMPs should consult a surgeon for further evaluation, because surgical repair remains the treatment of choice.[19]

Obstruction Gastric outlet obstruction is an increasingly rare complication of PUD. Only 5% of gastric outlet obstruction is caused by ulcerative disorders, which occur because of the surrounding edema caused by peptic ulcers in the antrum or duodenal region.[25] These patients typically present with the sensation of abdominal fullness, nausea, and vomiting and may have abdominal distension. Dehydration and electrolyte abnormalities may be present. EMPs should focus on correcting these imbalances, while relieving gastric distention with nasogastric tube suction.[25] Diagnosis is made through endoscopy because imaging is often inadequate. Admission is often required for intravenous (IV) hydration and serial abdominal examinations as the edema subsides. However, surgical intervention is often required.[25]

ESOPHAGEAL EMERGENCIES

Esophageal pain is notoriously difficult to distinguish from cardiac ischemia because of mirroring innervation to both structures.[26] Because of the high risk of mortality and morbidity associated with missed or delayed diagnosis of cardiac ischemia, EMPs should approach these patients with the assumption that the complaint is cardiac in nature. Esophageal disorders, if suspected, can be evaluated simultaneously.[26]

Food Bolus (Foreign Body) Impaction

Foreign body esophageal impaction (FBI) is a frequent complaint presenting to the ED. The incidence is roughly 13 per 100,000 persons, and it is associated with significant morbidity and risk for mortality secondary to esophageal perforation.[27,28] This presentation should be discussed as 2 distinct disorders: (1) true impaction of nonedible material, and (2) food bolus from nonsolid material obstructing the esophagus, because the management and risk for perforation differ.[29] The most common presentation is a patient with a poorly masticated meat bolus impaction that becomes lodged above a preexisting distal esophageal stricture (ring or malignant), esophageal peptic ulcer, or eosinophilic esophagitis (EoE).[27–29] This clinical presentation has a female predominance and the rate of incidence increases with age, particularly in patients more than 70 years old.[29]

Historical features that are consistent with FBI include sudden onset of dysphagia, odynophagia, chest pain, and sialorrhea.[27,29] Patients frequently report a sensation of discomfort referred to the suprasternal notch, but this cannot be used to predict the location of impaction.[29] The presence of wheezing, stridor, or dyspnea may indicate that the ingested foreign body is compromising the patient's respiratory effort and prompts the clinician to secure the airway.[27] Even in the absence of the aforementioned symptoms, these patients are at risk for aspiration because of their inability to tolerate secretions. This risk increases the urgency of foreign body removal.[27] On the more severe spectrum of this presentation, patients arrive to the ED with hypoxia, tachycardia, and hypertension caused by prolonged obstruction, resulting in airway compromise and extensive coughing.[29] Crepitus, tenderness, and erythema are associated physical examination findings suggestive of esophageal perforation (Boerhaave syndrome) in the oropharyngeal or proximal esophageal region.[29] These features make the diagnosis attainable on clinical presentation; however, further imaging and diagnostics are indicated to further stratify the presentation and evaluate the need for surgical intervention.[29]

A neck and chest radiograph can aid in the diagnosis of metallic versus soft material impaction.[29] Patients with ingestion of sharp objects or items with corrosive capacity (eg, batteries) should have emergent evaluation by a skilled endoscopist for removal.[27] The use of contrast (eg, barium or Gastrografin) is not recommended because it can coat the foreign body and complicate endoscopic evaluation as well as increasing the risk of aspiration in a patient already having difficulty clearing secretions.[29] Additional radiographic diagnostics with CT imaging of the chest and neck are typically reserved only for when the suspicion for rupture is high; these symptoms are discussed in detail later in this article.[29]

Management of this disorder is focused on passage or removal of the obstruction, either mechanically or medically, to reduce the risk of perforation and aspiration.[27,29] Indications for emergent endoscopic evaluation and removal are listed in **Box 4**.[27,29] If a patient reports a history of ingesting corrosive items or sharp materials, without evidence of radiographic presence in the esophagus, the clinician must consider endoscopic evaluation because there remains a risk for perforation in the remaining GI tract.[27] If there is suspicion of esophageal perforation, CT imaging and surgical consultation should be obtained.[27] However, if the impaction occurred within the past 24 hours, there is evidence to support better outcomes with the use of endoscopy

---

Box 4
Emergent indications for endoscopic FBI removal

- Aspiration risk: patient unable to tolerate secretions
- Ingestion of sharp objects: metal, pins, toothpicks, bones, and so forth
- Ingestion of corrosive items
  - Coin batteries
  - Lithium ion batteries
- Food bolus impaction present greater than 24 hours

as primary treatment before surgical intervention, even with the suggestion of perfo-ration.[27] Because the endoscopic evaluation and removal of FBI is best left to trained specialists, the focus here is on pharmacologic options available to ED providers. Because endoscopy has its own complications, pharmacologic management is an option in patients with uncomplicated FBI, especially if GI consultants are not readily available.[29] There are several options listed in **Table 2** that result in the relaxation of the lower esophageal sphincter and can facilitate the passage of the obstruction.[29–31] These agents have their own complications. In addition to discussing the risks and benefits of each modality with the patients, each facility should have a conversation with their GI consultants about whether they would prefer to be called before any trials of pharmacotherapy for possible immediate esophagogastroduodenoscopy (EGD). In summary, when presented with a patient with FBI, it is imperative to evaluate for airway patency, evaluate for symptoms indicating perforation, and be in contact with a skilled endoscopist to discuss medical versus endoscopic management.[29]

There are scenarios of ingested foreign bodies that do not pose significant increased risk for perforation (eg, coins, blunt objects) and are amenable to

Table 2
Pharmacotherapy options for the management of FBI

Medication Name	Dose/Route	Mechanism	Comments	Contraindications/SEs
Glucagon	0.25–0.5 mg IV	Decreases resting tone of LES	High risk of emesis warrants pretreatment with antiemetic	Hypersensitivity to glucagon, h/o insulinoma, pheochromocytoma. SEs: nausea, vomiting, diarrhea, rash, dry mouth
Diazepam	2.5–10 mg IV	Antispasmodic agent that relaxes LES	—	—
Nifedipine	10 mg sublingual liquid	Relaxes smooth muscle of LES	Successful use documented in case reports; no controlled study to support its routine use in FBI. Verapamil has been cited in successful case reports as well	May cause hypotension
Isosorbide	5 mg sublingual	Smooth muscle relaxation with reduction in LES pressure	Shown to be efficacious in reduction of LES tone in patients with achalasia but has not been studied or used in the management of acute food bolus impaction	May cause hypotension and should not be used in patients with bradycardia

Abbreviations: LES, lower esophageal sphincter; SEs, side effects.

conservative management as long as the object has passed into the stomach, the patient is asymptomatic, and the object is less than 2 cm in diameter.[27] These patients can be managed with repeat plain film imaging to evaluate for progression of the object through the GI tract, but endoscopic removal is subsequently indicated if the object fails to progress for more than 1 week.[27]

Pediatrics

Most patients (roughly 80%) requiring medical care for FBI are children.[32] EMPs must pay close attention to any historical clues of ingestion, because 30% may be asymptomatic.[32] Plain radiographs are useful in determining the location (upper esophageal sphincter, midesophagus at the aortic notch, lower esophageal sphincter) and type of foreign body and also can be used to differentiate a coin from a button battery.[32] EMPs should identify ingestion of a button battery because the recent increased production of lithium coin batteries has resulted in a 7-fold increase in major morbidity or mortality in children less than 4 years old.[32] Button lithium batteries can induce localized mucosal injury in 1 hour and damage all layers of the esophagus in as little as 4 hours, thus focus should be on removing the object as quickly as possible.[32]

Caustic Ingestions

Caustic solutions are easily available and ubiquitous in households as cleaning solutions, detergents, and other chemicals. Although caustic ingestions occur in patients of all ages, the morbidity and mortality are much more concerning and frequent in adults, because these are often nonaccidental.[33,34] Injuries caused by these ingestions can vary from minimal local inflammation to transmural necrosis and perforation requiring laparotomy and esophageal resection.[33] EMPs should prioritize stabilization of the patient as described earlier, with focus on the assessment of the airway, breathing, and circulation because concomitant injuries to the trachea or bronchus are ominous signs with a high mortality.[35] Although there is no consensus algorithmic approach to caustic ingestions, focus should be placed on resuscitation and evaluating for signs of peritonitis that suggest perforation and require emergent laparotomy.[34] If no evidence of perforation is present initially, the most appropriate next step is further evaluation by emergent endoscopy to assess for the level of gastric injury along with CT imaging to evaluate for the level of inflammation and associated extragastrointestinal injuries.[33–35] EMPs should not attempt to induce vomiting, use nasogastric suction, or attempt to neutralize the caustic ingestion because of the risk of precipitating more necrosis and placing the patient at risk for airway compromise.[35] This is a true GI emergency and a GI consultant should be contacted immediately after determining that the patient is stable. If no GI consultant is available, then transfer for endoscopy should be expedited.

Boerhaave Syndrome

Patients presenting with the clinical triad of chest pain, vomiting, and pneumomediastinum, without concern for foreign body impaction, can be presumed to have strain-induced esophageal rupture, or Boerhaave syndrome. Evidence of mediastinal, subdiaphragmatic, or subcutaneous air or a new pleural effusion on plain film is suggestive of esophageal perforation and thus indicates further radiographic evaluation with CT imaging.[27] There is no consensus algorithm for the management of Boerhaave syndrome, but several key steps can help establish appropriate disposition for these patients. When a patient presents with a clinical picture consistent with Boerhaave syndrome, CT imaging is integral in delineating the extent of the perforation.[27] If a patient is hemodynamically stable and able to tolerate secretions, the clinician can further evaluate for esophagomediastinal-thoracic communication and persistent extravasation with water-soluble contrast esophagram.[36] If this study shows that there is extravasation, the patient requires urgent surgical evaluation for primary repair versus resection.[36] This decision is largely based on the extent of the esophageal violation and should be left to the consulted surgeon.[36] If the water-soluble study does not show evidence of extravasation, these patients can typically be managed conservatively with observation and delayed EGD.[36] It is important to realize that most cases of esophageal perforation are not caused by Boerhaave syndrome, but are iatrogenic, from such procedures as endoscopy with esophageal dilation for stricture.

Esophagitis

Esophagitis should be suspected in patients presenting with the clinical picture of chest pain, odynophagia, dysphagia, and retrosternal pain.[37,38] Causes can include common reflux esophagitis (discussed at length earlier) to less common infectious processes listed in **Box 5**. In the absence of red flags listed in **Box 2**, reflux esophagitis can be managed conservatively with initiation of PPI and outpatient follow-up. Pill esophagitis frequently results in ulcers and is most often secondary to antibiotics and nonsteroidal antiinflammatory drugs.[38] This disorder can be managed with initiation of a PPI and removal of the causative agent when the patient is hemodynamically stable without red flags.[38]

Special Populations

Immunocompromised patients with esophagitis are at risk for a broadened differential of infectious disorders causing their discomfort.[39] They are also subject to subtle presentations of severe disorders and EMPs should have a high index of suspicion for esophagitis in any patient who is immunocompromised. The presence of any symptoms consistent with esophagitis should prompt exploration of possible infectious esophagitis.[39] These infectious causes include, but are not limited to, candida, herpes simplex virus (HSV), cytomegalovirus, human immunodeficiency virus (HIV), and tuberculous esophagitis and are historically known as acquired immunodeficiency syndrome–defining opportunistic infections if the patient is HIV positive. HIV infection should be suspected in patients thought to have infectious esophagitis without history of immunosuppression.[40] However, these patients are not only at risk for these infectious processes but can experience catastrophic complications from these disorders.[39] HSV esophagitis is rare in immunocompetent individuals, but treatment with

---

Box 5
Differential diagnosis of esophagitis

- Reflux esophagitis
- Pill esophagitis
- EoE
- Candidal esophagitis
- Herpes simplex virus esophagitis
- Cytomegalovirus esophagitis
- Human immunodeficiency virus esophagitis
- Tuberculous esophagitis

acyclovir can expedite resolution and decrease severity.[37] EMPs must maintain a high index of suspicion for infectious esophagitis in any patient with known immunosuppression, even those on low-dose glucocorticoid regimens, because evidence suggests that they too are at increased risk.[41]

Eosinophilic Esophagitis

EoE is an increasingly recognized risk factor for FBI and has been found in up to 33% of patients presenting with FBI. The chronic eosinophilic infiltration results in inflammation making the esophageal tissue fragile and inelastic.[27–29,42,43] This inflammation results in segmental or diffuse narrowing that predisposes to FBI.[42] Although this transmural eosinophilic infiltration results in more friable tissue and can present with primary presentation of esophageal rupture (these patients have increased risk for perforation from EGD and also from food bolus), spontaneous rupture caused by EoE is a rare occurrence.[27,28,36,42] Current evidence suggests that pharmacotherapy is unsuccessful in the management of FBI in patients with EoE.[43] A past medical history positive for GERD, atopy, seasonal allergies, or asthma should raise concern for EoE in the right clinical context of esophagitis symptoms.[27,36,44] Patients with a food bolus impaction in which underlying EoE is suspected should have urgent endoscopy. Early diagnosis of EoE with EGD biopsy can facilitate initiation of medical management with steroids and acid suppression to reduce inflammatory tissue remodeling and reduce risk for subsequent complications.[27,29,44]

PANCREATITIS

Acute pancreatitis (AP) is an important diagnosis to consider and recognize because providers often underdiagnose it in patients who present in the extremes of the disease spectrum.[45] The diagnosis is established when a patient has at least 2 of the 3 following criteria: (1) abdominal pain consistent with the disorder, (2) serum amylase/lipase level greater than 3 times the upper limit of normal, and/or (3) radiologic imaging to support the diagnosis.[46] This disease results in roughly 250,000 hospitalizations in the United States annually.[47] Although the mild form only portends a mortality of less than 1%, pancreatitis can carry a mortality of up to 47% if there is evidence of multiple organ system failure, and should be taken with the utmost seriousness.[48] Pancreatitis occurs after an initial insult from a broad list of possible causes, as listed in **Box 6**. The disorder occurs when pancreatic enzymes begin to digest pancreatic cell membranes, thus inducing the inflammatory cascade leading to hemorrhage, edema, ischemia, and necrosis.[48] Despite advances in medical care, as many as 30% of patients with AP progress to chronic pancreatitis.[48] The most common cause of AP is pancreatic obstruction (eg, gallstone pancreatitis), but EMPs should consider many of the other causes.[48,49] Medication-induced AP can be caused by a multitude of medications, the list being too extensive to cover completely in this article.[48] Several common causes that EMPs may encounter are listed in **Box 7**.[48]

This portion of the article briefly discusses the clinical presentation of pancreatitis, but also focuses on how to best stratify the broad spectrum of disease symptoms and highlights key features that EMPs must consider. Although the cardinal presentation associated with this presentation is abdominal pain, pancreatitis can present with a broad spectrum of disease from mild to extreme.[46] The location of pain in pancreatitis can vary from generalized abdominal discomfort, right upper quadrant (RUQ), and anywhere in between.[46,48] The most common description is constant discomfort located in the epigastric region.[47,48] A unique feature for pancreatic discomfort, explained by the organ's location in the retroperitoneum, is the patient's report of a

---

Box 6
Causes of pancreatitis

- Pancreatic duct obstruction
  - Gallstone
  - Mass lesion
- Alcohol
- Cystic fibrosis
- Endoscopic retrograde cholangiopancreatography
- Trauma
- Hypertriglyceridemia
- Medications
- Ischemia
- Autoimmune pancreatitis (Lupus, Sjögren)
- Genetics (PRSS!, SPINK1, CFTR)
- Posterior penetrating ulcer
- Infections
  - Bacterial: *Legionella*, *Leptospira*, *Mycoplasma*, *Salmonella*
  - Viral: mumps, Coxsackie, cytomegalovirus, echovirus, hepatitis B
  - Parasitic: *Ascaris*, *Cryptosporidium*, *Toxoplasma*
- Hypercalcemia/hyperparathyroidism
- Organophosphate poisoning
- Scorpion envenomation
- Idiopathic

---

deep, boring pain that often radiates to the back.[46] In cases in which biliary obstruction exists, some patients may be jaundiced.[48] Severe AP is characterized by significant necrosis along with intrapancreatic thrombosis and hemorrhage in addition to persistent single or multiple organ failure.[48] In patients with retroperitoneal hemorrhage, flank ecchymosis (Grey-Turner sign) and/or periumbilical ecchymosis (Cullen

---

Box 7
Medications and medication classes known to cause AP

- Angiotensin-converting enzyme inhibitors
- Statins
- Oral contraceptives/hormone replacement therapy
- Diuretics
- Highly active antiretroviral therapy
- Valproic acid
- Oral hypoglycemic agents
  - Metformin
  - DP4 inhibitors
  - GLP1 mimetics

sign) might be found on physical examination, but this is a late and rare finding in only about 3% of patients.[48] In addition, severe AP can present with fever, hypoxemia, tachycardia, and hypotension in addition to the cardinal symptoms.[48]

In order to fully understand the diagnostic strategy of AP, EMPs should be familiar with systemic and local complications associated with the disease, as listed in **Box 8**.[47,48] The complications listed in **Box 8** highlight the need for imaging in patients with moderate to severe AP because identification of local complications can affect management strategies.[47,48,50] Delayed complications, such as hemorrhagic pancreatitis associated with chronic pancreatitis and pseudoaneurysms, may present to the ED and providers must be familiar with their cause and management.[51]

Serum amylase level cannot be solely used to diagnose AP because of poor negative predictive value resulting from low sensitivity and specificity.[47] Because of these limitations, serum lipase level is the preferred laboratory test because it has increased sensitivity and specificity.[47] Providers should be aware that this laboratory value is nonspecific, as shown in **Box 9**.[47,52]

Patients with diabetes seem to have higher median serum lipase levels and may require setting cutoffs 3 to 5 times that of the upper limit of normal to maintain the same sensitivities and specificities as the nondiabetic population.[47] Other laboratory tests that may be abnormal depending on the cause of the AP include increased white blood cell count, bilirubin, serum alkaline phosphatase, aspartate aminotransferase, lactate dehydrogenase, and triglyceride levels.[50]

Given these limitations, the use of serum markers (lipase specifically) in diagnosing pancreatitis are of decreasing utility in the ED unless levels are many times greater than the upper limit of normal.[47] Therefore, if serum levels are equivocal and there is any suspicion for pancreatitis as the underlying cause of the patient's presentation,

---

Box 8
Complications of AP

Local complications:

- Regional fluid accumulation
- Pancreatic pseudocyst formation
- Necrotic tissue and fluid collection
- Walled-off necrosis
- Infected necrosis
- Hemorrhagic pancreatitis

Systemic complications

- Systemic inflammatory response syndrome (SIRS), secondary local fluid and necrosis becoming secondarily infected
- Splanchnic vein thrombosis
- Abdominal compartment syndrome
- Pseudoaneurysm
- Acute respiratory distress syndrome
- Acute exacerbation of underlying comorbidities (coronary artery disease and chronic lung disease)

Box 9
Nonpancreatic causes of increased serum lipase

- Renal insufficiency
- Appendicitis
- Small bowel obstruction
- Cholecystitis
- Malignant tumor producing lipolytic enzymes
- Esophagitis
- Hypertriglyceridemia
- Prolonged tourniquet time for blood draw
- Peritonitis

---

further work-up with contrast-enhanced CT (CECT) imaging may be indicated.[47] This decision should be weighed against the risk of radiation, the patient's age, the use and cost of resources, and the need for diagnosis based on severity of illness. CECT is not necessary or recommended to be performed while in the ED if the diagnosis is clear based on history, physical examination, and increased enzyme levels.[47] Pancreatic necrosis may take 48 to 72 hours to be detectable on CT scan after the onset of AP, and pseudocysts and pancreatic abscesses typically do not form for 4 to 5 weeks, respectively.[47,49] CECT is appropriate in searching for alternative diagnoses or to assess for the presence of complications. If present, pancreatic necrosis increases the associated mortality of AP from 1% to 23%.[50] The use of CECT is the gold standard for diagnosing AP, and can help EMPs to determine the need for antibiotics in the presence of necrosis.[50] Pancreatic necrosis can be identified on CECT by the presence of areas with no or low contrast enhancement caused by areas of microcirculatory failure.[51] CECT has an accuracy of 90% for detecting necrosis when the necrotic area is greater than 30% of the pancreas.[51] CECT has a sensitivity and specificity of 90% in the diagnosis of AP and abdominal MRI has similar figures.[47,53] With most AP diagnoses being caused by gallstone obstruction, RUQ ultrasonography is a valuable adjunct imaging modality that should be used often.[47] This modality is particularly important because evidence of gallstones should prompt surgical consultation for cholecystectomy given the risk of recurrent pancreatitis and biliary sepsis.[47] Gallstone pancreatitis is usually managed primarily via endoscopic retrograde cholangiopancreatography (ERCP) before consideration of surgical intervention.

EMPs should focus on the extent of the patient's acuity by assessing for the presence of systemic inflammatory response syndrome (SIRS) or end-organ dysfunction.[50] With this in mind, the Sequential Organ Failure Assessment (SOFA) score (**Table 3**), can be implemented in the ED as an initial assessment of predicted mortality and has more utility than the Ranson Criteria to help predict the severity of the presenting clinical picture.[50] A SOFA score of 9 or less correlates with 33% mortality, a score of 10 represents a mortality risk of roughly 40%, and a score of 11 or greater carries a risk of 80% mortality.[54]

However, in a busy ED, EMPs should focus on being able to evaluate for intrinsic patient-related characteristics, laboratory values, and radiographic evidence to assess for severe disease.[47] The BISAP (blood urea nitrogen [BUN], impaired mental status, SIRS criteria, age, pleural effusion) criteria, listed in **Box 10**, is a prognostic tool

Table 3
SOFA score

Organ System	Score: 1	2	3	4	5
Cardiovascular	No hypotension	MAP <70 mm Hg	Dopamine or dobutamine	Dopamine >5 μg/kg/min epinephrine <0.1 μg/kg/min or norepinephrine <0.1 μg/kg/min	Dopamine <0.1 μg/kg/min or >15 μg/kg/min or epinephrine >0.1 μg/kg/min or norepinephrine >0.1 μg/kg/min
Respiratory (Pao_2/Fio_2 mm Hg)	>400	400–300	300–200	200–100 (calculated with vent support)	<100 (calculated with vent support)
Renal (creatinine μmol/L)	<100	100–200	200–350	350–500	>500
Neuro (Glasgow Coma Scale)	15	14–13	12–10	9–7	<6
Hematologic (platelet count × 10^9/L)	>150	100–150	50–100	20–50	<20
Hepatic (bilirubin μmol/L)	<20	20–60	60–120	120–240	>240

SOFA score is calculated as the sum of the scores for the individual organs.
Abbreviations: Fio_2, fraction of inspired oxygen; MAP, mean arterial pressure.

Box 10
BISAP

- BUN level >25 mg/dL
- Impaired mental status: disorientation, lethargy, somnolence, coma, or stupor
- Two or more SIRS criteria
- Age >60 years
- Pleural effusion present

that can be used by EMPs to predict in-hospital mortality and help to more appropriately disposition the patient.[55]

This tool is easy to apply and, unlike the Ranson and modified Glasgow scoring systems, can be rapidly applied using information available to EMPs.[55] The patient receives 1 point for each criterion met. Patients with a score of less than or equal to 2 had an in-hospital mortality risk of less than 2%, with a significant increase in mortality with a score greater than 3, as shown in **Table 4**.[55]

Numerous risk factors put the patient at risk of severe AP, although many are nonspecific. Patients' vital signs and comorbid conditions are the most important factors in helping EMPs consider severe AP. Any evidence of organ failure or pancreatic necrosis automatically identifies severe AP.[47]

Necrotizing Pancreatitis

Patients found to have asymptomatic pseudocysts or extrapancreatic/pancreatic necrosis do not warrant intervention regardless of size, location, or extension.[47] However, for severe AP cases, EMPs must be able to recognize necrotizing and hemorrhagic pancreatitis as acutely life-threatening complications that likely require interventional consultation.[51] Necrotizing pancreatitis can occur in up to 15% of patients with severe AP.[51] With advancements in interventional technology, management of necrotizing AP now involves a multidisciplinary, graduated approach with interventional radiology, endoscopists, and surgical consultants.[51] Antibiotic usage is only indicated in cases of infected pancreatic necrosis, because evidence shows that there is no reduction in morbidity or mortality with antibiotics in sterile necrosis.[47,51] CECT can suggest infection of the necrotic tissue if there is presence of gas bubbles within the peripancreatic/pancreatic necrosis.[47,51]

Table 4	
Observed mortality based on BISAP score	
BISAP Score	Mortality (%)
0	0.1
1	0.5
2	1.9
3	5.3
4	12.7
5	22.5

Hemorrhagic Pancreatitis

Chronic pancreatitis is a disease typically characterized by pancreatic calcifications, steatorrhea, and diabetes mellitus, with the leading cause being chronic alcohol ingestion.[52] Patients with chronic pancreatitis may develop pseudoaneurysms as a result of the chronic inflammatory process of leaking digestive enzymes.[52] These pseudoaneurysms are at risk for rupture and hemorrhage; a rare, but life-threatening complication of chronic pancreatitis with a mortality of 90%.[52] This presentation is particularly difficult to diagnose because the hemorrhage from a ruptured pseudoaneurysm can bleed directly into the GI tract or pancreatic duct, mimicking a GI bleed and delaying the diagnosis.[52] The bleed may also penetrate the retroperitoneal or peritoneal space.[52] These various bleeding sites are important to isolate because management differs based on location.[52] CECT is the diagnostic tool of choice because it can identify the extent and location of the bleed and further describe anatomy that will benefit the interventionalists who will manage the case.[52] However, angiography is both 100% sensitive and an effective treatment modality because angioembolization has a success rate of 50% to 98% depending on the location of the bleed (splenic artery, 50% success rate; head of pancreas, 80% successful; 98% successful in visceral artery aneurysm).[52] Because of the risk of rebleeding after angioembolization, some evidence suggests that patients should have surgical ligation of aneurysmal bleeds after they are stabilized.[52]

Management of Acute Pancreatitis

Preventing hemoconcentration with IV hydration is the cornerstone of acute management of AP in the ED.[47,56] New evidence suggests that the previous American College of Gastroenterology 2013 guidelines recommendation of 250 to 500 mL/h rapid infusion technique was resulting in increased risk of sepsis, higher APACHE II scores, high fluid sequestration, and increased mortality.[56] These data suggest that a more controlled fluid repletion of 5 to 10 mL/kg/h results in better long-term outcomes in patients presenting with severe AP.[56,57]

For patients presenting with gallstone pancreatitis with evidence of persistent obstruction or ascending cholangitis, evidence suggests that early ERCP results in fewer complications and decreased progression to severe AP.[47] Evidence for early intervention is inconclusive for patients without evidence of persistent obstruction or ascending cholangitis; however, patients with mild AP and evidence of gallstones are likely to require cholecystectomy before discharge[47] (Fig. 1). A summary of the management goals for AP in the ED is listed in Box 11.[47,51,56–58]

Pearls

- EMPs must consider upper-GI bleeding in patients presenting with epigastric pain and dyspepsia.
- Empiric trial of PPI therapy in patients with uncomplicated PUD has shown improved symptoms and increased rate of ulcer healing.
- AP can have a wide spectrum of mortality and EMPs should use a SOFA score or BISAP criteria for appropriate disposition.
- Patients with sudden onset of dysphagia, odynophagia, chest pain, and sialorrhea should be considered to have food bolus impaction and to require involvement of GI specialists to help determine the appropriate management.

Pitfalls

- Do not overlook the possibility of acute coronary syndrome presenting solely with epigastric pain or other GI symptoms.

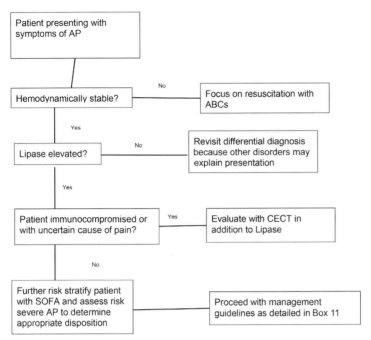

Fig. 1. Management algorithm for patients presenting with suspected AP. ABCs, airway, breathing, circulation.

- An increased serum lipase level is not specific for pancreatitis and numerous other serious intra-abdominal disorders are also on the differential.
- EMPs should be wary of serious causes of esophagitis when an immuno-compromised patient presents with dyspepsia, odynophagia, and/or dysphagia.

Box 11
Early goals of management in patients presenting with severe AP

IV hydration:
- Initial bolus of 1 L of crystalloid solution (preferably lactated Ringer)
- From 5 to 10 mL/kg/h (approximately 125 mL/h) with early use of pressors as needed with goal to maintain adequate urine output

RUQ ultrasonography evaluation in patients suspected to have obstructive disorders:
- Consult for ERCP within 24 hours if patient has concurrent ascending cholangitis or evidence of persistent obstruction

CECT for evaluation of acute complications:
- Evidence of necrotizing pancreatitis: consult interventionalist for percutaneous drain placement
- Evidence of infection of necrosis: initiate broad-spectrum antibiotics that have penetration of necrotic pancreatic tissue (eg, carbapenems, quinolones, and metronidazole)

REFERENCES

1. Macaluso C, McNamara R. Evaluation and management of acute abdominal pain in the emergency department. Int J Gen Med 2012;5:789–97.
2. Howell J, Eddy O, Lukens T, et al. Clinical policy: critical issues in the evaluation and management of emergency department patients with suspected appendicitis. Ann Emerg Med 2010;55:71–116.
3. Williams J, Sontag S, Schnell T, et al. Non-cardiac chest pain: the long-term natural history and comparison with gastroesophageal reflux disease. The Am J Gastroenterol 2009;104:2145–52.
4. NICE. Dyspepsia and gastrooesophageal reflux disease. NICE clinical guideline 184. 2014. Available at: https://www.nice.org.uk/guidance/cg184.
5. Malnick S, Melzer E, Attali M, et al. *Helicobacter pylori*: friend or foe? World J Gastroenterol 2014;20(27):8979–85.
6. Quan S, Frolkis A, Milne K, et al. Upper-gastrointestinal bleeding secondary to peptic ulcer disease: incidence and outcomes. World J Gastroenterol 2014; 20(46):17568–77.
7. Gomez J, Diehl A. Admission stool guaiac test: use and impact on patient management. Am J Med 1992;92:603–6.
8. Florent C. Progress with proton pump inhibitors in acid peptic disease: treatment of duodenal and gastric ulcer. Clin Ther 1993;15:14–21.
9. Konturek S, Brzozorksi T, Majka J, et al. Fibroblast Growth factor in gastroprotection and ulcer healing: interaction with sucralfate. Gut 1993;34(7):881–7.
10. Moayyedi P, Soo S, Deeks J, et al. Pharmacological interventions for non-ulcer dyspepsia. Cochrane Database Syst Rev 2006;(4):CD001960.
11. Sigterman K, Pinxteren B, Bonis P, et al. Short-term treatment with proton pump inhibitors, H2-receptor antagonists, and prokinetics for gastro-oesophageal reflux disease-like symptoms and endoscopy negative reflux disease [review]. Cochrane Database Syst Rev 2013;(5):CD002095.
12. Harmon R, Peura D. Evaluation and management of dyspepsia. Ther Adv Gastroenterol 2010;3(2):87–98.
13. Chan S, Maurice A, Davies S, et al. The use of gastrointestinal cocktail for differentiation gastro-oesophageal reflux disease and acute coronary syndrome in the emergency setting: a systematic review. Heart Lung Circ 2014;23(10):913–23.
14. Lichtenstein D, Cash B, Davilla R, et al. Role of endoscopy in the management of GERD. Gastrointest Endosc 2007;66(2):219–23.
15. di Pietro M, Alzoubaidi D, Fitzgerald R. Barrett's esophagus and cancer risk: How research advances can impact clinical practice. Gut and Liver 2014;8(4):356–70.
16. Apel D, Rieman J. Emergency endoscopy. Gastroenterol Hepatol 2000;14(3): 199–203.
17. Boonpongmanee S, Fleischer D, Pezzullo J, et al. The frequency of peptic ulcer as a cause of upper-GI bleeding is exaggerated. Gastrointest Endosc 2004; 59(7):788–94.
18. Bardou M, Benhaberou-Brun D, Le Ray I, et al. Diagnosis and management of nonvariceal upper gastrointestinal bleeding. Nat Rev Gastroenterol Hepatol 2012;9:97–104.
19. Taş I, Veli Ülger B, Önder A, et al. Risk factors influencing morbidity and mortality in perforated peptic ulcer disease. Ulusal Cer Derg 2014;31(1):20–5.
20. Sahin C, Alver D, Gulcin N, et al. A rare cause of intestinal perforation: ingestion of a magnet. World J Pediatr 2010;6(4):369–71.

21. Pitiakoudis M, Zezos P, Oikonomou A, et al. Spontaneous idiopathic pneumoperitoneum presenting as an acute abdomen: a case report. J Med Case Rep 2011; 5:86.
22. Iskandar M, Chory F, Goodman E, et al. Diagnosis and management of perforated duodenal ulcers following Roux-en-Y gastric bypass: a report of two cases and a review of the literature. Case Rep Surg 2015;2015:353468.
23. Grassi R, Romano S, Pinto A, et al. Gastro-duodenal perforations: conventional plain film, US, and CT findings in 166 consecutive patients. Eur J Radiol 2004; 50(1):30–6.
24. Gans S, Stoker J, Boermeester M. Plain abdominal radiography in acute abdominal pain; past, present, and future. Int J Gen Med 2012;5:525–33.
25. Graham D. Ulcer complications and their nonoperative treatment. In: Sleisenger M, Fordtran J, editors. Gastrointestinal diseases. 5th edition. Philadelphia: WB Saunders; 1993. p. 698.
26. Moore KL, Dalley AF. Clinically oriented anatomy. 4th edition. Baltimore (MD): Lippincott Williams & Wilkins; 1999.
27. Triadafilopoulos G, Roorda A, Akiyama J. Update on foreign bodies in the esophagus: diagnosis and management. Curr Gastroenterol Rep 2013;15:317.
28. Kirchner G, Zuber-Jerger I, Endlicher E, et al. Causes of bolus impaction in the esophagus. Surg Endosc 2011;25:3170–4.
29. Khayyat Y. Pharmacological management of esophageal food bolus impaction [review]. Emerg Med Int 2013;2013:924015.
30. Elson NR, Taylor IL. Nifedipine treatment of bolus esophageal obstruction. Gastrointest Endosc 1986;32(5):371–2.
31. Gelfond M, Rozen P, Gilat T. Isosorbide dinitrate and nifedipine treatment of achalasia: a clinical, manometric and radionuclide evaluation. Gastroenterology 1982; 83(5):963–9.
32. Kalyanshetter S, Patil S, Upadhya G. Button battery ingestion-case report and review. J Clin Diagn Res 2014;8(9):PD01–2.
33. Robustelli U, Bellotti R, Scardi F, et al. Management of corrosive injuries of the upper gastrointestinal tract: our experience in 58 patients. G Chir 2011;32(4): 188–93.
34. Tohda G, Sugawa C, Gayer C, et al. Clinical evaluation and management of caustic injury in the upper gastrointestinal tract in 95 adult patients in an urban medical center. Surg Endosc 2008;22:1119–25.
35. Dray X, Cattan P. Foreign bodies and caustic lesions. Best Pract Res Clin Gastroenterol 2013;27:679–89.
36. Jackson W, Mehendiratta V, Palazzo J, et al. Boerhaave's syndrome as an initial presentation of eosinophilic esophagitis: a case series. Ann Gastroenterol 2013; 26:166–9.
37. Marinho A, Bonfirm V, de Alencar L, et al. Herpetic esophagitis in immunocompetent medical student. Case Rep Infect Dis 2014;2014:930459.
38. Kim S, Jeong J, Kim J, et al. Clinical and endoscopic characteristics of drug-induced esophagitis. World J Gastroenterol 2014;20(31):10994–9.
39. Smith L, Ghangopadhyay M, Gaya D. Catastrophic gastrointestinal complication of systemic immunosuppression. World J Gastroenterol 2015;21(8):2542–5.
40. Branson B, Handsfield H, Lampe M, et al. Revised recommendations for HIV testing of adults, adolescents, and pregnant women in health-care settings. Morbidity Mortality Weekly Rep 2006;55(RR14):1–17.

41. Ozaki T, Yamashita H, Kaneko S, et al. Cytomegalovirus disease of the upper gastrointestinal tract in patients with rheumatic diseases: a case series and literature review. Clin Rheumatol 2013;32(11):1683–90.
42. Vernon N, Mohananey D, Ghetmiri E, et al. Esophageal rupture as a primary manifestation in eosinophilic esophagitis. Case Rep Med 2014;2014:673189.
43. Thimmapuram J, Oosterveen S, Grim R. Use of glucagon in relieving esophageal food bolus impaction in the era or eosinophilic esophageal infiltration. Dysphagia 2013;28:212–6.
44. Greenhawt M, Aceves S, Spergel J, et al. The management of eosinophilic esophagitis. J Allergy Clin Immunol Pract 2013;1(4):332–9.
45. Capelle M. Acute pancreatitis: etiology, clinical presentation, diagnosis and therapy. Med Clin North America 2008;92:889–923.
46. Tenner S, Baillie J, DeWitt J, et al. American College of Gastroenterology guideline: management of acute pancreatitis. Am J Gastroenterol 2013;108(9):1–16.
47. Jones M, Hall O, Kaye A, et al. Drug-induced acute pancreatitis: a review. The Ochsner J 2015;15:45–51.
48. Banks PA, Freeman ML. Practice guidelines in acute pancreatitis. Am J Gastroenterol 2006;101:2379–400.
49. Tonsi AF, Bacchion M, Crippa S, et al. Acute pancreatitis at the beginning of the 21st century: The state of the art. World J Gastroenterol 2009;15(24):2945.
50. Rosenberg A, Steensma E, Napolitano L. Necrotizing pancreatitis: new definitions and a new era in surgical management. Surg Infections 2015;16(1):1–13.
51. Chiang K, Chen T, Hsu J. Management of chronic pancreatitis complicated with a bleeding pseudoaneurysm. World J Gastroenterol 2014;20(43):16132–7.
52. Frank B, Gottlieb K. Amylase normal, lipase elevated: is it pancreatitis? A case series and review of the literature. Am J Gastroenterol 1999;94(2):463–9.
53. Balthazar EJ. Acute pancreatitis: assessment of severity with clinical and CT evaluation. Radiology 2002;223:603–13.
54. Ferreira F, Bota D, Bross A, et al. Serial evaluation of SOFA score to predict outcome in critically Ill patients. JAMA 2001;286(14):1754–8.
55. Wu B, Johannes R, Sun X, et al. The early prediction of mortality in acute pancreatitis: a large population-based study. Gut 2008;57(12):1698–703.
56. Mao E, Fei J, Peng Y, et al. Rapid hemodilution is associated with increased sepsis and mortality among patients with severe acute pancreatitis. Chin Med J 2010;123(13):1639–44.
57. Mao E, Tang Y, Fei J, et al. Fluid therapy for severe acute pancreatitis in acute response stage. Chin Med J 2009;122(2):169–73.
58. Wu B, Huang J, Gardner T, et al. Lactated ringer's solution systemic inflammation compared with saline in patients with acute pancreatitis. Clin Gastroenterol Hepatol 2011;9(8):710–7.

Evaluating the Patient with Right Upper Quadrant Abdominal Pain

 CrossMark

Jennifer Avegno, MD*, Matthew Carlisle, MD, MAS

KEYWORDS

- Abdominal pain • Pancreatitis • Cholecystitis • Cholelithiasis • Hepatitis
- Physical examination • Treatment • Diagnostic testing

KEY POINTS

- Review of anatomy and physiology of the right upper quadrant (RUQ) and common medical conditions causing pain in this area.
- Understanding key historical features, physical examination findings, and appropriate diagnostic testing used to evaluate the patient with RUQ pain.
- Strategies to approach evidence-based and appropriate treatment, management, and disposition decisions for common disorders of the right upper quadrant (RUQ).

Evaluation of the patient with acute RUQ pain requires a thorough understanding of the anatomy of that region as well as the physiology of proximal and remote organ systems. The anatomy of the RUQ is made up predominantly by the gastrointestinal system, including the liver, gallbladder, pancreas, and duodenum. The liver is the largest solid organ in the body and is divided anatomically into the larger right lobe and smaller left lobe by the falciform ligament, the quadrate lobe between the gallbladder and round ligament, and caudate lobe between the inferior vena cava, ligamentum venosum, and porta hepatis (**Fig. 1**).[1] Surgically, the liver is divided into 2 halves and 8 segments based on areas of liver parenchyma with vascular inflow, outflow, and biliary drainage—a segment of the hepatic artery, portal vein, hepatic vein, and biliary ductule.[2] The liver serves a multitude of functions that can be subdivided into clearance, storage, metabolism, and production (**Table 1**).[1,3]

The gallbladder is located on the undersurface of the right lobe of the liver and consists of the neck, body, and fundus. Its functions are to collect, concentrate, and secrete bile salts from the liver into the duodenum (**Fig. 2**).[1] Bile salts created in the

Disclosure Statement: The authors have nothing to disclose.
Section of Emergency Medicine, University Medical Center, Louisiana State University Health Sciences Center, 2000 Canal Street, Room 2720, New Orleans, LA 70112, USA
* Corresponding author.
E-mail address: Javegn@lsuhsc.edu

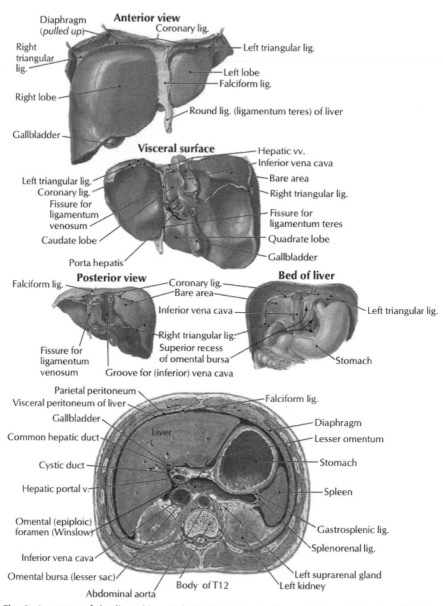

Fig. 1. Anatomy of the liver. (Copyright © 2016. Used with permission of Elsevier. All rights reserved. www.netterimages.com.)

liver through hepatic ducts are then refluxed into the gallbladder through the cystic duct. As the gallbladder is stimulated, the gallbladder contracts, secreting concentrated bile salts into the duodenum via the cystic duct to the common bile duct. These bile salts help to emulsify fats into globules that can be digested chemically.[3]

The pancreas is a retroperitoneal organ that consists of the head, neck, body, and tail, stretching from the duodenum to the spleen in the splenorenal ligament (**Fig. 3**).[1] The pancreas serves both endocrine and exocrine functions. The endocrine cells are

Table 1
Functions of the liver

Function	Substrate	Example
Clearance	Toxins	Medications Alcohol Ammonia
	Bacteria	Kupffer cells—specialized macrophages that phagocytize foreign material
	Bilirubin	Bilirubin is formed as a breakdown product as Kupffer cells phagocytize old red blood cells
Storage	Glycogen	Stored glucose—easily converted in time of hypoglycemia or stress
	Vitamins	A, D, E, K, B_{12}
	Essential elements	Iron, copper
Metabolism	Carbohydrate	Converts glycogen, monosaccharaides (such as fructose, galactose) to glucose that can be used by cells
	Amino acid	Transamination—converts nonessential amino acids to essential amino acids Deamination—eliminates excess amino acids
	Lipids	Creates lipoproteins to facilitate fat transport in the blood Uses beta-oxidation to break down fatty acids to usable products Creates bile salts to emulsify fats
Synthesis	Albumin	Helps to maintain oncotic pressure in vessels
	Clotting factors	I, II, V, VII, VIII, IX, X, XI
	Anticoagulation	Protein C, protein S, antithrombin

grouped into clusters known as the islets of Langerhans made up of beta cells that produce insulin, alpha cells that produce glucagon, and gamma cells that create somatostatin. These islets are located within exocrine lobules known as acini that drain into the common bile duct and directly into the duodenum via the main and accessory pancreatic ducts, respectively. The exocrine cells of the pancreas create proteases, lipases, and amylase that digest protein, fats, and carbohydrates. These cells also produce bicarbonate to neutralize the acidic environment in the duodenum created by the stomach.[4]

The digestive enzymes, bile salts, and some waste products created by the liver, gallbladder, and pancreas are ultimately secreted into the duodenum, the first portion of the small intestine. The duodenum is a mostly retroperitoneal organ that begins at the pylorus of the stomach and ends at the jejunum (the second portion of the small intestine) at the ligament of Treitz. It lies anterior to the pancreatic head and posterior to the gallbladder and quadrate lobe of the liver. The duodenum is divided anatomically into 4 parts—the superior, descending, inferior, and ascending (**Fig. 4**).[1] Although a majority of its function is digestive, the duodenal epithelium also provides an endocrine role through the secretion of secretin and cholecystokinin. These hormones are released in response to stomach acid and fat and stimulate the liver, gallbladder, and pancreas to release bile, lipases, proteases, amylase, and bicarbonate.[3]

DIFFERENTIAL DIAGNOSES OF RIGHT UPPER QUADRANT DISORDERS

Causes of RUQ pain may be found in the major organs of the anatomic area (liver, gallbladder, pancreas, small intestine), from other abdominal organs (renal, genitourinary), or from nonabdominal causes (pulmonary, cardiac, musculoskeletal, or other;

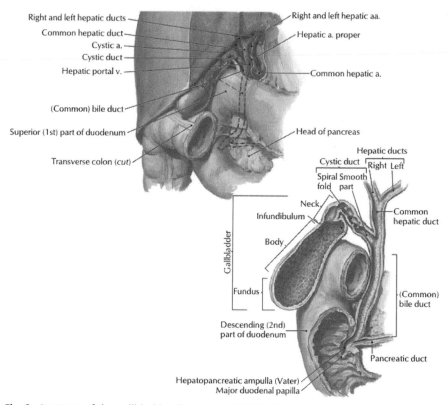

Right and left hepatic ducts
Common hepatic duct
Cystic a.
Cystic duct
Hepatic portal v.
(Common) bile duct
Superior (1st) part of duodenum
Transverse colon (cut)
Right and left hepatic aa.
Hepatic a. proper
Common hepatic a.
Head of pancreas
Hepatic ducts
Cystic duct
Right Left
Spiral Smooth
fold part
Neck
Infundibulum
Common hepatic duct
Body
Gallbladder
Fundus
(Common) bile duct
Descending (2nd) part of duodenum
Pancreatic duct
Hepatopancreatic ampulla (Vater)
Major duodenal papilla

Fig. 2. Anatomy of the gallbladder. (Copyright © 2016. Used with permission of Elsevier. All rights reserved. www.netterimages.com.)

Table 2). Differentiating a primary RUQ source from one outside often requires detailed history, physical examination, and appropriate testing.

Disorders of the Liver, Biliary System, Pancreas, and Small Intestine

Chronic liver disease is a frequent cause of morbidity, mortality, and presentations to the emergency department.[5] Liver disorders may be categorized as infectious or noninfectious, but the sequelae of both (particularly late in the course of disease) are often similar. Patients with primary hepatic disorders may present with localized RUQ pain, nausea, jaundice, abdominal distention with or without ascites, mental status changes/encephalopathy (if advanced), and skin changes, such as easy bruising and pruritus.

Infectious causes of liver disease are extremely common and should be considered in the patient with RUQ pain. Hepatitis A is transmitted through fecal–oral means and causes acute onset of nausea and vomiting, diarrhea, and jaundice. Hepatitis B spreads through sexual contact and blood transfusion and is highly contagious. More than 240 million people are estimated to be infected chronically worldwide, and it is responsible for more than 780,000 deaths per year, although vaccination has reduced the rate of new cases per year in the United States by 82%.[6–8] Chronic infection with hepatitis C (also spread through sexual contact and needle sharing) is also a major source of liver disease, and is a common cause of liver transplantation and cirrhosis.[9] Hepatitis C, unlike other infections, may be "silent"—that is, asymptomatic for many years until serious

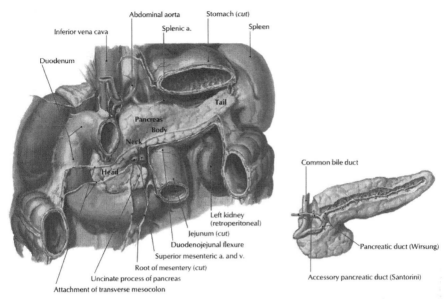

Fig. 3. Anatomy of the pancreas. (Copyright © 2016. Used with permission of Elsevier. All rights reserved. www.netterimages.com.)

symptoms develop. Hepatitis D (rare in the developed world) infects individuals who already have the hepatitis B virus, and leads to more severe disease and mortality; hepatitis E, in contrast, is generally a nonsevere and self-limiting infection with few sequelae in immunocompetent hosts. Other, less common infectious causes of liver disease

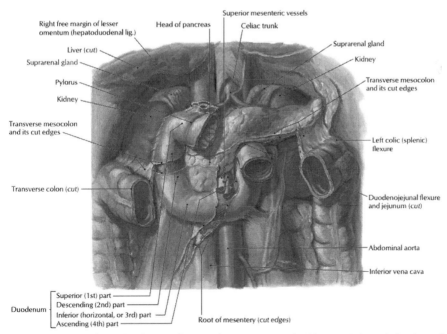

Fig. 4. Anatomy of the duodenum. (Copyright © 2016. Used with permission of Elsevier. All rights reserved. www.netterimages.com.)

Table 2 Differential diagnosis of right upper quadrant pain		
Right Upper Quadrant Structures	**Other Abdominal Sources**	**Nonabdominal**

Liver
 Infectious
  Hepatitis A, B, C, D, E
  Nonviral infections
 Alcoholic
 Autoimmune
 Toxin related
 Neoplastic
	Vascular
	 Aortic or splanchnic artery
	  dissection
	 Abdominal aortic aneurysm
	 Mesenteric ischemia
		Pulmonary
		 Pneumonia/effusion
		 Pulmonary embolus

Biliary system Cholelithiasis Cholecystitis Cholangitis Neoplastic	Renal Mass Stones	Cardiac Acute coronary syndrome Angina
Pancreas Pancreatitis Neoplastic	Genitourinary Ovarian torsion Complications of pregnancy	Musculoskeletal Abdominal or thoracic wall strain Rectus sheath hematoma
Intestinal Gastritis Peptic ulcer disease Obstruction	—	Other Herpes zoster

include amebic infections (single or multiple abscesses), pyogenic abscesses (usually from direct spread from a gallbladder source or hematogenous spread from infection elsewhere), and parasitic infestations. Patients with ascites from end-stage liver disease are also at risk for infectious peritonitis from a variety of pathogens.[10]

Direct toxic insults to the liver are often seen with alcohol consumption, and prescription and over-the-counter medications. Although a variety of medications including antibiotics, antiepileptics, and other analgesics can cause direct toxic effects on the liver, acetaminophen toxicity remains one of the most common and often fatal overdoses if not recognized or treated promptly.[11–13] Alcohol has a direct toxic and irreversible effect (acutely or through chronic use) on liver function, destroying hepatic cells and leading to cirrhotic changes or fatty infiltration. Alcohol-related liver disease is a significant contribution to morbidity and mortality in the United States, accounting for approximately 48% of cirrhosis-related deaths.[14,15]

Autoimmune inflammatory diseases of the liver may mimic other forms of hepatitis, but are not related to infection or alcohol use. Patients often present with vague symptoms of nausea, vomiting, weakness, dark urine, and jaundice. These disorders, chiefly primary biliary sclerosis and autoimmune hepatitis, often present with additional findings typical of rheumatologic disease, such as unusual rashes, joint pain, and myalgias. Finally, neoplastic disease of the liver—whether primary or metastatic—is a not uncommon presentation in the acute setting, and should be considered in the patient with chronic RUQ pain and symptoms consistent with hepatic dysfunction.[16]

Biliary Disorders

Gallbladder disease is responsible for a significant percentage of emergency department visits for abdominal pain, and gallstone disease alone is estimated to affect up to 25% of the population of the Western world.[16,17] Populations at higher risk for cholelithiasis include premenopausal and pregnant women, obesity and inactivity, the elderly, and patients with common chronic diseases such as hypercholesterolemia, diabetes, and cirrhosis.[18] Stones are formed from crystalline elements of bile (cholesterol, pigment, and/or calcium, primarily), and any impairment of emptying or filling of the gallbladder with bile contributes further to their formation.[19] Gallstones may be asymptomatic for some time, but it is estimated that each year 2% to 4% of patients become symptomatic.[17] Patients complain of often sharp, constant RUQ pain in intermittent attacks (biliary colic), which is owing to biliary duct dilation after a stone becomes impacted.

Cholelithiasis and choledocholithiasis (impaction of a stone at the common bile duct) should be distinguished from acute cholecystitis. In calculous cholecystitis, stones can lead to inflammation of the gallbladder and often bacterial infection, and is usually characterized by fever, nausea, and generally more ill appearance (and occasionally jaundice) associated with the typical symptoms of colic. Acalculous cholecystitis is most common in immunocompromised patients and has higher rates of morbidity and mortality.[20–22]

Cholangitis (infection or inflammation of the bile ducts) may be idiopathic (primary sclerosing cholangitis) or caused by bacteria or viruses; the vast majority are associated with concomitant stones. Infectious cholangitis usually originates in the duodenum, and is caused by common gut pathogens such as *Escherichia coli* and *Klebsiella*; immunocompromised patients are at greater risk and may present without obstructing stones. The classic Charcot's triad of fever, RUQ pain, and jaundice is classic for cholangitis but may be seen only 50% of the time.[23]

Other less common diseases are gallbladder cancers and primary sclerosing cholangitis. Biliary neoplasms are rare but are associated with high morbidity and mortality.[24] Patients may present with vague abdominal pain, malaise, or painless jaundice, pruritus, and weight loss. Most tumors are adenocarcinoma with origin in the gallbladder mucosa (cholangiocarcinoma), but can affect intrahepatic and extrahepatic ducts. Primary sclerosing cholangitis is associated with destruction of intrahepatic bile ducts, and disproportionately affects younger and female patients.

Pancreatic Disorders

Disorders of the pancreas are relatively common and are usually associated with biliary disease (gallstones) and/or environmental factors (alcohol abuse).[23,25] In the United States, acute pancreatitis—inflammation of the pancreas—is one of the leading GI causes of hospital admission, and a major cause of in-hospital mortality. Pancreatitis ranges from mild—responsive to fluids and amenable to outpatient treatment—to necrotic, and may involve fluid collections (pseudocyst or abscess). Patients generally present with acute onset of localized, constant midepigastric pain, often radiating to the back and associated with nausea/vomiting and decreased oral intake. Patients with abscess or necrotic pancreatitis often appear acutely ill. Severity of pancreatitis may be classified according to the Revised Atlanta classification (**Table 3**), which takes into account organ failure and the presence of systemic inflammatory response syndrome.[26] Most patients recover from an initial bout of pancreatitis; however, a small portion of patients go on to have recurrent episodes and develop chronic pancreatitis. Although the overall incidence is significantly lower than acute pancreatitis, the morbidity is significantly worse.[25,27]

Neoplastic disease of the pancreas is among the top 10 malignant causes of death.[28] Most cases arise from the head of the pancreas, and present with vague, nonlocalized symptoms such as pain, weight loss, and jaundice; patients are often diagnosed relatively late in the disease process.

Table 3
The revised Atlanta classification of acute pancreatitis severity

	Organ Failure	Local or Systemic Complications
Mild	None	None
Moderate	Resolves within 48 h (transient)	Present
Severe	Persistent (single or multiple)	Systemic inflammatory response syndrome One or more local complications

Adapted from Banks PA, Bollen TL, Dervenis C, et al. Classification of acute pancreatitis–2012: revision of the Atlanta classification and definitions by international consensus. Gut 2013;62(1):102; with permission.

Other Abdominal Pathology Presenting as Right Upper Quadrant Pain

Embryonic development guides the sensation of visceral pain, with foregut structures (stomach, biliary system, liver, pancreas, intestine) often localizing to the RUQ or mid-epigastric area.[29] Thus, disorders of the small intestine and stomach frequently present with RUQ pain. Specifically, gastritis and peptic and duodenal ulcers are often the source of midepigastric pain that involves the RUQ. Ulcer disease often presents with vague discomfort, nausea, and bloating; perforated ulcers are associated with more localized, sharp, severe pain radiating to the back (not unlike pancreatitis).[30] Abdominal disorders of every quadrant may also present with RUQ pain or radiation from the primary source, notably appendicitis and aortic pathologies. Classically, appendicitis in pregnancy was thought to present with RUQ pain owing to displacement by the uterus; however, this association is likely not as strong as previously thought.[31] However, inflamed appendices in variant anatomic locations may radiate to the RUQ and in some cases be the predominant area of pain.[32] Dissection of the aorta or its branches (especially the celiac artery) may also present with sharp RUQ pain.[33] Mesenteric ischemia and median arcuate ligament syndrome are additional vascular disorders that often produce vague upper abdominal symptoms with involvement of the RUQ.[34]

Genitourinary disease may also manifest as RUQ pathology. Renal masses and stones (anywhere from upper to lower tract) can cause flank pain that can radiate or be misinterpreted as RUQ in origin. Pelvic inflammatory disease is a risk factor for hepatic inflammation (Fitz–Hugh–Curtis syndrome) and should be considered when RUQ pain accompany cervicitis or infectious genital symptoms in women.[35] Several conditions of pregnancy may also present with RUQ pain, such as hemolysis, elevated liver enzymes, and low platelets (HELLP) syndrome, general discomfort owing to uterine enlargement, extrauterine pregnancy or ruptured ectopic.

Nonabdominal Causes of Right Upper Quadrant Pain

Several disorders of the thoracic, musculoskeletal, and dermatologic systems may present with RUQ pain as the predominant symptom. Acute coronary syndrome, like dissection, should always be considered in the workup of these patients, particularly in elderly women who are more likely to present with atypical complaints.[36] Any concomitant complaint of syncope, pain with exertion, or shortness of breath in a patient with cardiovascular risk factors should lead clinicians to consider testing for cardiac causes. Similarly, pulmonary disorders such as pneumonia (often localized to the right lower or middle lobe), pleural effusion, and pulmonary embolism may mimic RUQ pathology.[37] Diseases of the musculoskeletal system, whether adjacent to or distant (ie, of spinal origin) from the RUQ, may also be the etiology of pain in this area.[38]

Examination of the skin is paramount because herpes zoster commonly presents in the dermatome overlying the RUQ, but a visible rash may lag behind symptoms by several days.[39]

EVALUATION TOOLS IN THE WORKUP OF THE PATIENT WITH RIGHT UPPER QUADRANT PAIN
Physical Examination

As with most conditions, a thorough history and physical examination is important in making the proper diagnosis. An important feature to distinguish is the character of the RUQ pain—dull or poorly localized versus sharp and focal. Vaguely localized pain suggests a source with visceral innervation, and may be from a remote location such as the thorax (myocardial infarction), lower abdomen, or genitourinary system; it is generally poorly defined, predominantly midline, aching, diffuse, and accompanied by malaise and nausea.[29] Pain that is sharp and well-localized suggests direct somatic nerve irritation from that area (cholelithiasis, peptic ulcer disease [PUD], zoster). Sudden onset of pain associated with rebound or guarding raises the likelihood of an intraabdominal emergency, such as a vascular catastrophe (abdominal aortic aneurysm [AAA] or dissection), viscous perforation, or, more rarely, ovarian torsion or acute appendicitis. Intermittent symptoms with acute bouts of worsening pain may represent progression of disease (gallbladder stones, pancreatitis, liver failure), whereas chronic worsening complaints point toward a neoplastic or intrinsic organ cause (eg, chronic hepatitis). Aggravating or alleviating factors should be also considered. Pain worse after eating may be related to PUD, gallbladder stone disease, or mesenteric ischemia. Peritoneal conditions are often exacerbated with cough, moving, or walking. Associated systemic symptoms such as fever, jaundice, and weight loss may also be helpful in narrowing down the differential diagnosis (**Table 4**).

On physical examination, vital signs may give some clues to the diagnosis. Febrile patients, or those with systemic inflammatory response syndrome, are more likely to have an infectious process or acute manifestation of disease. Palpation of the abdomen may pinpoint the exact location of pain, as well as the presence or absence of peritoneal signs. Masses and RUQ organomegaly are best noted on deep palpation. Rebound tenderness and guarding may be assessed, but are relatively nonspecific findings for peritonitis.[40] The much-heralded "Murphy sign"—arrest of inspiration during RUQ palpation with fingers underneath the costal margin—had a sensitivity of

Table 4
Common signs and symptoms to assist in differentiation of right upper quadrant pain

	Common	Uncommon
Jaundice	Neoplasm: liver, pancreatic, and biliary Cholangitis Acute hepatitis End-stage liver disease/cirrhosis	Cholelithiasis Pancreatitis Intraabdominal or intrathoracic disorders
Localized pain	Cholelithiasis Pancreatitis Hepatitis Peptic ulcer disease Herpes zoster	Appendicitis (early) Mesenteric ischemia (early) Abdominal aortic aneurysm (unruptured) Acute coronary syndrome Pulmonary embolism
Fever	Cholangitis Liver abscess Peritonitis Pneumonia	Stone disease Ulcer disease

approximately 65% and specificity of 87% in a metaanalysis, but was not sufficient to make the diagnosis of cholecystitis alone.[40] Ascites and abdominal distention point to a hepatic etiology (whether primary or secondary).

Laboratory Testing

Specific laboratory tests may be useful to support a particular diagnosis in the workup of RUQ pain. A complete blood count may suggest infection if the WBC is elevated—although this is nonspecific and should not be used to exclude suspected conditions. Anemia may reflect a bleeding source (PUD) or be associated with chronic conditions (alcoholic cirrhosis). Platelet disorders and coagulopathies (noted on prothrombin time/partial thromboplastin time) also point to a hepatic source, because the liver is the production site for most coagulation factors; however, increased markers may not be as indicative of the degree of liver dysfunction as previously thought.[41]

A complete metabolic panel provides a great deal of useful information. Metabolic derangements can be helpful in pointing to the severity of disease, and in certain cases can suggest particular organ pathology (eg, glucose derangements in pancreatitis). Aminotransferase levels (aspartate aminotransferase and alanine aminotransferase) may be obtained to evaluate primary or secondary liver disease. Alanine aminotransferase is most specific for hepatic injury, but there is poor correlation between the severity of liver damage and enzyme values.[42] If the diagnosis of pancreatitis is considered, amylase and lipase levels may be obtained. Increased lipase levels show high specificity for acute pancreatitis; however, hyperamylasemia is present in a wide variety of other conditions.[43] Urine pregnancy test should always be ordered on women of reproductive age, and a basic urinalysis helps to support a renal or bladder etiology. Presentations that suggest a cardiac or vascular cause may also require measurement of cardiac enzymes, serum lactate (helpful as a marker of ischemia or sepsis severity), and blood typing if bleeding is suspected.

For infectious processes, cultures of blood and/or urine should be obtained. The Center for Disease Control and Prevention recommend hepatitis C virus testing for all adults born between 1945 and 1965, injection drug users, patients who received clotting factors before 1987, patients who received blood products before 1992, patients on hemodialysis, and patients with human immunodeficiency virus infection.[44] Because human immunodeficiency virus can predispose to and affect the severity of several RUQ disorders, testing should also be considered.

Imaging

Choosing the most appropriate and high-yield imaging modality is vital in the management of RUQ conditions. Optimizing available resources in the emergency department to make the initial diagnosis takes precedent over more detailed, thorough testing modalities that may be needed to plan definitive management. The maxim that ultrasound (US) is the initial study of choice in RUQ largely holds true for most disorders, but other imaging options should at least be considered in all but the most clearcut cases.

Plain Radiographs

Despite their speed, relatively low cost, and ubiquity, plain abdominal radiographs are of limited value in most disorders originating in the RUQ. Before the ready availability of US in the emergency department, plain radiographs were thought to have some usefulness in the diagnosis of cholelithiasis[45]; however, recent studies have found that abdominal radiographs primarily identify the cause of symptoms and/or change management in fewer than 10% of patients with acute abdominal pain, and very frequently do not obviate the need for further imaging.[45–47] Plain radiographs, either of the chest or abdomen, are probably most helpful when the origin of symptoms is suspected to be outside the RUQ, for example, pneumonia, pleural effusion, pulmonary embolism, PUD with perforation, or bowel obstruction.

Ultrasonography

RUQ US evaluation is a low-radiation, rapid, noninvasive, easily obtained test that can be performed at a patient's bedside and has been shown to be highly accurate in the hands of emergency physicians.[48] It is most helpful in the diagnosis of biliary tract disorders, such as cholelithiasis and cholecystitis. The American College of Radiology has published appropriateness criteria for the use of US (and other imaging modalities) in various scenarios of RUQ pain, and in every one US is rated as more appropriate than computed tomography (CT), MRI, or cholescintigraphy.[49] Acute cholelithiasis is generally easily seen on US owing to the bright (hyperechoic), round appearance of stones (one or multiple) within the gallbladder and often associated posterior shadowing below (Fig. 5). In addition to stones, cholecystitis presents with gallbladder wall thickening, pericholecystic fluid, and classically a sonographic Murphy's sign (localized pain over the gallbladder when the US transducer is applied; Fig. 6). Acalculous and emphysematous cholecystitis are also most easily diagnosed with US, as are less common benign and malignant gallbladder disorders.

Other biliary tree disorders can be evaluated readily by US. In the setting of RUQ pain with elevated liver function tests or bilirubin, RUQ US can evaluate the degree and location of biliary obstruction and/or dilation (intrahepatic, extrahepatic, or both). One exception to the superiority of US is in suspected choledocholithiasis, in which this modality is often less sensitive than MR cholangiopancreatography.[50] US is also helpful in diagnosing primary liver disorders, particularly masses/neoplasms, infections/abscesses, cirrhosis, and portal vein disease. Pancreatic US is useful to evaluate for gallstone-related pancreatic disease, and in the identification of acute or chronic pancreatitis. Masses and pseudocysts may also be identified, but generally CT is the preferred imaging study for these disorders.[50]

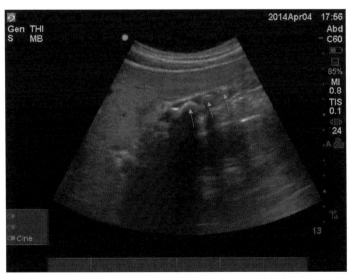

Fig. 5. Gallbladder with stones. Green arrows indicate stones with shadowing. (*Courtesy of* Christine Butts, MD, New Orleans, LA.)

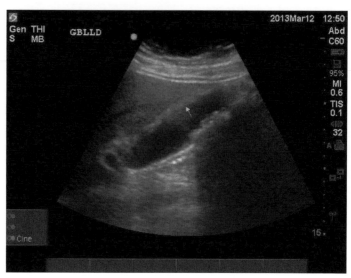

Fig. 6. Cholecystitis. Green arrow indicates gallbladder wall thickening. (*Courtesy of* Christine Butts, MD, New Orleans, LA.)

US may be helpful in diagnosing disorders that do not originate from the RUQ. Nephrolithiasis, pyelonephritis, renal masses, AAA, cardiac pathology, and ruptured ectopic pregnancy may be discovered either with conventional RUQ US or by expanding slightly the anatomic parameters for evaluation.[50,51]

Computed Tomography

CT imaging is, overall, the diagnostic modality of choice for undifferentiated abdominal pain, particularly those with fever and nonlocalized symptoms.[47,52] However, for most common biliary and hepatic disease, CT does not add any significant sensitivity or specificity over US, and comes at the cost of higher radiation and less portability.[53] Pancreatic diseases, however, are best evaluated with contrast-enhanced CT, and may show the degree of inflammation in pancreatitis, necrotizing features, pseudocysts, and masses (**Figs. 7** and **8**).[54–56] CT can also better delineate complicated biliary disorders, such as gas-forming processes, abscesses, hemorrhage, and perforation, and can be a second-line imaging modality when RUQ US fails to reveal a source of pain.[49]

CT is able to provide great sensitivity and specificity in diagnosing abdominal disorders distant to the RUQ; in particular, appendicitis, diverticulitis, and renal stone disease are well-delineated by this modality.[40,47] Vascular processes (aortic dissection, mesenteric ischemia, median arcuate ligament syndrome) and pulmonary disease (embolism, masses, infiltrates) are also best imaged with CT, but abdominal and chest studies may be necessary.

Other Imaging Modalities

Tests such as MRI, scintigraphy, and endoscopic or magnetic retrograde cholangiopancreatography (endoscopic retrograde cholangiopancreatography [ERCP]/MR cholangiopancreatography) are useful tools in the diagnosis of RUQ disorders, but are rarely indicated or available in the acute setting.[49,57] These studies are often time and labor intensive, with higher cost, and provide little additional information in an emergent patient. ERCP is helpful in the setting of gallstone pancreatitis, but in

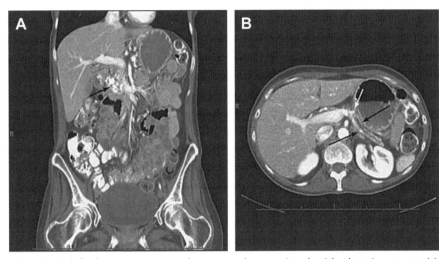

Fig. 7. Typical findings on computed tomography associated with chronic pancreatitis. Shown are pancreatic duct dilation (*long black arrows*) and intrapancreatic calcifications, which are also typical of chronic pancreatitis (*small black and white arrow*). (*From* Jensen EH, Borja-Cacho D, Al-Refaie WB, et al. Exocrine pancreas. Sabiston DC, Townsend CM. Sabiston textbook of surgery: the biological basis of modern surgical practice. Philadelphia: Elsevier Saunders; 2014; with permission.)

the absence of obstruction or cholangitis is not indicated in the acute or early disease course.[58]

MANAGEMENT AND TREATMENT OF RIGHT UPPER QUADRANT DISORDERS

As with any acute presentation of disease, resuscitation of an emergently ill patient takes precedence in RUQ disorders. Careful attention to airway and breathing

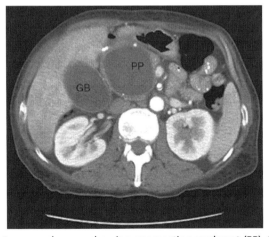

Fig. 8. Computed tomography scan showing pancreatic pseudocyst (PP). In this patient the pseudocyst was so large that compressed the common bile duct, causing obstructive jaundice. GB, gallbladder. (*From* Hemphill RR, Santen SA. Disorders of the Pancreas. In: Marx JA, Hockberger RS, Walls RM, et al, editors. Rosen's emergency medicine: concepts and clinical practice. Philadelphia: Elsevier/Saunders; 2014; with permission.)

difficulty (as direct sequela of the disease itself or as part of a systemic response) should be done first. Circulatory issues such as volume depletion are often major concerns in common diseases such as pancreatitis and severe biliary disease, but are not seen routinely in mild to moderate hepatic or gallbladder pathology.[59] Hypotension may prompt a workup for a severe infectious cause (cholangitis, appendicitis), perforated viscus, vascular etiology (AAA, mesenteric ischemia, dissection), or bleeding (in particular, a complication of cirrhosis). Resuscitation should be targeted carefully to the suspected condition, and there is no general superiority of 1 crystalloid over another.[60]

Pain control is critically important in the treatment of RUQ disorders. Patients in the emergency department are frequently undertreated based on long-held belief that appropriate analgesics will "mask" symptoms and decrease diagnostic ability, and that morphine and other opiates will cause dysfunction of the sphincter of Oddi and worsen gallstone or biliary pain. However, studies do not support any effect of withholding medications on improved clinical accuracy, nor is the effect of opiates on sphincter of Oddi clearly harmful.[61,62] Nonsteroidal antiinflammatory drugs may be used judiciously (if a bleeding disorder is not suspected) and antiemetics should be used in nauseated patients.

Surgical Treatment for Right Upper Quadrant Disorders

Gallstone disease generally requires cholecystectomy, but not always in the acute setting, and is not recommended for asymptomatic patients.[63] For cholecystitis and acute cholangitis, surgery may be needed, but generally after other interventions such as antibiotics and/or ERCP.[64] Biliary stenting, ERCP, or surgical intervention may be required in the setting of acute obstruction with cholangitis or where stone removal has failed, to decompress the biliary tree. Newly diagnosed malignancies of the biliary, hepatic, or pancreatic organs may require invasive biopsy or surgical resection; but again, this is rarely an emergent procedure (although admission for definitive diagnosis, staging, and management is often initiated in the emergency department).

Other intraabdominal disorders presenting with referred pain to the RUQ may require surgical interventions, particularly appendicitis, perforated viscus, and ruptured ectopic pregnancy. Vascular catastrophes (AAA, dissection, ischemia) necessitate immediate consultation with appropriate surgical specialists and emergent operative repair.

Medical Management of Right Upper Quadrant Disorders

Treatment of acute hepatitis varies widely depending on the type. Hepatitis A is self-limiting and requires supportive care only, generally as an outpatient. Hepatitis B and C may follow an indolent course, and patients may need to be admitted in the late stages of the disease when complications of fluid imbalance, coagulopathy, and encephalopathy occur. Novel antiviral therapies for hepatitis C have the potential to significantly decrease morbidity and the burden of this disease, with some new therapies considered curative.[65]

Acute pancreatitis requires targeted fluid resuscitation, close monitoring of electrolyte imbalance, proper nutrition (oral or parenteral, depending on disease severity), and modification of predisposing factors (if possible). Aggressive crystalloid administration of up to 250 to 500 mL/h is likely to be of most benefit within the first 12 to 24 hours, after which fluid requirements should be targeted to patient response and underlying status; antibiotics are reserved only for severe or necrotizing cases.[66] PUD, depending on the presence of complications (perforation and/or bleeding), may be managed outpatient with modification of lifestyle factors (avoidance of nonsteroidal antiinflammatory drugs), proton pump inhibitors, and consideration of *Helicobacter pylori* treatment; or may require admission for endoscopy and invasive intervention after resuscitation.[30,67] For disorders originating from the RUQ/midepigastrium for which patients are admitted, consultation with gastroenterologists (whether from the emergency department or soon after admission) is strongly recommended.

Other diseases not originating in the RUQ should be treated according to their specific process after general resuscitative efforts. Intraabdominal or thoracic infections such as pyelonephritis and pneumonia may require early institution of antibiotics. Pregnancy-related conditions should always be discussed with obstetrics/gynecologic consultants or close follow-up obtained for nonemergent patients.

SUMMARY

Disorders presenting with RUQ pain are frequently encountered in the emergency department, and vary considerably from benign to life threatening. Understanding the anatomy and physiology of the region (as well as that of contiguous and remote organ systems), historical clues, and physical examination findings is key to an appropriate, targeted approach to management and treatment.

REFERENCES

1. Hansen JT. Chapter 4: abdomen. Netter's clinical anatomy. 2nd edition. Philadelphia: Saunders; 2010. p. 488.
2. Juza RM, Pauli EM. Clinical and surgical anatomy of the liver: a review for clinicians. Clin Anat 2014;27(5):764–9.
3. Scanlon VC, Sanders T. Chapter 16: the digestive system. Essentials of anatomy and physiology. 7th edition. Philadelphia: F.A. Davis Company; 2015. p. 704.
4. Young W. The netter collection of medical illustrations: endocrine system. 2nd edition. Philadelphia: Elsevier Health Sciences; 2011. Available at: http://0-www.r2library.com.innopac.lsuhsc.edu/Resource/Title/1416063889. Accessed September 23, 2015.
5. Shaheen NJ, Hansen RA, Morgan DR, et al. The burden of gastrointestinal and liver diseases, 2006. Am J Gastroenterol 2006;101(9):2128–38.
6. Lozano R, Naghavi M, Foreman K, et al. Global and regional mortality from 235 causes of death for 20 age groups in 1990 and 2010: a systematic analysis for the Global Burden of Disease Study 2010. Lancet 2012;380(9859):2095–128.
7. World Health Organization. Hepatitis B fact sheet. Available at: http://www.who.int/mediacentre/factsheets/fs204/en/. Accessed September 15, 2015.
8. Hepatitis B FAQs for health professionals. Centers for Disease Control Media release. Available at: http://www.cdc.gov/hepatitis/hbv/hbvfaq.htm. Accessed September 15, 2015.
9. Davis GL, Albright JE, Cook SF, et al. Projecting future complications of chronic hepatitis C in the United States. Liver Transpl 2003;9(4):331–8.
10. Lata J. Spontaneous bacterial peritonitis: a severe complication of liver cirrhosis. World J Gastroenterol 2009;15(44):5505.
11. Larson AM, Polson J, Fontana RJ, et al. Acetaminophen-induced acute liver failure: results of a United States multicenter, prospective study. Hepatology 2005; 42(6):1364–72.
12. Shakil AO, Kramer D, Mazariegos GV, et al. Acute liver failure: clinical features, outcome analysis, and applicability of prognostic criteria. Liver Transpl 2000; 6(2):163–9.

13. Schiodt FV, Atillasoy E, Shakil AO, et al. Etiology and outcome for 295 patients with acute liver failure in the United States. Liver Transpl Surg 1999;5(1):29–34.
14. Gao B, Bataller R. Alcoholic liver disease: pathogenesis and new therapeutic targets. Gastroenterology 2011;141(5):1572–85.
15. Yoon Y-H. Liver cirrhosis mortality in the United States, 1970–2007 surveillance report #88(NIAAA homepage 2010). National Institute on Alcohol Abuse and Alcoholism. Surveillance report. Available at: http://pubs.niaaa.nih.gov/publications/surveillance88/Cirr07.htm. Accessed September 15, 2015.
16. Peery AF, Dellon ES, Lund J, et al. Burden of gastrointestinal disease in the United States: 2012 update. Gastroenterology 2012;143(5):1179–87.e1–3.
17. Gurusamy KS, Davidson BR. Gallstones. BMJ 2014;348:g2669.
18. Stinton LM, Shaffer EA. Epidemiology of gallbladder disease: cholelithiasis and cancer. Gut Liver 2012;6(2):172–87.
19. O'Connell K, Brasel K. Bile metabolism and lithogenesis. Surg Clin North Am 2014;94(2):361–75.
20. Knab LM, Boller AM, Mahvi DM. Cholecystitis. Surg Clin North Am 2014;94(2):455–70.
21. Ryu JK, Ryu KH, Kim KH. Clinical features of acute acalculous cholecystitis. J Clin Gastroenterol 2003;36(2):166–9.
22. Kalliafas S, Ziegler DW, Flancbaum L, et al. Acute acalculous cholecystitis: incidence, risk factors, diagnosis, and outcome. Am Surg 1998;64(5):471–5.
23. Privette TW Jr, Carlisle MC, Palma JK. Emergencies of the liver, gallbladder, and pancreas. Emerg Med Clin North Am 2011;29(2):293–317, viii–ix.
24. Wernberg JA, Lucarelli DD. Gallbladder cancer. Surg Clin North Am 2014;94(2):343–60.
25. Yadav D, Lowenfels AB. The epidemiology of pancreatitis and pancreatic cancer. Gastroenterology 2013;144(6):1252–61.
26. Banks PA, Bollen TL, Dervenis C, et al. Classification of acute pancreatitis–2012: revision of the Atlanta classification and definitions by international consensus. Gut 2013;62(1):102–11.
27. Braganza JM, Lee SH, McCloy RF, et al. Chronic pancreatitis. Lancet 2011;377(9772):1184–97.
28. Ryan DP, Hong TS, Bardeesy N. Pancreatic adenocarcinoma. N Engl J Med 2014;371(11):1039–49.
29. McNamara R, Dean AJ. Approach to acute abdominal pain. Emerg Med Clin North Am 2011;29(2):159–73, vii.
30. Tang RS, Chan FK. Therapeutic management of recurrent peptic ulcer disease. Drugs 2012;72(12):1605–16.
31. Mourad J, Elliott JP, Erickson L, et al. Appendicitis in pregnancy: new information that contradicts long-held clinical beliefs. Am J Obstet Gynecol 2000;182(5):1027–9.
32. Ong EMW. Ascending retrocecal appendicitis presenting with right upper abdominal pain: utility of computed tomography. World J Gastroenterol 2009;15(28):3576.
33. Obon-Dent M, Shabaneh B, Dougherty KG, et al. Spontaneous celiac artery dissection case report and literature review. Tex Heart Inst J 2012;39(5):703–6.
34. Bennett K, Rettew A, Shaikh B, et al. An easily overlooked cause of abdominal pain. J Community Hosp Intern Med Perspect 2014;4(5):25083.
35. Peter NG, Clark LR, Jaeger JR. Fitz-Hugh-Curtis syndrome: a diagnosis to consider in women with right upper quadrant pain. Cleve Clin J Med 2004;71(3):233–9.

36. Canto JG, Shlipak MG, Rogers WJ, et al. Prevalence, clinical characteristics, and mortality among patients with myocardial infarction presenting without chest pain. JAMA 2000;283(24):3223–9.
37. Gantner J, Keffeler JE, Derr C. Pulmonary embolism: an abdominal pain masquerader. J Emerg Trauma Shock 2013;6(4):280–2.
38. Cheyne G, Runau F, Lloyd DM. Right upper quadrant pain and raised alkaline phosphatase is not always a hepatobiliary problem. Ann R Coll Surg Engl 2014;96(1):118E–20E.
39. Brandt LJ. A 52-year-old man with right upper quadrant abdominal pain. Gastrointest Endosc 2010;72(4):807.
40. Liddington MI, Thomson WH. Rebound tenderness test. Br J Surg 1991;78(7): 795–6.
41. Mallett SV. Clinical utility of viscoelastic tests of coagulation (TEG/ROTEM) in patients with liver disease and during liver transplantation. Semin Thromb Hemost 2015;41(5):527–37.
42. Pratt DS, Kaplan MM. Evaluation of abnormal liver-enzyme results in asymptomatic patients. N Engl J Med 2000;342(17):1266–71.
43. Steinberg WM, Goldstein SS, Davis ND, et al. Diagnostic assays in acute pancreatitis. A study of sensitivity and specificity. Ann Intern Med 1985;102(5):576–80.
44. CDC Division of Viral Hepatitis and National Center for HIV/AIDS VH, STD, and TB Prevention. Testing recommendations for chronic hepatitis C virus infection. 2015. Available at: www.cdc.gov/hepatitis/hcv/guidelinesc.htm. Accessed September 1, 2015.
45. Eisenberg RL, Heineken P, Hedgcock MW, et al. Evaluation of plain abdominal radiographs in the diagnosis of abdominal pain. Ann Surg 1983;197(4):464–9.
46. Kellow ZS, MacInnes M, Kurzencwyg D, et al. The role of abdominal radiography in the evaluation of the nontrauma emergency patient. Radiology 2008;248(3): 887–93.
47. Stoker J, van Randen A, Lameris W, et al. Imaging patients with acute abdominal pain. Radiology 2009;253(1):31–46.
48. Summers SM, Scruggs W, Menchine MD, et al. A prospective evaluation of emergency department bedside ultrasonography for the detection of acute cholecystitis. Ann Emerg Med 2010;56(2):114–22.
49. Yarmish GM, Smith MP, Rosen MP, et al. ACR appropriateness criteria right upper quadrant pain. J Am Coll Radiol 2014;11(3):316–22.
50. Spence SC, Teichgraeber D, Chandrasekhar C. Emergent right upper quadrant sonography. J Ultrasound Med 2009;8(4):479–96.
51. Rodgerson JD, Heegaard WG, Plummer D, et al. Emergency department right upper quadrant ultrasound is associated with a reduced time to diagnosis and treatment of ruptured ectopic pregnancies. Acad Emerg Med 2001;8(4):331–6.
52. Shuman WP, Ralls PW, Balfe DM, et al. Imaging evaluation of patients with acute abdominal pain and fever. American College of Radiology. ACR Appropriateness Criteria. Radiology 2000;215 Suppl:209–12.
53. van Randen A, Lameris W, van Es HW, et al. A comparison of the accuracy of ultrasound and computed tomography in common diagnoses causing acute abdominal pain. Eur Radiol 2011;21(7):1535–45.
54. Koo BC, Chinogureyi A, Shaw AS. Imaging acute pancreatitis. Br J Radiol 2010; 83(986):104–12.
55. Townsend C, Beauchamp R, Evers B, et al. Sabiston textbook of surgery. 19th edition. Philadelphia: Elsevier Health Sciences; 2012. Available at: www. r2library.com/Resource/Title/1437715605. Accessed May 10, 2015.

56. Marx J. Rosen's emergency medicine. 8th edition. Philadelphia: Elsevier Health Sciences; 2014. Available at: www.r2library.com/Resource/Title/1455706051. Accessed May 10, 2015.
57. Eckenrode AH, Ewing JA, Kotrady J, et al. HIDA scan with ejection fraction is over utilized in the management of biliary dyskinesia. Am Surg 2015;81(7):669–73.
58. Fogel EL, Sherman S. ERCP for gallstone pancreatitis. N Engl J Med 2014;370(2): 150–7.
59. Wu BU, Banks PA. Clinical management of patients with acute pancreatitis. Gastroenterology 2013;144(6):1272–81.
60. Burdett E, Dushianthan A, Bennett-Guerrero E, et al. Perioperative buffered versus non-buffered fluid administration for surgery in adults. Cochrane Database Syst Rev 2012;(12):CD004089.
61. Thomas SH, Silen W, Cheema F, et al. Effects of morphine analgesia on diagnostic accuracy in emergency department patients with abdominal pain: a prospective, randomized trial. J Am Coll Surg 2003;196(1):18–31.
62. Thompson DR. Narcotic analgesic effects on the sphincter of Oddi: a review of the data and therapeutic implications in treating pancreatitis. Am J Gastroenterol 2001;96(4):1266–72.
63. Illige M, Meyer A, Kovach F. Surgical treatment for asymptomatic cholelithiasis. Am Fam Physician 2014;89:468–70.
64. Cooper JJ. Biliary tract disorders. In: Adams JG, editor. Emergency medicine: clinical essentials. 2nd edition. Philadelphia: Elsevier; 2013. p. 361–9.
65. Dieperink E, Pocha C, Thuras P, et al. All-cause mortality and liver-related outcomes following successful antiviral treatment for chronic hepatitis C. Dig Dis Sci 2014;59(4):872–80.
66. Yokoe M, Takada T, Mayumi T, et al. Japanese guidelines for the management of acute pancreatitis: Japanese guidelines 2015. J Hepatobiliary Pancreat Sci 2015; 22(6):405–32.
67. Palmer K. Acute upper gastrointestinal bleeding. Medicine 2011;39(2):94–100.

Lower Abdominal Pain

David J. Carlberg, MD[a],*, Stephen D. Lee, MD[b],
Jeffrey S. Dubin, MD, MBA[a,c]

KEYWORDS

- Review • Appendicitis • Diverticulitis • Crohn's disease • Ulcerative colitis
- Inflammatory bowel disease

KEY POINTS

- Diseases of the lower abdominal tract usually cause lower abdominal pain but, because of the path of the colon, can cause pain throughout the abdomen.
- Computed tomography (CT) is useful for evaluating lower abdominal tract disease; because of radiation and contrast risks, its use should be avoided when alternatives exist.
- Ultrasonography and MRI may be alternatives to CT, but have drawbacks including variable sensitivity (ultrasonography) and availability (MRI and sometimes ultrasonography).
- Appendicitis generally requires admission and operative intervention.
- Diverticulitis and inflammatory bowel disease can frequently be managed on an outpatient basis, but may require admission and surgical consultation.

It is important for the emergency physician to have a sound understanding of diseases of the lower intestinal tract. Although most frequently presenting with lower abdominal pain, appendicitis, colitis, and diverticulitis can cause pain throughout the abdomen as the colon runs through all 4 quadrants. The track of the colon also means that these diseases cause both peritoneal and retroperitoneal symptoms. This article focuses on the key diagnostic and management issues pertaining to appendicitis, inflammatory bowel disease, and diverticulitis. Infectious and ischemic colitis are discussed elsewhere.

ACUTE APPENDICITIS
Epidemiology

Acute appendicitis shows significant variability in age, race, gender, and seasonality. The peak incidence occurs between 10 and 19 years of age.[1,2] The incidence is lowest

Disclosure Statement: The authors have nothing to disclose.
[a] Department of Emergency Medicine, MedStar Georgetown University Hospital, 3800 Reservoir Road, NW, G-CCC, Washington, DC 20007, USA; [b] Department of Emergency Medicine, University of Maryland School of Medicine, 110 South Paca Street, 6th Floor, Suite 200, Baltimore, MD 21201, USA; [c] Department of Emergency Medicine, MedStar Washington Hospital Center, 110 Irving Street, NW, Washington, DC 20010, USA
* Corresponding author.
E-mail address: david.carlberg@gunet.georgetown.edu

between 0 and 4 years and older than 50 years.[1,2] Appendicitis affects both men and women with a slight predominance in men[1,2] and is more common in Caucasians and Hispanics than it is in African Americans or Asians.[2] Appendicitis has seasonal variability as well, with a higher incidence in summer months.[1–5]

Perforation rates are greatest at the extremes of age; patients less than 4 years old and greater than 60 years old develop perforation in 60% to 70% of cases. In comparison, perforation rates are 20% to 30% between 5 and 29 years of age.[2]

The incidence of negative appendectomy has decreased significantly with the advent of computed tomography (CT). Although the classically accepted negative appendectomy rate was 15% to 25%, recent negative appendectomy rates are as low as 1.7%.[6] The dependence on CT to drive operative intervention means the rate of imaging has increased significantly. At one institution, between 1990 and 2007 the percentage of patients undergoing CT before appendectomy went from 1% to 97.5%.[6]

Disparities

Racial and economic disparities are common in acute appendicitis. However, causes for these disparities have not been determined and may be due to accelerated disease progression, delayed presentation to medical care, and/or provider bias. A retrospective review of approximately 1.6 million appendectomies performed in the United States between 2003 and 2011 showed that African American patients were more likely to have acute complications than Caucasian patients. Also, patients with public insurance were more likely to have acute complications than those with private.[7]

A pediatric retrospective study that adjusted for age, perforation, hospital type, use of laparoscopy, insurance status, household income, and time from admission to appendectomy showed that African American children were more likely than Caucasian children to experience a complication.[8] African American and Hispanic children were more likely than Caucasian children to present with perforation (27% and 31% vs 23%).[8]

Symptoms

Classic appendicitis
Approximately 50% of acute appendicitis cases demonstrate the classic presentation of poorly localized periumbilical pain migrating to the right lower quadrant associated with anorexia, low-grade fever, and leukocytosis.[9] Rebound (69.5%), guarding (47.6%), psoas sign (12.6%), and obturator sign (7.7%) may or may not be present.[10,11] No single historical component or examination finding is sufficient for ruling in or out appendicitis. Migrating pain, rigidity, and the psoas sign are most specific for appendicitis.[10]

Atypical appendicitis
Unusual locations of the appendix within the abdomen may lead to atypical findings on examination. Retrocecal and retroileal appendicitis does not cause the classic migratory pain. Retrocecal appendicitis may present with right-sided low back pain. Tenderness and guarding may be decreased or absent because of protection from the overlying colon. Psoas sign may be present.[9] Uncomplicated appendicitis causing hip pain and a limp owing to psoas irritation have also been reported.[12] Retroileal appendicitis may present with nonspecific and hard to localize discomfort. Because of ileal irritation, vomiting and diarrhea may predominate.[9] Pelvic appendicitis may cause pain in the left lower quadrant. If the appendix abuts the bladder or ureter, it

may cause dysuria, urgency, and pyuria, and if the appendix abuts the rectum, it may cause defecation urgency and diarrhea.[10,13]

Stump appendicitis in a postappendectomy patient can occur if the base of the appendix was not identified and fully removed during initial appendectomy. Stump appendectomy is the treatment of choice.[14]

Special populations

Classic presentations are less common at the extremes of age and in gravid females. In pregnancy, the uterus may displace the appendix upwards toward the costal margin, causing pain in the right upper quadrant in up to 55% of late pregnancy appendicitis cases.[15] Diagnosing appendicitis is challenging in pregnancy because nausea, vomiting, anorexia, and leukocytosis are common in both normal pregnancy and appendicitis.[15,16] Ruptured appendicitis becomes more common as pregnancy progresses, possibly because appendicitis is more difficult to diagnose in this group.[16]

Children are also a challenging population. One study in the pre-CT era showed a missed appendicitis rate of 28% in children younger than 13 years. Misdiagnoses included gastroenteritis, respiratory infection, sepsis, and urinary tract infection. Misdiagnosed patients were more often younger, with a mean age of 5.3 versus 7.9 years for those diagnosed correctly. Misdiagnosed patients were more likely to have constipation, diarrhea, dysuria, and onset of vomiting before pain.[17]

The elderly are a high-risk group. One study reported that less than one-third of those older than 60 years present with the classic symptoms of fever, elevated white blood cell count, anorexia, and right lower quadrant pain.[18] Additionally, the elderly (>68 years) are more likely to have a delayed presentation, presenting 50 hours into symptoms compared with the nonelderly, who presented at 31 hours.[19] This is troubling because 1 study reported that 29% (7 of 24) of those over 55 years had perforated appendicitis within 36 hours of symptom onset, compared with 7% (13 of 188) of those 55 and under. By 48 hours into symptoms, 71% of those older than 55 years had perforated.[20]

Mimics

Mesenteric adenitis is the second most common cause of right lower quadrant pain and occurs more often in children. Because mesenteric adenitis is idiopathic, and because acute appendicitis can cause enlarged and inflamed mesenteric lymph nodes, visualization of a noninflamed appendix is required to make the diagnosis.[21,22]

Two other common mimics of acute appendicitis are omental infarction and epiploic appendagitis. These entities can be difficult to differentiate on CT, but differentiation is not important because both are benign and self-limited. Epiploic appendagitis is present in 1% of patients with suspected appendicitis.[21,22]

Infectious processes (especially *Yersinia*, *Campylobacter*, and *Salmonella*) and inflammatory processes (Crohn's disease) in the terminal ileum and cecum can also mimic acute appendicitis.[21,22] A more comprehensive list of appendicitis mimics is shown in **Box 1**.[21,22]

Diagnosis

Making the diagnosis of acute appendicitis can sometimes be simple, requiring only a history and physical examination. Other times, it can be extremely challenging, requiring laboratory testing, layered diagnostic imaging, consultant input, and shared decision making with the patient.

Box 1
Appendicitis mimics

Gastrointestinal mimics

- Mesenteric adenitis
- Epiploic appendagitis
- Omental infarction
- Infectious enterocolitis
- Inflammatory enterocolitis
- Ischemic enterocolitis
- Right-sided diverticulitis
- Ileocecal intussusception

Genitourinary mimics

- Pelvic inflammatory disease and tuboovarian abscess
- Hemorrhagic ovarian cyst
- Ovarian torsion
- Mittelschmerz
- Ectopic pregnancy
- Ureterolithiasis

Musculoskeletal mimics

- Rectus sheath hematoma
- Abdominal wall abscess
- Endometrial implants from prior uterine surgery
- Metastatic disease

Data from van Breda Vriesman AC, Puylaert JB. Mimics of appendicitis: alternative nonsurgical diagnoses with sonography and CT. AJR Am J Roentgenol 2006;186:1103–12; and Shin LK, Jeffrey RB. Sonography and computed tomography of the mimics of appendicitis. Ultrasound Q 2010;26:201–10.

Laboratory testing

Laboratory tests are a useful tool in the diagnosis of appendicitis; they increase or decrease the probability of appendicitis, but they are not sensitive enough to rule out appendicitis nor are they specific enough to rule it in.

A large metaanalysis reported the sensitivity of a white blood cell count of >10,000 cells/mm^2 to be 83%. The sensitivity of PMN ratio greater than 75% is 66% to 87%. A band count of greater than 700 cells/μL is 28% sensitive.[23] C-reactive protein (CRP) begins to increase approximately 8 to 12 hours after the onset of inflammation and peaks between 24 and 48 hours; therefore, CRP is not useful in early appendicitis. When CRP is greater than 10 mg/L, its sensitivity is 65% to 85%. CRP is predictive of perforated appendicitis, but with advanced imaging so ubiquitous, the utility of CRP for this purpose is limited.[23]

Imaging

With the advent of CT, negative appendectomies have dropped significantly, especially in women 18 to 45 years of age.[24] However, with concerns about ionizing radiation, efforts to minimize exposure and subsequent cancer risk should be employed. Ultrasonography (US) and MRI used in appropriate clinical circumstances reduce this risk but have their own challenges.[24]

Computed tomography

CT is the most accurate radiographic study for the diagnosis of appendicitis. An adult study from an academic medical center showed a sensitivity of 98.5%, a specificity of 98%, and a negative predictive value of 99.5%.[25] Metaanalyses and community-based, non–protocol-driven studies have not been as generous, with sensitivities as low at 87%.[26,27] A pediatric study of 128 CT images showed a sensitivity of 96% and a specificity of 97%.[28] The sensitivity and specificity of CT are more consistent and reproducible than US, likely owing to intraoperator variability with US.[24]

Low-dose CT may be a reasonable option in the evaluation of suspected appendicitis. One Korean study showed the sensitivity and specificity of low dose CT to be the same as standard dose; however, the CT reader's level of confidence for the diagnosis of acute appendicitis was reduced. If nondiagnostic, low-dose CT may need to be followed by a standard CT.[24,29] Low-dose CT can deliver 75% less radiation than standard CT.[24] The ability of low-dose CT to evaluate for other pathology may be limited.[29]

The two largest risks with CT are ionizing radiation and acute kidney injury from intravenous (IV) contrast. An estimate of the attributable risk of all cancers from 1 adult CT of the abdomen and pelvis is 3 in 5000. The risk in neonates is estimated at 7 in 5000.[30]

When choosing among CT contrast options (IV and enteral), the emergency physician must weigh study optimization, emergency department (ED) throughput, and contrast risk. For adults with suspected appendicitis, the authors recommend CT with IV contrast only. The adult emergency medicine, surgery, and radiology literature shows that CT with IV contrast alone is comparable with CT with IV and enteral contrast.[31–34] Eliminating oral contrast can decrease time to CT, disposition, operating room, and discharge.[34,35] Kepner and associates[34] showed a 2-hour decrease in duration of stay in those with a negative CT.

Although there is not enough evidence to forego enteral contrast in pediatrics,[30] one study showed that 27.5% of children with oral contrast studies did not have the contrast reach the terminal ileum. Vomiting occurred in 19.3% of those with appendicitis and in 12.9% without. CT accuracy was no different between the 2 groups.[32]

If IV contrast administration is moderate to high risk, it is reasonable to obtain a noncontrast CT. The small degradation in study quality does not generally decrease sensitivity to the point of rendering the study nondiagnostic.[30]

Ultrasonography

US is an appealing alternative to CT because it lacks ionizing radiation. When US is readily available, the authors recommend it as the initial imaging choice in children, young adults, and pregnant women. Unfortunately, US is operator dependent and non-visualization of the appendix is common.[24,36] Nonvisualization rates are as high as 75.6%.[37,38] Compared with general sonographers, pediatric sonographers are more frequently able to identify the appendix.[38] Patient size and build may play a role in the diagnostic ability of US, with visualization more difficult in larger patients.[28,38,39]

It is unclear whether an US that visualizes the appendix and is read as negative is sufficient to rule out appendicitis. A 2014 pediatric study showed a sensitivity of 99.5% with complete visualization, but a 2011 study that looked at children and adults showed a sensitivity of 81.7% with complete visualization.[37,40] A Dutch study reported 18 false negatives among 105 US read as appendix visualized and negative for appendicitis.[41] Based on the available literature, the authors do not recommend terminating an appendicitis workup after a negative US.

The strategy of performing US first, followed by CT if the US results are negative or nondiagnostic has yielded good results. Sensitivity has ranged from 95% to 100% and the CT rate has ranged from 17.9% to 39.7%.[24,42]

The ability of emergency physicians to perform bedside US for appendicitis has been studied with mixed results.[43,44] It is unclear if the time required to perform the study combined with the variable sensitivity and specificity make US for appendicitis worthwhile for the emergency physician to perform.

MRI

Although MRI is less well-studied than CT, the authors recommend MRI as a reasonable alternative in the evaluation of suspected appendicitis. MRI, like CT, allows for visualization of the appendix and several other intraabdominal and extraabdominal structures; however, MRI does not require ionizing radiation, making it an appealing study in children and pregnant women. The drawbacks to MRI include availability, study time, and cost.[24] The availability and study time are institution dependent; one institution has a pediatric protocol that achieved a median time from request to scan of 71 minutes and a median imaging duration of 11 minutes.[45]

Several MRI studies show sensitivity of greater than 95% in adults and children; however, one study did report a sensitivity as low as 85%.[24,45,46] Specificities range from 93% to 100%.[24,45,46]

MRI seems to be reliable in pregnancy. A metaanalysis reported a sensitivity of 80% (95% CI, 44%–98%) for MRI performed after US. The results were similar for CT. Of note, 3 of the MRI studies reviewed used gadolinium, which is generally avoided in pregnant patients.[47] MRI evaluation may be reader dependent, with a sensitivity of 89% when read by general radiologists and 97% when read by radiologists with MRI expertise.[46] Gadolinium can enhance MRI image quality in children.[48]

Imaging recommendations

- The physician must weigh risks and benefits of testing modalities.
- When risk from radiation exposure is low, CT with IV with or without enteral contrast is the preferred choice.
- When the differential diagnosis has a high risk of morbidity or mortality, CT with IV contrast (with or without enteral contrast) is the preferred choice.
- CT without IV contrast is reasonable, especially when IV contrast poses a moderate to high risk.
- When ionizing radiation is a concern, a tiered approach to imaging should be tailored to the imaging modalities available.
- In children and young adults, US is a good first step. If suspicion for appendicitis still exists despite a negative or indeterminate study, MRI or CT is recommended.[45,49–51]
- In pregnancy, consider starting with US and, if negative, moving to MRI.[47]
- Consultation with obstetrics and general surgery can be useful, especially because the true sensitivity of MRI in pregnancy is still unclear.[24]

Decision rules

Many decision rules exist to aid evaluation for suspected appendicitis. The Alvarado score and the pediatric appendicitis score take into account history and physical examination findings as well as leukocytosis and neutrophilia. The appendicitis inflammatory response score takes these findings and CRP into account.[52,53]

These rules are generally not sufficient to rule out appendicitis owing to the high number of false negatives.[52–55] A study in Thailand found 2 of 15 low-risk patients with appendicitis.[56] Another study showed a 4.7% miss rate with appendicitis inflammatory response and a 9.7% miss rate for Alvarado.[57]

Treatment

Beyond providing an initial antibiotic dose in acute appendicitis, the emergency physician has little role in the overall treatment of the disease. However, patients and families often have questions about possible next steps, so it is important for the emergency physician to have an understanding of treatment options.

Surgical treatment

Laparoscopic appendectomy has become the most frequent procedure for acute appendicitis in the United States, with 75% of appendectomies in 2011 performed laparoscopically. Laparoscopic appendectomy has fewer complications, a lower mortality rate, and a shorter hospital stay than open appendectomy.[58] Brief delays (<24 hours) to appendectomy have not shown increased complications or worse outcomes.[59–61]

Antibiotic treatment

The effectiveness of antibiotic treatment alone for appendicitis continues to be evaluated. Studies have strict inclusion/exclusion criteria and require hospital admission for serial examinations.[62] Although the antibiotics only approach is reported to be safe, there are a significant number of treatment failures and recurrent appendicitis cases. In adults, treatment failure ranges from 4.8% to 9.2%, and recurrent appendicitis ranges from 4.4% to 22.7%.[63–69] In the pediatric literature, treatment failure ranges from 8.3% to 16.7% and recurrent appendicitis ranges from 2.4% to 8.3%.[70–72]

Although 1 pediatric study showed a recurrence rate of only 1 in 22, 5 patients (22.3%) had an appendectomy because of recurrent abdominal pain. Although none of these 5 patients had recurrent appendicitis, the study highlights the challenge of managing abdominal pain in patients with possibly recurrent appendicitis.[71] Children managed with antibiotics alone had a quicker return to school and everyday activities. Their parents took less time off work.[73]

Based on available data, antibiotic therapy alone cannot be recommended as preferred or equal to appendectomy, but it is likely safe in the appropriately selected patient who weighs risks and benefits and wishes to avoid surgery or has a contraindication to surgery.

Antibiotic choice

Antibiotic prophylaxis is recommended for uncomplicated appendicitis before appendectomy, and antibiotic treatment is recommended for complicated appendicitis.[74] Antibiotics should be initiated in the ED and should cover gram-negative aerobes, enteric gram-positive streptococci, and anaerobes. Antipseudomonal activity is not required for mild or moderate community acquired infection.[75] See **Box 2** for specific antibiotic recommendations.[75]

INFLAMMATORY BOWEL DISEASE

Inflammatory bowel diseases (IBD)—Crohn's disease and ulcerative colitis (UC)—are incurable, lifelong diseases. Inflammation and ulceration of the intestines are the hallmarks of IBD. In Crohn's disease, the entire gastrointestinal tract is involved, whereas

---

Box 2
Antibiotic selection for acute appendicitis

- Previously healthy pediatric patients
  - Ertapenem
  - Meropenem
  - Imipenem–cilastatin
  - Ticarcillin–clavulanate
  - Piperacillin–tazobactam
  - Metronidazole plus ceftriaxone, cefotaxime, ceftazidime, or cefepime
- Well-appearing, healthy, immunocompetent adult patients
  - Cefoxitin
  - Ertapenem
  - Moxifloxacin
  - Metronidazole plus ciprofloxacin, levofloxacin, cefazolin, cefuroxime, ceftriaxone, or cefotaxome
- Systemically ill, immunosuppressed, or elderly adult patients
  - Imipenem–cilasatin
  - Meropenem
  - Doripenem
  - Piperacillin–tazobactam
  - Metronidazole plus ciprofloxacin, levofloxacin, cefepime, or ceftazidime
- Not recommended
  - Clindamycin (resistance)
  - Ampicillin–sulbactam (resistance)
  - Cefotetan (resistance)
  - Aminoglycosides (toxicity)

Data from Solomkin JS, Mazuski JE, Bradley JS, et al. Diagnosis and management of complicated intra-abdominal infection in adults and children: guidelines by the surgical infection society and the infectious diseases society of America. Clin Infect Dis 2010;50:133–64.

UC is limited to the colon and rectum. Crohn's disease causes full-thickness inflammation, whereas UC only causes mucosal inflammation.

Epidemiology

IBD has a prevalence of 348 per 100,000 persons in the United States. UC is more prevalent at 202 per 100,000 compared with Crohn's disease at 146 per 100,000. IBD is more frequent in Caucasians. IBD is a disease of older people, with patients older than 50 years 3 times more likely to carry the diagnosis than younger patients. Women are more likely to have Crohn's disease.[76] UC is more frequent in men.[77] First-degree relatives have a 5% to 15% chance of developing Crohn's disease over their lifetimes.[78] Smoking is associated with increased prevalence and severity of Crohn's disease, as well as higher rates of hospitalization. In UC, smoking does not exacerbate the disease and may be protective.[79]

Clinical Presentation

IBD is difficult to diagnose de novo in the ED. Most patients are not diagnosed for months to years after symptom onset. Emergency physicians should not be expected to make the definitive diagnosis of inflammatory disease; however, they should be aware of the signs and symptoms and refer discharged patients to gastroenterology if IBD is suspected.

To properly manage those with a known diagnosis of IBD, the emergency physician must have an understanding of the common clinical conditions and complications of UC and Crohn's disease. **Table 1** compares and contrasts common intestinal presentations and complications of UC and Crohn's disease,[80] and **Table 2** shows common extraintestinal manifestations of IBD, which are seen in 25% to 40 % of patients.[81]

Management

Patients with IBD may require imaging in the ED to assess for obstruction, abscess, or toxic megacolon. Many patients, especially those with Crohn's disease, undergo extensive imaging during their lifetimes so avoidance of ionizing radiation from additional CT scans is important. Plain radiographs for evaluating obstruction or megacolon are preferred to CT. In centers with experience, perianal US can be done instead of CT if evaluation for perianal abscess is needed.[82] MR enterography is preferred to CT for small bowel evaluation in patients with Crohn's disease with suspected bowel obstruction or strictures.[83] For patients who can tolerate fluids and do not require hospitalization, MR enterography may be deferred to the outpatient arena.

Table 1
Inflammatory bowel disease intestinal manifestations

	Ulcerative Colitis	Crohn's Disease
Common Findings		
Fever, abdominal pain, diarrhea, rectal bleeding, weight loss, malnutrition Note that fever is common and although this does not always indicate sepsis, clinicians should be concerned.	Diarrhea and bleeding more frequent • Very ill-appearing patient heightens concern for toxic megacolon	Abdominal pain more frequent • Vomiting is uncommon and when present raises concern for strictures and small bowel obstruction
Perianal disease	Absent	Frequent
Abdominal mass	Absent	Common
Locations	Colon and rectum only	Entire gastrointestinal tract at risk but most (2/3 of patients) have only colon/ileum disease
Complications		
Toxic megacolon	Uncommon • Ill patient, abdominal distention should raise concern	Absent
Strictures	Infrequent	Common • Vomiting should raise concern for severe stricture and small bowel obstruction
Fistulas	Absent	Common • Enteroenteric • Enterocutaneous
Colon cancer	Common	Less common

Adapted from Podolsky D. Inflammatory bowel disease. N Engl J Med 2002;347:417–29. Copyright © 2002 Massachusetts Medical Society. Reprinted with permission from Massachusetts Medical Society.

Table 2
Extra-intestinal manifestations of inflammatory bowel disease

System	Manifestation
Musculoskeletal	Monoarthritis or polyarthritis, ankolysing spondylitis, osteoporosis
Skin	Erythema nodosum, pyoderma gangrenosom, psoriasis
Ocular	Uveitis, episcleritis
Hepatobiliary	Cholelithiasis, hepatitis, primary sclerosing cholangitis, cholangiocarcinoma
Renal	Nephrolithiasis

Adapted from Levine JS, Burakoff R. Extraintestinal manifestations of inflammatory bowel disease. Gastroenterol Hepatol (N Y) 2011;7:235–41; with permission.

ED CT for UC patients has been shown unnecessary in more than one-half of patients. Its utility increases in UC patients with any of the following features: vomiting without diarrhea, absence of rectal bleeding, and gastrointestinal surgery during the previous month. In UC patients without colectomy whose primary symptoms are pain and/or diarrhea and/or bleeding, CT is unlikely to show clinically significant findings.[84]

Emergency Department Treatment

Hospitalization is recommended for patients with severe UC, defined as 6 or more bloody stools per day, fever of 37.8°C or greater, hemoglobin of less than 10.5 g/dL, heart rate of greater than 90 bpm, and erythrocyte sedimentation rate of greater than 30 mm/h.[85,86] These patients should receive IV fluids and steroids (methylprednisolone 60 mg or hydrocortisone 400 mg, daily).[85,87] Toxic patients, especially those with megacolon, are treated with broad spectrum antibiotics and should have a surgical consultation. For patients with less severe disease, outpatient treatment is recommended. Outpatient medications are detailed in **Table 3**.[85]

Mild to moderate Crohn's disease can be managed on an outpatient basis. Patients with perianal fistulas are treated with antibiotics (ciprofloxacin/metronidazole) and avoidance of steroids. Perianal abscesses require drainage. Patients with ileal inflammation require oral steroids (budesonide 9 mg/d or prednisolone 40 mg/d). Ill patients with fever, weight loss, intestinal obstruction, or volume depletion require hospitalization and IV fluids with or without antibiotics depending upon toxicity.[85]

Although immune modulators (methotrexate, thiopurines) and anti-tumor necrosis factor therapy (infliximab) are used for UC and Crohn's disease resistant to

Table 3
Outpatient medication management of ulcerative colitis

Isolated Proctitis	Mesalamine suppositories
Left-sided colitis	Mesalamine enemas Consider 5-aminosalicylate @ 2 g/d
Diffuse colitis	Mesalamine enemas 5-aminosalicylate @ 4 g/d
Continued symptoms despite above medication compliance	Oral steroids

Data from Burger D, Travis S. Conventional medical management of inflammatory bowel disease. Gastroenterology 2011;140:1827–37.

conventional therapy, these medications have many side effects and initiation of therapy and monitoring should be managed by gastroenterologists. **Table 4** shows side effects of common IBD medications.[88–90] Patients with Crohn's and UC suffer from recurrent flares. These may be owing to medication resistance, medication noncompliance, or adverse effects of other medications; for example, nonsteroidal antiinflammatory drugs should be avoided in IBD.[91]

Crohn's disease patients often require multiple surgeries over their lifetimes owing to complications from abscesses and strictures. The use of biologic drugs has greatly improved treatment of resistant disease; however, they have significant adverse effects. Emergency physicians should ask patients about use of such medications because their symptoms may be complications of medications rather than IBD.

Finally, for IBD patients under the care of a gastroenterologist or primary care physician, the emergency physician should coordinate care with that doctor because many of these patients can be managed safely as outpatients.

DIVERTICULITIS

Diverticula are mucosal and serosal outpouchings of the bowel wall, typically colonic, that likely form due to increased intraluminal pressure, altered gut motility, and/or a disordered colonic microenvironment.[92] Diverticula are vulnerable to becoming occupied or abraded by a fecalith, which can lead to inflammation, infection, and/or perforation, causing diverticulitis.[93]

Epidemiology

Incidence and risk factors
The incidence of diverticulosis increases with age. Diverticuli may be present in up to 60% of adults 60 years or older. Risk of progression to diverticulitis ranges from 4% to

Table 4
Side effects of medications for inflammatory bowel disease

Medication or Medication Class	Side Effects

Biologics (anti-tumor necrosis factor-alpha)—infliximab, adalimumab, certolizumab	Opportunistic infections
	    Tuberculosis (pulmonary and extrapulmonary)
	    Fungal infections
	    Parasitic infection
	    Varicella zoster
	    Cytomegalovirus
	    Epstein-Barr virus
	Lymphoma
	Progressive multifocal leukoencephalopathy

Ciprofloxacin	Tendon rupture, tendonitis
Cyclosporine and tacrolimus	Renal toxicity, hypertension, gingival hyperplasia
Methotrexate	Hepatotoxicity, nausea/vomiting, pulmonary fibrosis
Metronidazole	Nausea, dysgeusia, peripheral neuropathy
Salicylates (mesalamine)	Diarrhea, nausea, vomiting, headache, thrombocytopenia
Steroids	Growth retardation (pediatrics), osteoporosis, hyperglycemia/diabetes, immunosuppression
Thiopurines (immunomodulators) azathioprine, 6-mercaptopurine, thioguanine	Pancreatitis, nausea/vomiting, hepatotoxicity, bone marrow suppression

Data from Refs.[88–90]

25%.[94–96] Risk factors for diverticular disease include a Western (low-fiber) diet, smoking, medications affecting bowel integrity (eg, nonsteroidal antiinflmmatory drugs, aspirin, steroids), obesity, and advancing age.[94] Hereditary diseases that affect motility or connective tissue may increase the risk of developing diverticula.[94] There is a higher prevalence of right-sided diverticula in Asians, although the etiology of this difference remains unclear.[97]

Age

Older patients, particularly those over 50 years, tend to present with more colonic diverticula, the majority of which are found in the sigmoid colon.[95] A majority of younger patients with diverticulitis are obese (63%–96%; relative risk of approximately 2), with the mechanism theorized to be the production of proinflammatory cytokines from adipose tissue.[98] Recurrence rates in two metaanalyses were higher in younger patients (approximately 30% in patients <50 vs approximately 18% in patients >50 years),[99,100] although a retrospective study of 1441 patients by Unlu and colleagues[101] did not reach this same conclusion, showing no difference in the recurrence rate. Younger patients require admission less frequently (11% of those <40 years).[98] Patients under 50 years had lower rates of complicated diverticulitis compared with older patients (22.0% vs 38.8%, respectively).[98] Older patients (>55 years) were less likely to present with fever.[102]

Gender

Younger patients with diverticulitis tend to be male (58.6% of those <50 years; 77% of those <40 years), and older patients tend to be female (57.6% of those >50 years).[99] An ED-based study found similar ratios, with females accounting for 69% of those 65 years and older.[96]

Diagnosis

Clinical evaluation

The clinical diagnosis of acute diverticulitis can be challenging. In the ED, the classic triad of abdominal pain, fever, and leukocytosis occurs in only 10% of cases.[102] Frequency of signs and symptoms of diverticulitis are listed in **Table 5**.[102]

In one ED study, three of the strongest associated features, focal left lower quadrant tenderness, absence of vomiting, and CRP greater than 50 mg/L, were present in only 24% of those clinically suspected to have diverticulitis.[103] External validation of these features as a potential decision rule showed good specificity (98%), but poor sensitivity (36%).[104] Although it is prudent to consider diverticulitis in the differential of

Table 5 Signs and symptoms of diverticulitis	
Sign/Symptom	%
Isolated left lower quadrant pain	42
Nausea	31
Diarrhea	19
Prior diverticulitis	18
Fever	14
Vomiting	9

Data from Iyer R, Longstreth G, Kawatkar A, et al. Acute colonic diverticulitis: diagnostic evidence, demographic and clinical features in three practice settings. J Gastrointestin Liver Dis 2014;23: 379–86.

any patient with abdominal pain and gastrointestinal complaints, no individual feature or triad of features seems to have a high clinical utility.

Computed tomography and other imaging modalities

CT findings of diverticulitis include diverticulosis with bowel wall thickening and pericolic fat stranding. Phlegmon, extraluminal gas, abscess, stricture, and fistula may also be present.[105,106] One significant advantage of CT is its ability to demonstrate complicated diverticulitis (eg, abscess, perforation), which might lead to inpatient or surgical management.[92] CT is also helpful in identifying alternative diagnoses with similar presentations. CT sensitivity for diverticulitis is 91% and specificity is 77%.[107] Comparatively, US had a sensitivity of 84% to 85%, but a wide range of specificities from 80% to 93%, suggesting variability in US technique.[107,108] MRI has a sensitivity of 83% and specificity of 81%.[107]

Given that CT is likely to be the most efficient and readily available imaging option in many ED settings, the benefits of imaging must be weighed against the risks of radiation exposure and contrast administration. Although surgical practice guidelines recommend CT, noting that the severity on CT correlates with risk of outpatient treatment failure, there may be a subset of patients with mild symptoms who do not necessitate imaging, because only 3.8% of those with isolated lower abdominal pain with no fever or leukocytosis have severe diverticulitis on CT.[105,108,109]

Management

Antibiotics

Antibiotic use in the treatment of diverticulitis is targeted toward coverage of gram-negative organisms and anaerobes. There is no advantage of IV over oral antibiotics for uncomplicated diverticulitis.[92] Commonly recommended antibiotic choices are listed in **Table 6**.[109]

Recent studies have suggested that antibiotics may not be necessary in uncomplicated diverticulitis, reporting no differences in recovery time, complications, need for surgery, or recurrence compared with placebo.[92,108,109] However, many practice guidelines still recommend the use of antibiotic treatment, and those that do not recommend antibiotics for everyone still recommend their use in pregnancy, sepsis, and immunosuppression.[105,110] Further study is needed before antibiotic-free treatment for mild diverticulitis is universally adopted.

Indications for admission

Inpatient admission with bowel rest and IV antibiotic therapy is recommended for patients who are older, septic, immunocompromised, or with multiple comorbidities, as

Table 6 Antibiotic treatment options for diverticulitis	
Mild Disease	**Inpatient or Severe Illness**
Ciprofloxacin + metronidazole	Piperacillin/tazobactam
Trimethoprim/sulfamethoxazole	Moxifloxacin
Amoxicillin/clavulanate	Tigecycline
—	Ticarcillin/clavulanate
—	Carbapenems

Data from Wilkins T, Embry K, George R. Diagnosis and management of acute diverticulitis. Am Fam Physician. 2013;87:612–20.

well as those who require procedural intervention (eg, perforation, abscess). Those who cannot tolerate oral fluids or those with poor self-care, limited home support, or follow-up may also benefit from admission.[105]

Indications for surgery

Historically, uncomplicated diverticulitis patients were instructed to follow-up for possible elective colectomy; however, this practice is no longer routine or required. It was noted in one guideline that 18 patients would need an elective colectomy to prevent one emergent surgery for recurrent diverticulitis.[105] Patients with multiple episodes of acute diverticulitis do not automatically require surgical consultation, because they are not at increased risk for morbidity and mortality.[105] Additionally, the majority of patients with complicated disease on presentation often have no prior history of diverticulitis.[108]

Patients with abscess, perforation, diffuse peritonitis, fistula, stricture, or failure of antibiotic treatment have been managed with urgent surgical therapy, ranging from laparoscopic lavage to colonic resection.[92,94,110] However, in stable patients, abscess management has trended toward interventional percutaneous drainage over primary surgical intervention.

Abscess formation occurs in 15% to 20% of diverticulitis cases.[105] Abscesses less than 2 to 3 cm are small enough to consider outpatient antibiotic therapy, because readmission rates in these patients are similar to those in patients without abscesses.[106] Many smaller abscesses resolve without drainage.[105] Patients who do not improve clinically and those with larger abscesses frequently require a percutaneous drain. Those with abscesses greater than 5 cm are more likely to fail medical therapy.[105] Continuing or worsening infection requires surgical consultation.

Discharge considerations: diet and exercise

A high-fiber diet is recommended by the American Society of Colon and Rectal Surgeons.[92] Insoluble fiber plays a role in increasing bulk and decreasing bowel transit time, thus decreasing the intraluminal pressure thought to contribute to the development of diverticula.[97] Interestingly, a Swedish study noted that non-Western immigrants had a lower risk of hospitalization from diverticular disease than native Swedes, although the immigrants' diverticulitis risk slowly increased over time spent in the country, presumably owing to adoption of a Western diet.[111]

Historically, patients were told to avoid foods containing seeds, nuts, and corn owing to concerns they may lodge in a diverticulum and result in inflammation and/or bleeding[94]; however, Strate and colleagues[112] did not show any association between diverticulitis and the consumption of these foods.

Probiotics, theorized to help reduce abnormal gut flora that might promote inflammation, are not associated with a significant reduction in recurrence of diverticulitis, although they are associated with reductions in abdominal pain, bloating, and fever.[92]

Obese men and women have a greater risk of developing diverticulitis and diverticulitis recurrence.[92,113] Similarly, those who are more physically active have a lower diverticulitis risk.[94] Counseling regarding physical activity and weight reduction may prove beneficial in selected patients.

SUMMARY

The evaluation and management of lower intestinal disease, although often straightforward, frequently requires a nuanced approach by the emergency physician. CT allows for remarkable visualization of abdominal organs and has spared countless individuals surgery; however, it puts patients at risk for ionizing radiation and kidney injury. When evaluating lower intestinal disease, the emergency physician should attempt to spare patients from the risks of CT whenever feasible, whether through shared decision making, serial examination, close follow-up, or alternate imaging modalities.

Once a presumed or confirmed diagnosis is made, appropriate treatment should be initiated. Appendicitis should be admitted and will usually require surgery. IBD can frequently be discharged after hydration, pain control, nausea control, and a discussion with the patient's gastroenterologist. Diverticulitis may or may not require admission and may or may not require surgical or percutaneous intervention.

PEARLS AND PITFALLS

- Appendicitis presents atypically up to 50% of the time and pain may occur throughout the abdomen and pelvis, or even the hip.
- Antibiotic treatment alone for acute appendicitis should be performed in an inpatient setting that allows for frequent abdominal examination and rapid identification of treatment failure.
- Avoid nonsteroidal medications for IBD because these agents can exacerbate the disease.
- CT for UC is generally not necessary when the primary symptoms are pain, bleeding, or diarrhea.
- Be suspicious of opportunistic infection in IBD patients on biologic medications.
- Clinical diagnosis of diverticulitis is challenging, because no individual symptom or triad is particularly prevalent.
- CT is highly sensitive for diverticulitis, but some patients with presumed mild disease may not require imaging.
- Complicated or severe diverticulitis warrants admission and possible surgical consultation.
- Diverticulitis related abscesses less than 2 to 3 cm may not need inpatient therapy; abscesses greater than 5 cm will likely require intervention.

REFERENCES

1. Al-Omran M, Mamdani M, McLeod RS. Epidemiologic features of acute appendicitis in Ontario, Canada. Can J Surg 2003;46:263–8.
2. Luckmann R, Davis P. The epidemiology of acute appendicitis in California: racial, gender, and seasonal variation. Epidemiology 1991;2:323–30.
3. Zangbar B, Rhee P, Pandit V, et al. Seasonal variation in emergency general surgery. Ann Surg 2016;263(1):76–81.
4. Ilves I, Fagerström A, Herzig KH, et al. Seasonal variations of acute appendicitis and nonspecific abdominal pain in Finland. World J Gastroenterol 2014;20:4037–42.
5. Stein GY, Rath-Wolfson L, Zeidman A, et al. Sex differences in the epidemiology, seasonal variation, and trends in the management of patients with acute appendicitis. Langenbecks Arch Surg 2012;397:1087–92.
6. Raja AS, Wright C, Sodickson AD, et al. Negative appendectomy rate in the era of CT: an 18-year perspective. Radiology 2010;256(2):460–5.
7. Bliss LA, Yang CJ, Kent TS, et al. Appendicitis in the modern era: universal problem and variable treatment. Surg Endosc 2015;29:1897–902.
8. Zwintscher NP, Steele SR, Martin MJ, et al. The effect of race on outcomes for appendicitis in children: a nationwide analysis. Am J Surg 2014;207:748–53.
9. Humes DJ, Simpson J. Acute appendicitis. BMJ 2006;333:530–4.

10. Wagner JM, McKinney WP, Carpenter JL. Does this patient have appendicitis? JAMA 1996;276:1589–94.
11. Berry J, Malt R. Appendicitis near its centenary. Ann Surg 1984;200:567–75.
12. Waseem M, Raja A, Al-Husayni H. Hip pain in a child: myositis or appendicitis? Pediatr Emerg Care 2010;26:431–3.
13. Puskar D, Bedalov G, Fridrih S, et al. Urinalysis, ultrasound analysis, and renal dynamic scintigraphy in acute appendicitis. Urology 1995;45:108–12.
14. Artul S, Daud M, Abboud N, et al. Stump appendicitis: a challenging diagnosis. BMJ Case Rep 2014. Available at: http://casereports.bmj.com/content/2014/bcr-2014-206775.full.pdf.
15. Pastore PA, Loomis DM, Sauret J. Appendicitis in pregnancy. J Am Board Fam Med 2006;19:621–6.
16. Flexer SM, Tabib N, Peter MB. Suspected appendicitis in pregnancy. Surgeon 2014;12:82–6.
17. Rothrock SG, Skeoch G, Rush JJ, et al. Clinical features of misdiagnosed appendicitis in children. Ann Emerg Med 1991;20:45–50.
18. Storm-Dickerson TL, Horattas MC. What have we learned over the past 20 years about appendicitis in the elderly? Am J Surg 2003;185:198–201.
19. Segev L, Keidar A, Schrier I, et al. Acute appendicitis in the elderly in the twenty-first century. J Gastrointest Surg 2015;19:730–5.
20. Augustin T, Cagir B, Vandermeer TJ. Characteristics of perforated appendicitis: effect of delay is confounded by age and gender. J Gastrointest Surg 2011;15:1223–31.
21. van Breda Vriesman AC, Puylaert JB. Mimics of appendicitis: alternative nonsurgical diagnoses with sonography and CT. AJR Am J Roentgenol 2006;186:1103–12.
22. Shin LK, Jeffrey RB. Sonography and computed tomography of the mimics of appendicitis. Ultrasound Q 2010;26:201–10.
23. Shogilev DJ, Duus N, Odom SR, et al. Diagnosing appendicitis: evidence-based review of the diagnostic approach in 2014. West J Emerg Med 2014;15:859–71.
24. Smith MP, Katz DS, Lalani T, et al. ACR appropriateness criteria® right lower quadrant pain–suspected appendicitis. Ultrasound Q 2015;31:85–91.
25. Pickhardt PJ, Lawrence EM, Pooler BD, et al. Diagnostic performance of multidetector computed tomography for suspected acute appendicitis. Ann Intern Med 2011;154:789–96.
26. van Randen A, Bipat S, Zwinderman AH, et al. Acute appendicitis: meta-analysis of diagnostic performance of CT and graded compression US related to prevalence of disease. Radiology 2008;249:97–106.
27. Huynh V, Lalezarzadeh F, Lawandy S, et al. Abdominal computed tomography in the evaluation of acute and perforated appendicitis in the community setting. Am Surg 2007;73:1002–5.
28. Abo A, Shannon M, Taylor G, et al. The influence of body mass index on the accuracy of ultrasound and computed tomography in diagnosing appendicitis in children. Pediatr Emerg Care 2011;27:731–6.
29. Kim K, Kim YH, Kim SY, et al. Low-dose abdominal CT for evaluating suspected appendicitis. N Engl J Med 2012;26(366):1596–605.
30. Howell JM, Eddy OL, Lukens TW, et al. Clinical policy: critical issues in the evaluation and management of emergency department patients with suspected appendicitis. Ann Emerg Med 2010;55:71–116.

31. Anderson SW, Soto JA, Lucey BC, et al. Abdominal 64-MDCT for suspected appendicitis: the use of oral and IV contrast material versus IV contrast material only. AJR Am J Roentgenol 2009;193:1282–8.

32. Laituri CA, Fraser JD, Aguayo P, et al. The lack of efficacy for oral contrast in the diagnosis of appendicitis by computed tomography. J Surg Res 2011;170: 100–3.

33. Drake FT, Alfonso R, Bhargava P, et al. Enteral contrast in the computed tomography diagnosis of appendicitis: comparative effectiveness in a prospective surgical cohort. Ann Surg 2014;260:311–6.

34. Kepner AM, Bacasnot JV, Stahlman BA. Intravenous contrast alone vs intravenous and oral contrast computed tomography for the diagnosis of appendicitis in adult ED patients. Am J Emerg Med 2012;30:1765–73.

35. Levenson RB, Camacho MA, Horn E, et al. Eliminating routine oral contrast use for CT in the emergency department: impact on patient throughput and diagnosis. Emerg Radiol 2012;19:513–7.

36. Parks NA, Schroeppel TJ. Update on imaging for acute appendicitis. Surg Clin North Am 2011;91:141–54.

37. D'Souza N, D'Souza C, Grant D, et al. The value of ultrasonography in the diagnosis of appendicitis. Int J Surg 2015;13:165–9.

38. Trout AT, Sanchez R, Ladino-Torres MF, et al. A critical evaluation of US for the diagnosis of pediatric acute appendicitis in a real-life setting: how can we improve the diagnostic value of sonography? Pediatr Radiol 2012;42:813–23.

39. Al-Ajerami Y. Sensitivity and specificity of ultrasound in the diagnosis of acute appendicitis. East Mediterr Health J 2012;18:66–9.

40. Ross MJ, Liu H, Netherton SJ, et al. Outcomes of children with suspected appendicitis and incompletely visualized appendix on ultrasound. Acad Emerg Med 2014;21:538–42.

41. Leeuwenburgh MM, Stockmann HB, Bouma WH, et al. A simple clinical decision rule to rule out appendicitis in patients with nondiagnostic ultrasound results. Acad Emerg Med 2014;21:488–96.

42. Toorenvliet BR, Wiersma F, Bakker RF, et al. Routine ultrasound and limited computed tomography for the diagnosis of acute appendicitis. World J Surg 2010;34:2278–85.

43. Sivitz AB, Cohen SG, Tejani C. Evaluation of acute appendicitis by pediatric emergency physician sonography. Ann Emerg Med 2014;64:358–64.

44. Lam SH, Grippo A, Kerwin C, et al. Bedside ultrasonography as an adjunct to routine evaluation of acute appendicitis in the emergency department. West J Emerg Med 2014;15:808–15.

45. Kulaylat AN, Moore MM, Engbrecht BW, et al. An implemented MRI program to eliminate radiation from the evaluation of pediatric appendicitis. J Pediatr Surg 2015;50(8):1359–63.

46. Leeuwenburgh MM, Wiarda BM, Jensch S, et al. Accuracy and interobserver agreement between MR-non-expert radiologists and MR-experts in reading MRI for suspected appendicitis. Eur J Radiol 2014;83:103–10.

47. Basaran A, Basaran M. Diagnosis of acute appendicitis during pregnancy: a systematic review. Obstet Gynecol Surv 2009;64:481–8.

48. Rosines LA, Chow DS, Lampl BS, et al. Value of gadolinium-enhanced MRI in detection of acute appendicitis in children and adolescents. AJR Am J Roentgenol 2014;203:W543–8.

49. Srinivasan A, Servaes S, Peña A, et al. Utility of CT after sonography for suspected appendicitis in children: integration of a clinical scoring system with a staged imaging protocol. Emerg Radiol 2015;22:31–42.

50. Poortman P, Oostvogel HJ, Bosma E, et al. Improving diagnosis of acute appendicitis: results of a diagnostic pathway with standard use of ultrasonography followed by selective use of CT. J Am Coll Surg 2009;208:434–41.

51. Atema JJ, Gans SL, Van Randen A, et al. Comparison of imaging strategies with conditional versus immediate contrast-enhanced computed tomography in patients with clinical suspicion of acute appendicitis. Eur Radiol 2015;25:2445–52.

52. Mandeville K, Pottker T, Bulloch B, et al. Using appendicitis scores in the pediatric ED. Am J Emerg Med 2011;29:972–7.

53. Kollár D, McCartan DP, Bourke M, et al. Predicting acute appendicitis? A comparison of the Alvarado score, the appendicitis inflammatory response score and clinical assessment. World J Surg 2015;39:104–9.

54. Pogorelić Z, Rak S, Mrklić I, et al. Prospective validation of alvarado score and pediatric appendicitis Score for the diagnosis of acute appendicitis in children. Pediatr Emerg Care 2015;31:164–8.

55. Kulik DM, Uleryk EM, Maguire JL. Does this child have appendicitis? A systematic review of clinical prediction rules for children with acute abdominal pain. J Clin Epidemiol 2013;66:95–104.

56. Apisarnthanarak P, Suvannarerg V, Pattaranutaporn P, et al. Alvarado score: can it reduce unnecessary CT scans for evaluation of acute appendicitis? Am J Emerg Med 2015;33:266–70.

57. de Castro SM, Ünlü C, Steller EP, et al. Evaluation of the appendicitis inflammatory response score for patients with acute appendicitis. World J Surg 2012;36:1540–5.

58. Masoomi H, Nguyen NT, Dolich MO, et al. Laparoscopic appendectomy trends and outcomes in the United States: data from the nationwide inpatient sample (NIS), 2004-2011. Am Surg 2014;80:1074–7.

59. Schnüriger B, Laue J, Kröll D, et al. Introduction of a new policy of no nighttime appendectomies: impact on appendiceal perforation rates and postoperative morbidity. World J Surg 2014;38:18–24.

60. United Kingdom National Surgical Research Collaborative, Bhangu A. Safety of short, in-hospital delays before surgery for acute appendicitis: multicentre cohort study, systematic review, and meta-analysis. Ann Surg 2014;259:894–903.

61. Drake FT, Mottey NE, Farrokhi ET, et al. Time to appendectomy and risk of perforation in acute appendicitis. JAMA Surg 2014;149:837–44.

62. Flum DR. Clinical practice. Acute appendicitis–appendectomy or the "antibiotics first" strategy. N Engl J Med 2015;372:1937–43.

63. Salminen P, Paajanen H, Rautio T, et al. Antibiotic therapy vs appendectomy for treatment of uncomplicated acute appendicitis: the APPAC randomized clinical trial. JAMA 2015;313:2340–8.

64. Hansson J, Körner U, Khorram-Manesh A, et al. Randomized clinical trial of antibiotic therapy versus appendicectomy as primary treatment of acute appendicitis in unselected patients. Br J Surg 2009;96:473–81.

65. Park HC, Kim MJ, Lee BH. Antibiotic therapy for appendicitis in patients aged ≥80 years. Am J Med 2014;127:562–4.

66. Park HC, Kim MJ, Lee BH. The outcome of antibiotic therapy for uncomplicated appendicitis with diameters ≤ 10 mm. Int J Surg 2014;12:897–900.

67. Kaminski A, Liu IL, Applebaum H, et al. Routine interval appendectomy is not justified after initial nonoperative treatment of acute appendicitis. Arch Surg 2005;140:897–901.
68. Kırkıl C, Yiğit MV, Aygen E. Long-term results of nonoperative treatment for uncomplicated acute appendicitis. Turk J Gastroenterol 2014;25:393–7.
69. McCutcheon BA, Chang DC, Marcus LP, et al. Long-term outcomes of patients with nonsurgically managed uncomplicated appendicitis. J Am Coll Surg 2014; 218:905–13.
70. Svensson JF, Johansson R, Kaiser S, et al. Recurrence of acute appendicitis after non-operative treatment of appendiceal abscess in children: a single-centre experience. Pediatr Surg Int 2014;30:413–6.
71. Svensson JF, Patkova B, Almström M, et al. Nonoperative treatment with antibiotics versus surgery for acute nonperforated appendicitis in children: a pilot randomized controlled trial. Ann Surg 2015;261:67–71.
72. Armstrong J, Merritt N, Jones S, et al. Non-operative management of early, acute appendicitis in children: is it safe and effective? J Pediatr Surg 2014; 49:782–5.
73. Horst JA, Trehan I, Warner BW, et al. Can children with uncomplicated acute appendicitis be treated with antibiotics instead of an appendectomy? Ann Emerg Med 2015;66:119–22.
74. Andersen BR, Kallehave FL, Andersen HK. Antibiotics versus placebo for prevention of postoperative infection after appendicectomy. Cochrane Database Syst Rev 2005;(3):CD001439.
75. Solomkin JS, Mazuski JE, Bradley JS, et al. Diagnosis and management of complicated intra-abdominal infection in adults and children: guidelines by the surgical infection society and the infectious diseases society of America. Clin Infect Dis 2010;50:133–64.
76. Betteridge JD, Armbruster SP, Maydonovitch C, et al. Inflammatory bowel disease prevalence by age, gender, race, and geographic location in the U.S. military health care population. Inflamm Bowel Dis 2013;19:1421–7.
77. Cosnes J, Gower-Rousseau C, Seksik P, et al. Epidemiology and natural history of inflammatory bowel diseases. Gastroenterology 2011;140:1785–94.
78. Sorrentino D, Avellini C, Geraci M, et al. Tissue studies in screened first-degree relatives reveal a distinct Crohn's disease phenotype. Inflamm Bowel Dis 2014; 20:1049–56.
79. Roberts H, Rai SN, Shannon KV, et al. Hospital discharges for Crohn's disease in States with high smoking prevalence. J Clin Gastroenterol 2014;48:650–1.
80. Podolsky D. Inflammatory bowel disease. N Engl J Med 2002;347:417–29.
81. Levine JS, Burakoff R. Extraintestinal manifestations of inflammatory bowel disease. Gastroenterol Hepatol (N Y) 2011;7:235–41.
82. Maconi G, Tonolini M, Monteleone M, et al. Transperineal perineal ultrasound versus magnetic resonance imaging in the assessment of perianal Crohn's disease. Inflamm Bowel Dis 2013;19:2737–43.
83. Cheriyan DG, Slattery E, McDermott S, et al. Impact of magnetic resonance enterography in the management of small bowel Crohn's disease. Eur J Gastroenterol Hepatol 2013;25:550–5.
84. Gashin L, Villafuerte-Galvez J, Leffler DA, et al. Utility of CT in the emergency department in patients with ulcerative colitis. Inflamm Bowel Dis 2015;21: 793–800.
85. Burger D, Travis S. Conventional medical management of inflammatory bowel disease. Gastroenterology 2011;140:1827–37.

86. Truelove SC, Witts LJ. Cortisone in ulcerative colitis; final report on a therapeutic trial. Br Med J 1955;2:1041–8.
87. Kornbluth A, Sachar DB, Practice Parameters Committee of the American College of Gastroenterology. Ulcerative colitis practice guidelines in adults: American College of Gastroenterology, Practice Parameters Committee. Am J Gastroenterol 2010;105:501–23.
88. Stallmach A, Hagel S, Bruns T. Adverse effects of biologics used for treating IBD. Best Pract Res Clin Gastroenterol 2010;24:167–82.
89. Rogler G. Gastrointestinal and liver adverse effects of drugs used for treating IBD. Best Pract Res Clin Gastroenterol 2010;24:157–65.
90. Triantafillidis JK, Merikas E, Georgopoulos F. Current and emerging drugs for the treatment of inflammatory bowel disease. Drug Des Devel Ther 2011;5: 185–210.
91. Guslandi M. Exacerbation of inflammatory bowel disease by nonsteroidal anti-inflammatory drugs and cyclooxygenase-2 inhibitors: fact or fiction? World J Gastroenterol 2006;12:1509–10.
92. Morris AM, Regenbogen SE, Hardiman KM, et al. Sigmoid diverticulitis: a systematic review. JAMA 2014;311:287–97.
93. Heise CP. Epidemiology and pathogenesis of diverticular disease. J Gastrointest Surg 2008;12:1309–11.
94. Razik R, Nguyen GC. Diverticular disease: changing epidemiology and management. Drugs Aging 2015;32:349–60.
95. Parks TG. Natural history of diverticular disease of the colon. A review of 521 cases. Br Med J 1969;4:639–42.
96. Schneider E, Singh A, Lidor A, et al. Emergency department presentation, admission, and surgical intervention for colonic diverticulitis in the United States. Am J Surg 2015;210:404–7.
97. Korzenik JR. Case closed? Diverticulitis: epidemiology and fiber. J Clin Gastroenterol 2006;40(Suppl 3):S112–6.
98. Pilgrim S, Hart A, Speakman C. Diverticular disease in younger patients - is it clinically more complicated and related to obesity? Colorectal Dis 2013;15: 1205–10.
99. Katz LH, Guy DD, Lahat A, et al. Diverticulitis in the young is not more aggressive than in the elderly, but it tends to recur more often: systematic review and meta-analysis. J Gastroenterol Hepatol 2013;28:1274–81.
100. van de Wall BJ, Poerink JA, Draaisma WA, et al. Diverticulitis in young versus elderly patients: a meta-analysis. Scand J Gastroenterol 2013;48:643–51.
101. Unlu C, van de Wall BJ, Gerhards MF, et al. Influence of age on clinical outcome of acute diverticulitis. J Gastrointest Surg 2013;17:1651–6.
102. Iyer R, Longstreth G, Kawatkar A, et al. Acute colonic diverticulitis: diagnostic evidence, demographic and clinical features in three practice settings. J Gastrointest Liver Dis 2014;23:379–86.
103. Laméris W, van Randen A, Boermeester M, et al. A clinical decision rule to establish the diagnosis of acute diverticulitis at the emergency department. Dis Colon Rectum 2010;53:896–904.
104. Kiewiet J, Andeweg C, Boermeester M, et al. Alimentary tract: external validation of two tools for the clinical diagnosis of acute diverticulitis without imaging. Dig Liver Dis 2014;46:119–24.
105. Feingold D, Steele S, Rafferty J, et al. Practice parameters for the treatment of sigmoid diverticulitis. Dis Colon Rectum 2014;57:284–94.

106. Jackson J, Hammond T. Systematic review: outpatient management of acute un-complicated diverticulitis. Int J Colorectal Dis 2014;29:775–81.
107. Liljegren G, Chabold A, Wickbom M, et al. Acute colonic diverticulitis: a system-atic review of diagnostic accuracy. Colorectal Dis 2007;9:480–8.
108. Humes D, Spiller R. Review article: the pathogenesis and management of acute colonic diverticulitis. Aliment Pharmacol Ther 2014;39:359–70.
109. Wilkins T, Embry K, George R. Diagnosis and management of acute diverticu-litis. Am Fam Physician 2013;87:612–20.
110. Vennix S, Morton D, Hahnloser D, et al. Systematic review of evidence and consensus on diverticulitis: an analysis of national and international guidelines. Colorectal Dis 2014;16:866–78.
111. Hjern F, Johansson C, Mellgren A, et al. Diverticular disease and migration–the influence of acculturation to a Western lifestyle on diverticular disease. Aliment Pharmacol Ther 2006;23:797–805.
112. Strate LL, Liu YL, Syngal S, et al. Nut, corn, and popcorn consumption and the incidence of diverticular disease. JAMA 2008;300:907–14.
113. Bose KP, Khorshidi I, Southern WN, et al. The impact of ethnicity and obesity on the course of colonic diverticulitis. J Clin Gastroenterol 2013;47:160–4.

Anorectal Complaints in the Emergency Department

Christina Lynn Tupe, MD*, Thuy Van Pham, MD

KEYWORDS

- Anorectal • Hemorrhoids • Anal fissures • Anal abscesses • Pruritus ani
- Anal foreign bodies • Anal cancer • STI

KEY POINTS

- Thorough history and physical can help distinguish between different types of anorectal complaints.
- Most anorectal complaints can be managed conservatively, but it is imperative to know when to consult surgeons.
- The most common anorectal complaints that present to the emergency department are rectal bleeding, rectal mass, and rectal discomfort, which are often caused by hemorrhoids, anal fissures, and anal abscesses.

INTRODUCTION

Patients with anorectal complaints commonly seek medical care in emergency departments (EDs), but they might not be forthcoming with their history because they are embarrassed. Moreover, because of the sensitive nature of the complaint, patients tend to present later in the course of their illness. However, physicians with an awareness of patients' reticence about the condition can elicit important information that facilitates the diagnostic process.

Anorectal conditions can be differentiated based on the presenting symptoms, their onset, frequency, and character, their recurrence, and systemic manifestations. The physical examination requires optimal positioning, adequate visualization, and a digital rectal examination (DRE) followed by anoscopy when clinically indicated. Grucela and colleagues[1] documented that physicians' diagnostic accuracy with anorectal conditions is about 50%, which emphasizes the need for them to become more familiar with the history and clinical findings associated with various anorectal complaints.

Disclosure: The authors have nothing to disclose.
Department of Emergency Medicine, University of Maryland School of Medicine, 110 South Paca Street, 6th Floor, Suite 200, Baltimore, MD 21201, USA
* Corresponding author.
E-mail address: ctupe@umem.org

Emerg Med Clin N Am 34 (2016) 251–270
http://dx.doi.org/10.1016/j.emc.2015.12.013
emed.theclinics.com

The anorectal area is the transition point from the rectosigmoid portion of the intestines to the skin (**Fig. 1**). The transition occurs at the dentate line. The first 1 to 2 cm distal to the dentate line constitute the anal canal. Distal to the anal canal is the anal verge, which has the appearance of normal external skin, with hair follicles, glands, and subcutaneous tissue. Proximal to the dentate line, the pleats of the rectum form the rectal ampulla with multiple crypts. Tissues distal and proximal to the dentate line have different embryonic origins and therefore have different blood supplies and innervation. The rectum above the dentate line is supplied by the superior hemorrhoidal artery, which is a branch off the inferior mesenteric artery and drains into the portal system through the internal hemorrhoidal plexus; the area below the dentate line is supplied by the middle and inferior hemorrhoidal arteries and drains into the systemic circulation via the external hemorrhoidal plexus. Tissue proximal to the dentate line is insensate, whereas sensation distal to the dentate line is supplied by the pudendal nerve and pelvic branches of S3 and S4 nerve roots.

HEMORRHOIDS
Pathophysiology

Hemorrhoids are a common source of discomfort and rectal bleeding, affecting 10 million to 23 million people. About half of them are symptomatic.[2] Hemorrhoids are downward displacements of the anal cushions. These cushions are formed from loose connective tissue, smooth muscle, and arterial and venous vessels. Hemorrhoids form when these supporting structures deteriorate, leading to venous dilatation, vascular thrombosis, and inflammation.[3]

Hemorrhoids are classified as either external or internal, based on their location below or above the dentate line (**Fig. 2**). External hemorrhoids are located below the dentate line and arise from the inferior hemorrhoidal plexus. They are innervated by

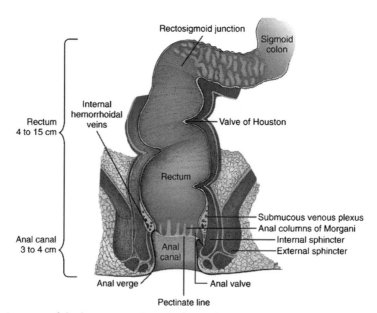

Fig. 1. Anatomy of the lower gastrointestinal tract. (*From* Coates WC. Anorectal procedures. In: Roberts JR, Hedges JR, eds. Clinical procedures in emergency medicine, 5th ed. Philadelphia: Elsevier, 2010; with permission.)

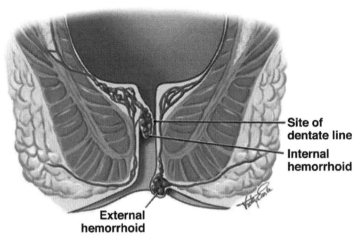

Fig. 2. Anatomy of internal and external hemorrhoids. (*Courtesy of* Iain Cleator, MD, Vancouver, BC, Canada; with permission.)

somatic nerves, so they may be painful when they occur. Internal hemorrhoids are located above the dentate line and arise from the superior hemorrhoidal plexus. They are innervated by visceral nerves and are usually painless.

Patients with a history of constipation and prolonged straining are at risk for hemorrhoidal disease. Those with diarrhea may also develop hemorrhoids as a result of recurrent straining. Pregnancy is also a significant risk factor for hemorrhoids, which usually resolve after giving birth.

Clinical Features

Patients with hemorrhoids usually complain of rectal bleeding associated with bowel movements. This bleeding is often painful with external hemorrhoids or painless with internal hemorrhoids. The bleeding is usually described as bright red blood seen in the toilet bowl or on wiping after a bowel movement. Melena is not consistent with hemorrhoidal disease. Hemorrhoids can be associated with a feeling of rectal fullness and perineal irritation. External hemorrhoids can present as a tender mass that make it uncomfortable for the patient to sit. They can cause an acute onset of pain caused by thrombosis. Thrombosed hemorrhoids are easily visualized on examination (**Fig. 3**). Acute thrombosis appears as a blue, tender mass. An internal hemorrhoid is difficult to appreciate on inspection unless it is prolapsed from the rectum (**Fig. 4**). A prolapsed hemorrhoid appears different from the perianal skin. Internal hemorrhoids are not easily palpated on a DRE unless they are enlarged or thrombosed. They are graded based on the Goligher classification (**Table 1**). When an internal hemorrhoid cannot be reduced, it becomes incarcerated and strangulated, which can lead to gangrenous changes.[3]

Management

When a patient presents with a history and physical examination consistent with hemorrhoidal disease, the primary treatment is directed at symptom control. In rare instances, patients present with significant rectal bleeding that necessitates resuscitation; in these cases, additional work-up and surgical evaluation are warranted. Most patients are hemodynamically stable and require neither laboratory

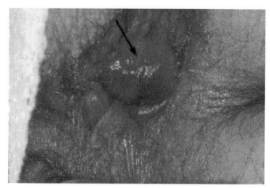

Fig. 3. Thrombosed external hemorrhoids (*arrow*). (*From* Pfenninger JL, Zainea GG. Common anorectal conditions. Obstet Gynecol 2001;98(6):1130–9; with permission.)

analyses nor imaging. Some patients have a prolonged history of rectal bleeding from hemorrhoids, which can lead to symptomatic anemia. In these cases, a complete blood count may be appropriate to assess the hemoglobin level.

Patients with hemorrhoids should be directed to start a high-fiber diet. This change can reduce symptoms by 50% but might take up to 6 weeks for full effect.[3] In addition, patients should maintain adequate hydration and use stool softeners to avoid constipation and straining. For symptomatic relief, patients should take sitz baths 2 to 4 times a day. Topical corticosteroid creams can be used, but patients should be instructed to not use them beyond a few days because of the risk of skin breakdown.

Patients with internal hemorrhoids of grade 1, 2, or 3 can be treated conservatively with sitz baths, fiber supplementation, laxatives, and adequate hydration after reduction of the hemorrhoids during the physical examination. They should be referred to a surgery service as an outpatient. Patients with grade 4 internal hemorrhoids have a high risk of thrombosis and should be seen by a surgeon in the ED.

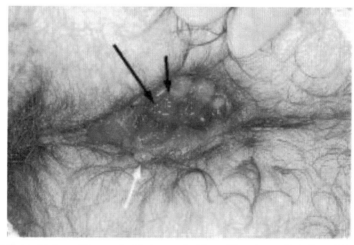

Fig. 4. Prolapsed internal hemorrhoids (*arrows*). (*From* Pfenninger JL, Zainea GG. Common anorectal conditions. Obstet Gynecol 2001;98(6):1130–9; with permission.)

Table 1	
Goligher criteria for internal hemorrhoids	
Grade 1	Bleed but do not prolapse
Grade 2	Prolapse through the anus on straining but spontaneously reduce
Grade 3	Prolapse through the anus on straining or exertion and require manual replacement into the anal canal
Grade 4	Irreducible

Immunocompetent adult patients who have had acutely thrombosed hemorrhoids for less than 72 hours may undergo clot excision in the ED for symptomatic relief. There are few data about the benefits of excision versus conservative management in the ED, but excision might provide more rapid pain relief.[4] After 72 hours, the pain from the procedure may exceed the relief provided. This procedure is not intended for patients with hemodynamic instability, liver disease, or coagulopathy; for those who are immunocompromised; or for children.[5] Patients undergoing surgical excision should be placed in the prone or lateral decubitus position. Using tape, the buttocks can be spread and the hemorrhoid should be identified. The skin under and above the hemorrhoid should be anesthetized with lidocaine 1% with epinephrine. Once the skin is adequately anesthetized, make an elliptical excision radially from the anal orifice. After exposing the underlying thrombosis, remove the clot with forceps or direct pressure. Place gauze between the buttocks, and instruct the patient to remove it during their first sitz bath at home. The patients should have a follow-up appointment with an outpatient surgery service within 48 hours or should return to the ED if outpatient surgical consultation is unavailable or if they experience persistent pain or bleeding. Patients with persistent, symptomatic hemorrhoids should be referred to a surgeon to discuss further procedures, both nonsurgical and surgical.

ANAL FISSURES
Pathophysiology

An anal fissure is a split in the anoderm distal to the dentate line. These fissures are more common in young adults, both male and female, than in other age groups.[6] Anal fissures start with the passage of a hard stool, which tears the anoderm, causing spasm of the internal sphincter. Patients typically experience a fear of defecation and the subsequent spasm. The spasm promotes mucosal ischemia, which delays healing.[6] Most anal fissures occur in the posterior midline, 10% to 15% occur in the anterior midline, and less than 1% occur in the lateral position.[3] Patients with lateral fissures should have a work-up to consider other causes of the injury, such as Crohn disease, malignancy, or human immunodeficiency virus (HIV).[7] Fissures are considered chronic when they fail to resolve in 6 to 8 weeks.

Clinical Features

Patients with anal fissures complain of intense pain with defecation and bright red blood noted after a bowel movement. They might also report anal spasms, described as pain in the anorectal area after a bowel movement.[3] These spasms correspond with spasm of the sphincter muscle, which impairs healing of the fissure. On physical examination, the lower end of the fissure can be identified once the buttock is gently separated (**Fig. 5**). A skin tag from previous episodes of anal fissures might also be identified. Patients experience considerable pain on DRE because of the fissure and spasm.

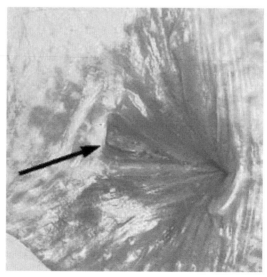

Fig. 5. Anal fissure (*arrow*). (*From* Pfenninger JL, Zainea GG. Common anorectal conditions. Obstet Gynecol 2001;98(6):1130–9; with permission.)

Management

The primary goal of therapy in anal fissures is to relax the anal sphincter, which allows patients to break the cycle of fear of defecation and anal pain. Patients should use a bulking agent as well as warm sitz baths for symptomatic relief. The area should be kept clean and dry. Warm water has been reported to reduce anal pressure.[3] Bulking agents and mild laxatives can help regularize bowel movements and have been shown to be 87% effective by 3 weeks for acute anal fissure and can decrease recurrence from 68% to 16%.[6] Rectal suppositories with local anesthetic and corticosteroids can be beneficial. Some patients prefer to use a cream rather than a rectal suppository. In the ED, the primary goal is to initiate sitz baths, laxatives, topical anesthetics, and corticosteroids. If dietary and lifestyle modifications do not resolve symptoms, patients might require further therapies such as topical nitroglycerin or topical calcium channel blockers, which are typically initiated by a primary care physician or gastroenterologist. Topical nitroglycerin (0.2%) used 2 or 3 times a day can be effective but is limited by the side effect of headache. Topical calcium channel blockers such as nifedipine (2%) and diltiazem (2%) have also been used successfully and usually have fewer side effects than topical nitrates.[6,8,9] Patients can also be referred for botulism (Botox) treatments, which have shown efficacy similar to topical nitroglycerin.[6] If conservative methods do not work, patients need outpatient consultation for surgical treatment such as lateral internal sphincterotomy.

ANORECTAL ABSCESSES/CRYPTITIS
Pathophysiology

Anorectal abscesses begin as an infection in the anal glands that tracks through the planes of the anorectal region. An infection localized to the anal gland is called cryptitis. An infection that presents at the anal verge is a perianal abscess. The infection can also track between the internal and external sphincters to the ischiorectal space. When the suppurative process tracks between the inner and outer muscles of the anorectal wall, it is referred to as an intersphincteric abscess. A supralevator abscess arises from cryptoglandular anal disease or from a primary abdominal infection (**Fig. 6**). Anorectal abscesses occur most commonly in middle-aged men and patients with hemorrhoids, diabetes, previous surgery, inflammatory bowel disease, and rectal trauma.[5] Anorectal abscesses can be caused by aerobic or anaerobic organisms, but most patients have mixed flora (72% in the series studied by Brook and Frazier[10]).

Clinical Features

Patients usually present with persistent, throbbing anal pain, which can be aggravated by defecation. Patients might also complain of swelling, drainage, or bleeding in the anal region. Although systemic symptoms such as fever and chills might present later in the course of the disease, initially they are usually absent. Cryptitis presents similarly, with anal pain and indurated papillae found on rectal examination. If cryptitis progresses, a perianal abscess can develop. Perianal abscesses present as localized pain and swelling at the anal verge. Ischiorectal abscesses more commonly cause buttock pain and can present with an indurated, painful mass in the buttock region. Intersphincteric abscesses produce pain in the anal canal and a painful, boggy area of fluctuance palpable on rectal examination. Supralevator abscesses are difficult to diagnosis on physical examination. They can present with perirectal pain, leukocytosis, and fever. On DRE, a fullness may be palpable near the sacrum.

Management

The treatment of anorectal abscesses is incision and drainage (I&D). If the anal gland has a focal area of inflammation without abscess formation, cryptitis is present. This cryptitis is treated with laxatives and sitz baths, but it may require outpatient surgical

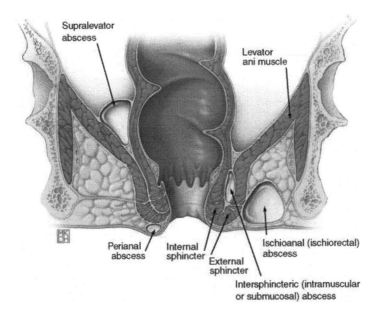

Fig. 6. Anorectal abscess. (*From* Pfenninger JL, Zainea GG. Common anorectal conditions. Obstet Gynecol 2001;98(6):1130–9; with permission.)

referral for gland excision if conservative management fails or if the abscess recurs. Most patients with superficial anorectal abscesses without systemic signs of illness can undergo I&D in the ED without further diagnostic imaging; however, in patients with systemic signs of illness or concern for deeper infection, computed tomography (CT) is the most usefully imaging modality. Ultrasonography can identify more superficial abscesses, such as perirectal and ischiorectal abscesses, but deeper infections require a CT scan for evaluation. If the CT scan is negative and there is still a high suspicion for an anorectal abscess, MRI should be used for evaluation.[5] When the clinician is concerned about a deeper infection or if the patient has systemic signs of illness or is immunocompromised, surgical consultation should be requested in the ED, in anticipation of I&D in the operating room.

To drain a superficial perirectal abscess in the ED, the area can be visualized by using tape or another health care provider to retract the buttocks. Induce local anesthesia with lidocaine 1%. The incision should be made close to the anal verge, making sure to avoid the anal sphincter. As in traditional I&D procedures, practitioners should break up loculations. Wound cultures are usually unnecessary unless there is concern about infection with a nontraditional organism, such as in immunocompromised patients. Antibiotics are not routinely required unless the patient is immunocompromised, is diabetic, or has extensive cellulitis. After I&D, patients should perform sitz baths 3 or 4 times a day. Patients should have close follow-up after I&D with an outpatient practitioner and should be instructed to return to the ED if the pain worsens or if fever or bleeding occurs. Patients with supralevator abscesses should have surgical consultation in the ED for treatment of the primary suppurative process. Patients with abscesses should receive close follow-up with a surgeon, given that 50% to 75% of patients develop a fistula after abscess drainage.[11]

ANORECTAL FISTULA

Anal fistulas usually result from cryptoglandular infection and can present as either abscess or infection. Other causes of fistulas include Crohn disease, proctitis, foreign body, anal surgery, infections, and malignancy.[7] Patients may present with drainage of blood, pus, or stool from any area in the perianal region. Fistulas can be intermittently painful or itchy. Patients who present with a fistula warrant an evaluation for inflammatory bowel disease, most commonly Crohn disease. Fistulas can have an extensive tract, which is best evaluated with MRI or endoscopic ultrasonography. Patients with fistulas should be referred to a specialist for treatment including nonsurgical and surgical management.

PILONIDAL ABSCESSES/CYSTS
Pathophysiology

Pilonidal disease affects approximately 70,000 Americans annually and is most common in young men (adolescence to mid-20s).[12,13] The pilonidal cyst occurs as a midline pit between the upper part of the gluteal clefts (always in this location). It usually contains a hair follicle or other debris, which is seen at the opening of the pit. Patients who have excess hair growth, poor hygiene, a family history of the disease, and those who are sedentary and obese are prone to getting pilonidal cysts and abscesses. These cysts are usually formed by an inflammatory reaction from an ingrown hair follicle, which is susceptible to infection.[12] Patients usually experience repeated episodes of inflammation and infection, followed by resolution.

Clinical Findings

Pilonidal cysts can be asymptomatic, but pain and swelling in the sacrococcygeal region often prompt patients to seek relief in an ED. Patients may also describe drainage or bleeding from the area. On physical examination, patients have a cyst at the top of the gluteal cleft in the midline. If infected, the patient might have cellulitis or a painful fluctuant mass associated with hair debris and usually with multiple draining tracts (**Fig. 7**).

Management

If a patient presents with an abscess, the primary treatment is I&D. When this approach is chosen, midline incisions should be avoided because they tend to heal poorly. Following the first I&D of an acute pilonidal abscess, the healing rate is approximately 60% and the risk of recurrence is decreased if the inflammatory debris is removed.[13] The patient should have a follow-up evaluation within 48 hours. The patient should be instructed to maintain local hygiene, to use sitz baths, and to shave the area at intervals of 2 to 3 weeks for several months.[11] There is no role for antibiotics for a simple pilonidal abscess; however, patients who have an overlying cellulitis, are immunosuppressed, or are systemically ill should receive antibiotics covering gram-positive skin flora.[13] Patients who have a recurrence and require multiple I&Ds should be referred to a surgeon as outpatients.

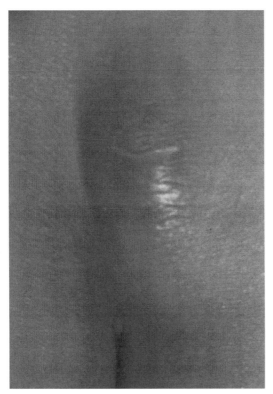

Fig. 7. Pilonidal abscess. (*From* De Parades V, Bouchard D, Janier M, et al. Pilonidal sinus disease. J Visc Surg 2013;150(4):237–47; with permission.)

PROCTALGIA FUGAX

Proctalgia fugax is a gastrointestinal disorder that causes severe, self-limiting anorectal pain usually lasting 5 seconds to 90 minutes. Patients experience this fleeting and recurring pain over weeks, with no pain between episodes. Although this is a diagnosis of exclusion in the ED, it is important to have an awareness of the condition. It has several triggers, including sexual activity, stress, constipation, defecation, and menstruation.[14,15] This disease affects women more than men, most commonly between the ages of 30 and 60 years, with a prevalence of 4% to 18% in the general population.[7] Proctalgia fugax is thought to be caused by spasm of the internal anal sphincter or compression of the pudendal nerve.[7] Given the fleeting nature of the pain, patients usually do not require medications; however, those with severe symptoms might get relief with topical treatments such as nitroglycerin or diltiazem. Nonpharmacologic agents such as biofeedback have been shown to be effective as well.

PRURITUS ANI
Pathophysiology

Pruritus ani is a burning or itching sensation in the perianal region. Approximately 1% to 5% of the general population is affected by this condition; most people do not seek medical care for it. It is the second most common anorectal disease, after hemorrhoids. It affects men more than women, in a ratio of 4 to 1.[5,16] Primary, or idiopathic, pruritus ani has no discernible cause, whereas secondary pruritus ani has an underlying cause (**Table 2**).[7,17] Approximately 50% to 90% of cases are idiopathic.[16] Symptoms of mild irritation, itchiness, or burning usually start insidiously but the condition may progress to intolerable soreness and itchiness. It is hypothesized that pruritus ani is caused by the activation of a self-propagating cycle of itchiness in the perianal area, leading to scratching and excoriations causing skin injury, which induces both an inflammatory and pruritus response, leading to further scratching, excoriation, and skin injury.[18]

Table 2 Secondary causes of pruritus ani	
Mechanical	Fecal soiling (ie, diarrhea), tight undergarment, trauma (ie, scratching), hemorrhoids, anal fissures/fistulas, gynecologic problems (atopic vaginitis, discharge)
Dermatitis	Eczema, inverse psoriasis, atopic, lichen planus, scleroderma, erythema multiforme, herpetiformis, lichen planus
Infection	Pinworms (*Enterobius vermicularis*), erythrasma (*Corynebacterium minutissimum*), sexually transmitted diseases (condyloma, herpes, syphilis, gonorrhea), *Candida albicans*
Systemic	Diabetes, cholestasis, lymphoma, leukemia, pellagra, renal failure, thyrotoxicosis, HIV/AIDS, hypothyroidism, vitamin A deficiency, vitamin D deficiency, iron deficiency, obesity, hyperhidrosis, hidradenitis
Inflammatory	Inflammatory bowel diseases
Malignancy	Bowen disease, squamous cell carcinoma, melanoma, perianal Paget disease
Medications[a]	Colchicine, neomycin
Dietary[a]	Coffee, tea, soda, chocolate, tomatoes, citrus, dairy

Abbreviation: AIDS, acquired immunodeficiency syndrome.
[a] Associations have been made, but no evidence suggests causation.

Clinical Findings

A common clinical classification used to stage pruritus ani is based on the physical examination of the skin (**Table 3**).[16,18] The physical examination usually yields normal results but might reveal excoriation marks, hemorrhoids, anal fissures, or other inciting lesions. If the examining clinician is concerned about pinworms, the tape test can be used to search for eggs. First, the perianal region should be examined by direct visualization with a bright light 2 to 3 hours after the patient is asleep. Then, first thing in the morning, before the patient bathes, transparent tape is used to collect a sample from the perianal region and the sample can be evaluated under a microscope for the presence of pinworm eggs. In addition, samples from underneath a patient's fingernails can be examined.[19]

Management

The work-up for patients with pruritus ani varies based on the presenting symptoms. For acute complaints in the ED, a thorough physical examination may be all that is necessary to rule out obvious inciting factors such as dermatitis, trauma, and infection. However, for subacute and especially chronic pruritus ani, patients might require further work-up, including complete blood count, comprehensive metabolic panel (to assess renal and liver function and bilirubin), thyroid-stimulating hormone, and HIV, which can all be done on an outpatient basis.[17] Patients who have had symptoms for more than 2 or 3 weeks and who have not responded to outpatient therapy can be referred to outpatient dermatology for biopsy because of the risk of malignancy.[18]

Most patients present with idiopathic pruritus ani. For these cases, treatment is symptomatic. Initially, the focus is on maintaining dry, clean, and intact perianal skin.[5,17] The use of medicated soap is discouraged. Instead, topical barriers such as zinc oxide, Kerodex, or hydrocortisone cream can be used to reduce inflammation.[5,17] Topical anesthesia is also discouraged because it might mask the disease.[17] Once symptoms improve, topical barriers can be replaced with cornstarch or talc powder.[17] Dietary changes may be attempted, but there is not sufficient evidence to suggest causation. Patients should be instructed to wear loose-fitting clothing. For secondary pruritus ani, treat the underlying cause. Systemic diseases can be controlled and infections can be treated. Low-dose capsaicin cream has been shown to be effective in intractable pruritus ani.[17,20] Treatment options are summarized in **Table 4**.[5,17,18]

In severe and resistant cases, treatment methods have included injecting methylene blue into the sensory nerve bundles of the perianal area, sclerotherapy, radiation therapy, and even surgical procedures.[17] These procedures are not done in the ED.

Table 3 Pruritus ani stages	
Stages	**Skin Findings**
0	Normal, intact
1	Red, inflamed
2	White, lichenified skin
3	Lichenified skin, coarse ridges, possible ulcerations

Adapted from Smith LE. Perianal dermatological disease. In: Gordon PH, Nivatvongs S, editors. Principles and practice of surgery for the colon, rectum, and anus. 3rd edition. New York: Informa Healthcare USA; 2007. p. 247–59.

Table 4	
Treatment options for idiopathic pruritus ani	
Zinc-oxide–based ointments, Berwick solution	Leave on skin for 1 wk
Hydrocortisone cream, 1%	—
Capsaicin cream, 0.006%	—

PROLAPSE

Pathophysiology

Rectal prolapse is the protrusion of the rectal wall through the anal orifice (**Fig. 8**). The prolapse might be of partial or full thickness, involving the mucosa walls. It is a rare condition, affecting less than 0.5% of the general population.[21] It is most common in children less than 3 years of age, especially those with cystic fibrosis or malnutrition, and in elderly patients.[5] In the elderly population, women are more often affected than men. In 3% of affected women, pelvic organs are often involved, leading to uterine or vaginal prolapse, rectocele, cystocele, urethrocele, or enterocele.[21]

Rectal prolapse is usually caused by constipation, bowel dysfunction (massive diarrhea), fecal incontinence, and complications from rectal ulceration.[21]

Clinical Findings

Patients generally present with nonspecific complaints such as fullness in the rectal area, pain, rectal bleeding, constipation, abdominal pain, or fecal incontinence.[21] On physical examination, rectal prolapse might be mistaken for a prolapsed hemorrhoid. Careful evaluation for incarceration, thrombosis, and strangulation is imperative because the management strategy depends on the diagnosis.

Management

If any sign of ischemia is evident, a general surgeon should be consulted for possible reduction in an operating room. These masses tend to be large, painful, and immobile, with dusky discoloration. If ischemia has not occurred, manual reduction can be attempted in the ED. Applying gentle pressure to the mass while rolling the walls

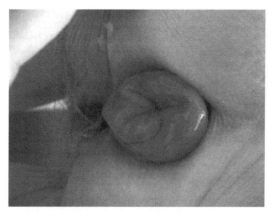

Fig. 8. Rectal prolapse. (*From* Hull T, Zutshi M. Pathophysiology, diagnosis, and treatment of defecatory dysfunction. In: Raz S, Rodriguez LV. Female urology. 3rd edition. Philadelphia: Elsevier, 2008; with permission.)

inward may be sufficient.[5,21] For patients with significant edema, the application of granulated sugar might reduce the edema by causing desiccation of the mucosa.[22] Procedural sedation might be necessary, depending on the patient. If the reduction is successful, patients may be discharged home with follow-up in an outpatient general surgery clinic. It is important to send patients home with a stool softener, fiber supplements, and instructions to stay hydrated in order to prevent constipation, which could trigger another prolapse.[5,21]

FOREIGN BODIES/TRAUMAS
Pathophysiology

Rectal trauma is uncommon, being responsible for 0.1% to 1.1% of all colorectal injuries, but it is associated with high morbidity and mortality.[23] Penetrating injury constitutes 80% of rectal trauma, whereas blunt trauma is the cause of 6.2% of cases.[23,24] Most penetrating trauma is the result of shootings, and motor vehicle collisions are the cause of a third of all blunt injuries.[23,24] Iatrogenic causes of rectal injuries have a 2.5% incidence. Most rectal trauma occurs in young men; this is attributed to higher rates of trauma in this population.[23]

Rectal foreign body injury is well recognized but underreported. Reliable epidemiologic data are not available.[25,26] Everything from bottles to vibrators to fruits and vegetables to tools have been documented in the literature.[27] Rectal foreign bodies generally result from autoeroticism or sexual stimulation, but sexual assault, voluntary insertion, and nonsexual insertion for issues such as pruritus ani or constipation have all been reported.[27,28] There have been case reports of prisoners hiding weapons in their rectums and psychiatric patients purposely putting sharp objects in their rectums, with the intention of injuring the clinicians performing rectal examinations.[5,27]

Clinical Findings

Assessment of rectal trauma involves a combination of clinical, endoluminal, and radiographic studies. A complete secondary survey should be performed to assess for pelvic fractures, perineal or transpelvic penetration, and rectal or urethral bleeding.[25] A DRE has long been recommended as part of the secondary survey, but studies have shown that it has a sensitivity of 37% for detecting decreased rectal tone, 33% for detecting rectal wall injury, and 5% for detecting free rectal bleeding.[25,29] Rigid proctosigmoidoscopy is mandatory in the assessment of rectal injury because of its higher sensitivity for detecting extraperitoneal injuries. This procedure is usually performed by surgical or gastrointestinal teams, not by emergency care providers.[23,24] Radiography is neither sensitive nor specific in detecting injuries but may detect free air or foreign objects. CT has both high sensitivity and high specificity and thus is the gold standard.[25] If contrast is necessary, water-soluble triple contrast (oral, rectal, and intravenous) should be used to obtain the best image.[25] The 5 grades of rectal injury defined by the Organ Injury Scale developed by the American Association for the Surgery of Trauma are listed in **Box 1**.

The main difficulty in the assessment of rectal foreign bodies is getting the history from the patient. Because of the sensitive nature of the topic, patients often delay their presentations and have nonspecific complaints of rectal pain, rectal fullness, rectal bleeding, abdominal pain/discomfort, or constipation.[5] Lateral and anteroposterior plain films of the abdomen and pelvis help to identify the number, size, shape, location, and orientation of the foreign body. Plain films do not visualize fish bone, plastic,

> **Box 1**
> **Rectal injury grading system, American Association for the Surgery of Trauma**
>
> I. Hematoma. Contusion of hematoma without devascularizationLaceration. Partial thickness laceration
>
> II. Laceration less than 50% circumference
>
> III. Laceration. Laceration greater than 50% circumference
>
> IV. Laceration. Full-thickness laceration with extension into the perineum
>
> V. Vascular. Devascularized segment
>
> *Adapted from* Moore EE, Cogbill TH, Malangoni MA, et al. Organ injury scaling, II: pancreas, duodenum, small bowel, colon, and rectum. J Trauma 1990;30:1428; with permission.

candle, thin glasses, or organic material.[28] A chest film is also indicated to rule out free air. CT scans are rarely indicated but might be necessary to localize nonradiopaque objects or if a complication is suspected. Complications from foreign objects include rectal or colonic perforation, intestinal obstruction, hemorrhage, deep mucosal tears, abscesses, and peritonitis.[5]

Management

For patients with rectal trauma, a colorectal or general surgeon needs to be consulted for further management. These patients might have multiple concomitant injuries that require attention.

For patients who have foreign bodies above the rectosigmoid junction, or for those in whom a complication is suspected, emergent surgical consultation is necessary. When a foreign body is palpable during a DRE and it is located below the rectosigmoid junction, the emergency care provider may attempt to remove it. Most patients have attempted to remove the object at home, likely causing edema and muscular spasm. Multiple removal techniques have been described: enemas, anal dilatation followed by digital extraction, surgical forceps, obstetric forceps, and balloon catheters with balloon inflation.[5] The use an anoscope or a sigmoidoscope may aid in direct visualization and thus prevent iatrogenic injuries.[26] The anal sphincter can be relaxed by inducing an anal block with local 1% lidocaine or 0.5% bupivacaine, or procedural sedation might aid in the procedure.[5] An anal block is induced by injecting a local anesthetic in the subcutaneous tissue circling the anus in a radius of 2.5 cm, with the goal of blocking the inferior rectal nerve. Factors that predict failure of transanal extraction include objects more than 10 cm in length, hard or sharp objects, migration to the sigmoid, or a duration of more than 2 days.[25,26]

It is of utmost importance to arrange for proctosigmoidoscopy after a foreign body is removed from the rectum to assess for mucosal tears, bleeding, and bowel injury and for any residual foreign bodies if the foreign body is removed in the ED. Patients in whom mucosal injury is confirmed must be kept for observation.[25,26]

RECTAL SEXUALLY TRANSMITTED INFECTIONS
Pathophysiology

Sexually transmitted infections (STIs) are a major health concern, with an incidence of approximately 15 million cases annually in the United States and 333 million cases worldwide.[30–32] Anorectal involvement is common and its incidence is increasing. Anorectal STIs are usually the result of anal receptive intercourse or oroanal sexual contacts; however, they can spread from the genital region.[30] Although anal receptive intercourse is commonly associated with men who have sex with men, it is more widely practiced in absolute numbers by heterosexual couples.[30]

Clinical Findings/Management

STIs are often asymptomatic, or present with nonspecific symptoms. Common complaints of anorectal STIs include anal pain, tenesmus, urgency, purulent discharge or drainage, and bleeding.[30] Anorectal STIs are diagnosed in the same way as other STIs. Coinfection is common and should be considered in all patients affected with an STI. HIV transmission is facilitated by any STI. Coinfection with HIV may alter the infectiveness of the STI. For instance, gonococcal infection increases the infectiveness of HIV; syphilis is associated with decreased CD4 count and increased viral load.[30,33] In addition to these common STIs, patients with HIV/acquired immunodeficiency syndrome (AIDS) are susceptible to other anorectal diseases once their CD4 cell count declines to less than 500 cells/mm.[3] This patient population is prone to atypical infections, including cytomegalovirus, *Mycobacterium avium* complex (MAC), human papilloma virus (HPV), and human herpes virus 8 (HHV 8).[30] HPV and HHV 8 can both lead to cancer, anal intraepithelial neoplasia and Kaposi sarcoma, respectively.[30] CMV and Kaposi sarcoma are both AIDS-defining diseases.

Table 5 lists the most common STIs, their clinical presentations, and their management in the ED (**Box 2**).[30]

PROCTITIS
Pathophysiology

Proctitis is the inflammation of the rectal mucosa within 15 cm of the dentate line; it can extend into the proximal colon as well. It can be acute or chronic, and it is usually secondary to another disease process. It occurs predominantly in adults, affects men more than women, and has a higher incidence in Jewish persons.[35] It has many causes (**Table 6**). Up to 20% of cases of acute proctitis can be linked to radiation therapy.[36,37]

Proctitis starts as an inflammatory response to an irritant, with mucosal cell loss, eosinophilia, and endothelial edema, but this acute reaction can turn into fibrosis of connective tissue and endarteritis of the arterioles, leading to tissue ischemia that causes mucosal friability, bleeding, ulcerations, strictures, or fistula.[35]

Clinical Findings

Patients often present with nonspecific complaints of anal irritation, itching, burning, and tenesmus. The physical examination findings may be nonspecific, but signs of inflammation, including mucosal erythema and mucosal friability, are often found. Specific findings may be present from specific causes; for example, groups of vesicles in patients who have herpes simplex virus or painless chancres in patients with syphilis. Patients are often Hemoccult positive as a result of the inflammatory process.

Management

Supportive and symptomatic care is the mainstay treatment of acute proctitis. Once other life-threatening conditions have been excluded, management includes sitz baths, antispasmodic medications, stool softeners, and a high-fiber diet.[35] If the cause of the proctitis is known, it should be treated. Antibiotics are indicated for infectious causes, antivirals for viral causes. Steroid enemas and suppositories may be necessary for autoimmune causes to quell the inflammatory reaction.[35] For radiation proctitis, steroid enemas and/or sucralfate may alleviate some of the discomfort.[35] It is

Table 5
Common anorectal STIs, their presentations, and their management

	Clinical Findings	Diagnosis	Management
Chlamydia trachomatis	Most commonly asymptomatic (serotype D–K), or mild proctitis with tenesmus, pain, and/or discharge	Mucosa can be normal to erythematous and friable; diagnosis with PCR	Azithromycin 1000 mg PO × 1 or doxycycline 100 mg BID × 7 d (concomitant treatment of gonorrhea with ceftriaxone)
	LGV (serotypes L1–L3) produces more aggressive proctitis with anal, perianal, or rectal ulcerations, purulent anal discharge, tenesmus, lower abdominal pain and cramping; patients may present with perirectal abscesses, anal fissures, and fistula formation[38]	For LGV, rectal biopsy	LGV: doxycycline 100 mg BID × 21 d
Neisseria gonorrhoeae	84% are latent and asymptomatic; pruritus ani, constipation, mucopurulent or bloody anal discharge, pain, and tenesmus	Mucosa can be normal to erythematous and friable; diagnosis with PCR	Ceftriaxone 250 mg IM × 1 (treatment of coinfection with chlamydia with azithromycin)
Treponema pallidum	Primary: asymptomatic, chancre, proctitis, or pseudotumors Secondary: condyloma lata, rectal mass, mucous patches, skin rash, fever, and/or lymphadenopathy Tertiary: gummatous lesions	Dark field visualization of *T pallidum* (especially useful in patients with HIV[a]), VDRL or RPR	Primary or secondary: benzathine penicillin G 2.4 million units (PCN allergic: doxycycline, tetracycline, ceftriaxone)
Human papillomavirus	Condyloma acuminatum, raised lesions, rectal bleeding or discharge, pain, pruritus ani	Physical examination reveals lesion; anoscope to assess extension into anal canal. Biopsy to confirm diagnosis if needed	Condyloma removal: tangential excision, cryotherapy, fulguration. (recurrence 20%–30%) Topical creams: podophyllin, dichloroacetic acid, imiquimod

(*continued on next page*)

Table 5
(continued)

	Clinical Findings	Diagnosis	Management
Herpes simplex virus	Anorectal pain, constipation, tenesmus, pruritus, difficulty initiating micturition, sacral paresthesia, posterior thigh pain, fever, inguinal lymphadenopathy, small vesicles, ulcerations or friable mucosa	Cell culture or PCR viral DNA polymerase chain	Acyclovir, famciclovir, valacyclovir × 7–10 d[33,34]

Abbreviations: BID, twice a day; IM, intramuscular; LGV, lymphogranuloma venereum; PCR, polymerase chain reaction; PCN, penicillin; PO, by mouth; RPR, rapid plasma regain; VDRL, Venereal Disease Research Laboratory test.

[a] Patients with HIV are more likely to have false-negative results.

important that patients with proctitis have appropriate follow-up with a colorectal surgeon or gastroenterologist.

RECTAL CANCER

Colon and rectal cancer are the third most common cancer in both men and women, with an incidence of 6% per year for the general population in the United States.[38] Adenocarcinoma accounts for 98% of cases of colon and rectal cancer. Lymphoma, carcinoid, and sarcoma represent the other 2%. Approximately 20% of colon cancers develop in the cecum, another 20% in the rectum, and an additional 10% in the rectosigmoid junction.[38] Approximately 25% of colon cancers develop in the sigmoid colon.[39] The American Cancer Society estimates that colorectal cancer will account for 8% of cancer deaths in men and 9% of cancer deaths in women during 2015.[38]

Clinical Findings

Rectal bleeding is the most common symptom of rectal cancer, occurring in up to 60% of patients.[39] Other symptoms include change in bowel habits (most commonly diarrhea), occult bleeding, abdominal pain, malaise, and pelvic pain. Late symptoms that increase concern for metastatic disease include back pain, nerve trunk involvement, jaundice, and peritonitis from bowel perforation.[39] However, many cancers are asymptomatic and are discovered during DREs or proctoscopic screening examinations.

Box 2
Anorectal lesions found in patients with AIDS

Cytomegalovirus

MAC

Anal intraepithelial neoplasia

Kaposi sarcoma

| Table 6 | |
Causes of proctitis	
Sexually transmitted diseases (anal intercourse)	Chlamydia, gonorrhea, lymphogranuloma venereum, herpes
Radiation	Can be delayed up to years after initial treatment
Medications	Antibiotics
Autoimmune	Crohn disease, ulcerative colitis, celiac
Iatrogenic	Chemicals, rectal instrumentation, trauma
Idiopathic	Most common

Management

In the ED, an initial work-up should be targeted at ruling out life-threatening disease processes. This work-up can include DRE and basic blood work, including complete metabolic panel and complete blood count, to assess kidney, liver, electrolyte, and blood count abnormalities. CT might be warranted to rule out intra-abdominal causes of rectal bleeding.[39] For stable patients without clinically significant bleeding or bowel obstruction, the work-up for colorectal cancer can be pursued as outpatients. The management of rectal cancer requires a multidisciplinary team approach, including colorectal surgery, medical oncology, and radiation oncology. Most of these patients can be treated on an outpatient basis. The need for hospitalization depends on the patient's clinical stability and need for acute care.

SUMMARY

Patients commonly present to the ED with anorectal complaints. Most of these complaints are benign and can be managed conservatively; however, there are a few anorectal emergencies that clinicians must be aware of in order to prevent further complications. The history and physical examination are especially important so that critical disorders can be recognized and specific treatment plans can be determined. It is important to maintain a broad differential diagnosis of anorectal disease and to distinguish benign from serious processes.

REFERENCES

1. Grucela A, Salinas H, Khaitov S, et al. Prospective analysis of clinician accuracy in the diagnosis of benign anal pathology: comparison across specialties and years of experience. Dis Colon Rectum 2010;53:47–52.
2. Thornton SC. Hemorrhoids. Medscape; 2014. Available at: http://emedicine.medscape.com/article/775407-overview#a7.
3. Schubert MC, Sridhar S, Schade RR, et al. What every gastroenterologist needs to know about common anorectal disorders. World J Gastroenterol 2009;15:3201–9.
4. Greenspon J, Williams SB, Young HA, et al. Thrombosed external hemorrhoids: outcome after conservative or surgical management. Dis Colon Rectum 2004;47:1493–8.
5. Glauser J, Katz J. Anorectal emergencies. Emerg Med Rep 2014;35(10):113–22.
6. Higuero T. Update on the management of anal fissure. J Visc Surg 2015;152:S37–43.
7. Foxx-Orenstein AE, Umar SB, Crowell MD. Common anorectal disorders. Gastroenterol Hepatol (N Y) 2014;10:294–301.

8. Pfenninger JL, Zainea GG. Common anorectal conditions. Obst Gynecol 2001; 98:1130–9.

9. Pfenninger JL, Zainea GG. Common anorectal conditions: Part II. Lesions. Am Fam Physician 2001;64:77–88.

10. Brook I, Frazier EH. The aerobic and anaerobic bacteriology of perirectal abscesses. J Clin Microbiol 1997;35:2974–6.

11. Burnstein M. Managing anorectal emergencies. Can Fam Physician 1993;39: 1782–5.

12. de Parades V, Boucharf D, Janier M, et al. Pilonidal sinus disease. J Visc Surg 2013;150:237–47.

13. Steele SR, Perry WB, Mills S, et al. Practice parameters for the management of pilonidal disease. Dis Colon Rectum 2013;56:1021–7.

14. Jeyarajah S, Chow A, Ziprin P, et al. Proctalgia fugax, an evidence-based management pathway. Int J Colorectal Dis 2010;25:1037–46.

15. Jeyarajah S, Purkayastha S. Five things to know about proctalgia fugax. Can Med Assoc J 2013;185(5):417.

16. Smith LE. Perianal dermatological disease. In: Gordon PH, Nivatvongs S, editors. Principles and practice of surgery for the colon, rectum, and anus. 3rd edition. New York: Informa Healthcare USA; 2007. p. 247–59.

17. Breen E, Bleday R. Approach to the patient with anal pruritus. Uptodate; 2015.

18. Song S-G, Kim S-H. Pruritus ani. J Korean Soc Coloproctol 2011;27:54–7.

19. Parasites: enterobiasis. Centers for Disease Control. Available at: http://www.cdc.gov/parasites/pinworm/. Accessed July 22, 2015.

20. Lysy J, Sistiery-Ittah M, Israelit Y, et al. Topical capsaicin—a novel and effective treatment for idiopathic intractable pruritus ani: a randomised, placebo controlled, crossover study. Gut 2003;52:1323–6.

21. Bordeianou L, Hicks CW, Kaiser AM, et al. Rectal prolapse: an overview of clinical features, diagnosis, and patient-specific management strategies. J Gastrointest Surg 2014;18:1059–69.

22. Shaikh MH, Shah B, Sahu S, et al. Highlighting the role of nonsurgical (conservative) method in the management of complete rectal prolapse in an Indian male. Int J Stud Res 2013;3:54–6.

23. Barkley S, Khan M, Garner J. Rectal trauma in adults. Trauma 2013;15:3–15.

24. Merlino J, Reynolds H. Management of rectal injuries. Semin Colon Rectal Surg 2004;15:95–104.

25. Ayantunde AA. Approach to the diagnosis and management of retained rectal foreign bodies: clinical updates. Tech Coloproctol 2013;17:13–20.

26. Ayantunde AA, Oke T. A review of gastrointestinal foreign bodies. Int J Clin Pract 2006;60:735–9.

27. Anderson KL, Dean AJ. Foreign bodies in the gastrointestinal tract and anorectal emergencies. Emerg Med Clin North Am 2011;29:369–400.

28. Pinto A, Miele V, Pinto F, et al. Rectal foreign bodies: imaging assessment and medicolegal aspects. Semin Ultrasound CT MRI 2015;36:88–93.

29. Shlamovitz GZ, Mower WR, Bergman J, et al. Poor test characteristics for the digital rectal examination in trauma patients. Ann Emerg Med 2007;50:25–33.

30. Assi R, Hashim PW, Reddy VB, et al. Sexually transmitted infections of the anus and rectum. World J Gastroenterol 2014;20:15262–8.

31. Sultan S. Sexually transmissible infections of the anus and the rectum. Rev Prat 2008;58:1793–801.

32. Cates W. Estimates of the incidence and prevalence of sexually transmitted diseases in the United States. American Social Health Association Panel. Sex Transm Dis 1999;26:S2–7.

33. Kofoed K, Gerstoft J, Mathiesen LR, et al. Syphilis and human immunodeficiency virus (HIV)-1 coinfection: influence on CD4 T-cell count, HIV-1 viral load, and treatment response. Sex Transm Dis 2006;33:143–8.

34. American Cancer Society. Cancer facts & figures 2015. American Cancer Society. Available at: http://www.cancer.org/acs/groups/content/@editorial/documents/document/acspc-044552.pdf. Accessed April 21, 2015.

35. Irizarry L, Yarde I. Acute proctitits. 2014. Available at: http://emedicine.medscape.com/article/775952-overview. Accessed July 30, 2015.

36. Greaves AB. The frequency of lymphogranuloma venereum in persons with perirectal abscesses, fistulae in ano, or both. With particular reference to the relationship between perirectal abscesses of lymphogranuloma origin in the male and inversion. Bull World Health Organ 1963;29:797–801.

37. Workowski KA, Berman S, Centers for Disease Control and Prevention (CDC). Sexually transmitted diseases treatment guidelines, 2010. MMWR Recomm Rep 2010;59:1–110.

38. Giovannucci E, Wu K. Cancers of the colon and rectum. In: Schottenfeld D, Fraumeni J, editors. Cancer epidemiology and prevention. 3rd edition. Oxford University Press; 2006. p. 806–40.

39. Cagir B, Trostle DR. Rectal cancer. 2015. Available at: http://emedicine.medscape.com/article/281237-overview. Accessed July 15, 2015.

The Vomiting Patient
Small Bowel Obstruction, Cyclic Vomiting, and Gastroparesis

Jumana Nagarwala, MD[a,b,*], Sharmistha Dev, MD, MPH[c,1], Abraham Markin, MD[a,d]

KEYWORDS

- Small bowel obstruction • Cyclic vomiting • Cannabinoid hyperemesis
- Gastroparesis • Prokinetic agents

KEY POINTS

- Small bowel obstructions represent 15% of emergency department visits for acute abdominal pain and can be associated with significant morbidity and mortality if unrecognized and untreated.
- Computed tomography scans have become the mainstay of diagnosis, and management should be designed to correct physiologic and electrolyte disturbances, allow bowel rest, and remove the source of the obstruction.
- Cyclic vomiting syndrome is a poorly understood condition characterized by recurrent episodes of intense vomiting, which is treated acutely with antiemetics, fluids, and electrolyte replacement, although, among adults, cannabinoid may represent a previously under-recognized cause.
- Gastroparesis is a chronic motility disorder of the stomach that involves delayed gastric emptying without evidence of mechanical obstruction.
- First-line therapy in the emergency department is the use of metoclopramide, but domperidone, erythromycin, and antiemetics are also often used, and interventional therapy should be reserved for refractory cases.

Disclosures: None.
Funding sources: None.
Conflicts of interest: None.
[a] Department of Emergency Medicine, Henry Ford Hospital, 2799 West Grand Boulevard, CFP-258, Detroit, MI 48202, USA; [b] Department of Emergency Medicine, Wayne State University School of Medicine, Detroit, MI, USA; [c] Departments of Emergency Medicine and Internal Medicine, University of Michigan, Ann Arbor, MI, USA; [d] Department of Internal Medicine, Henry Ford Hospital, 2799 West Grand Boulevard, Detroit, MI 48202, USA
[1] Present address: Taubman Center B1 354 1500 E. Medical Center Drive, SPC 5303, Ann Arbor, MI 48109.
* Corresponding author. Department of Emergency Medicine, Henry Ford Hospital, 2799 West Grand Boulevard, Clara Ford Pavillion-#263, Detroit, MI 48202.
E-mail address: Jnagarw1@hfhs.org

Emerg Med Clin N Am 34 (2016) 271–291
http://dx.doi.org/10.1016/j.emc.2015.12.005
0733-8627/16/$ – see front matter © 2016 Elsevier Inc. All rights reserved.

emed.theclinics.com

APPROACH TO VOMITING PATIENTS

Vomiting and abdominal pain are among the most common complaints for which patients present to the emergency department. **Box 1** lists the differential diagnoses for vomiting. A thorough history, physical examination, and evaluation in the emergency department can help narrow the differential diagnosis for a more certain diagnosis.

Box 1
Differential diagnosis for vomiting

Abdominal causes
  Mechanical obstruction
  Motility disorders
  Acute appendicitis
  Acute cholecystitis
  Acute hepatitis
  Acute mesenteric ischemia
  Crohn disease
  Gastric and duodenal ulcer disease
  Pancreatitis and pancreatic neoplasms
  Peritonitis and peritoneal carcinomatosis
  Retroperitoneal and mesenteric disorders
  Acute cholecystitis
  Acute hepatitis
  Acute mesenteric ischemia
  Crohn disease
  Gastric and duodenal ulcer disease
  Pancreatitis and pancreatic neoplasms
  Peritonitis and peritoneal carcinomatosis
  Retroperitoneal and mesenteric disorders

Drugs

Infectious causes
  Acute gastroenteritis
  Systemic infections

Metabolic and endocrine causes
  Acute intermittent porphyria
  Addison disease
  Diabetic ketoacidosis
  Hypoparathyroidism/hyperparathyroidism
  Hyperthyroidism
  Pregnancy

Nervous system causes
  Demyelinating disorders
  Hydrocephalus
  Intracerebral lesions
  Labyrinthine disorders
  Meningitis
  Migraine headaches
  Seizure disorders

Other causes
  Anxiety and depression
  Cardiac disorders
  Collagen vascular diseases
  Paraneoplastic syndromes
  Postoperative states
  Eating disorders

This article focuses on 3 specific entities that have become increasingly prevalent: small bowel obstruction (SBO), cyclic vomiting, and gastroparesis.

SMALL BOWEL OBSTRUCTION
Introduction

SBO is one of the true emergencies encountered in the emergency department. It is defined as a failure of progression of food and bowel contents through the small intestine[1] and is secondary to functional or mechanical causes. In SBOs, the main concerns arise from systemic effects of electrolyte and fluid abnormalities and increased intestinal tract pressure.

A functional SBO is caused by an intestinal motility disorder. Typically, neurogenic causes lead to atony of intestinal muscles and malfunction of peristalsis, often referred to as adynamic or paralytic ileus.[2] The primary causes of functional SBOs are listed in **Box 2**. Although the exact cause of paralytic ileus is unknown, it is suspected to result from the synergistic effect of autonomic dysfunction, endocrine response, and inflammatory mediators.[3]

A mechanical obstruction occurs secondary to a physical impediment to the flow of intestinal matter as a result of intraluminal, intramural, and extramural causes.[1] This condition can be further classified as simple or complicated. A simple obstruction is caused by a blockage at 1 or 2 points of the intestine, without vascular compromise. A complicated or strangulated obstruction leads to intestinal ischemia. A partial obstruction occurs when gas or liquid stool is still capable of moving forward past a narrowing of the intestine.

SBOs are responsible for 15% of all emergency department visits for acute abdominal complaints.[2] Approximately 300,000 laparotomies are performed to relieve SBOs, costing the health care industry about $2.3 billion annually.[4,5] The incidence of SBOs in patients who have not had previous abdominal surgery is reported to be between 0.1% and 5% but those with previous surgery have an incidence as high as 15%.[2,6] This risk increases with each laparotomy that is performed, with recurrence rates as high as 30% at 30 years.[7]

Although 15% of partial SBOs require surgery, up to 85% of complete SBOs require surgery. The presence of ischemic bowel can increase mortality 10-fold. In the past 50 years, overall mortality from SBOs has decreased from 25% to 5%.[8]

Pathophysiology

In SBOs, there is a disruption in the patency of the bowel, causing gradual accumulation of fluids. An initial increase in peristalsis produces an increase in intraluminal pressure. As the pressure approaches the systolic blood pressure, venous blood flow

Box 2
Main causes of functional SBO
Abdominal surgery
Major trauma
Shock
Infection
Medications
Metabolic derangements
Renal colic

decreases to the bowel wall and adjacent mesentery, resulting in a decrease in absorption of fluids, electrolytes, and lymphatic drainage. This process eventually leads to ischemia and necrosis of the bowel with a mounting concern for perforation.[1] In a closed-loop obstruction, in which a segment of bowel is obstructed at 2 sites and rotates around an adhesion or hernia opening, this course is more sudden.[2]

SBOs can generate significant volume depletion and electrolyte abnormalities. Dehydration is the result of the prevention of reabsorption of intestinal contents from the colon, the loss of fluids because of vomiting and reduced intake, and progressive bowel wall edema. The most common electrolyte abnormalities with SBOs are hyponatremia and hypokalemia. Initially, metabolic alkalosis develops because of volume loss, reabsorption of bicarbonate, and a loss of chloride by the renal proximal tubule. However, as the bowel becomes more ischemic, metabolic acidosis may develop.[9,10] In addition, the stasis of intestinal matter can cause an overgrowth of bacterial intestinal flora proximal to the obstruction, causing feculent emesis. As the bowel infarcts, there is a translocation of bacteria and toxins across the bowel wall and eventual perforation.[11,12]

In a functional SBO, it is suspected that there is an activation of neural reflexes involving the sympathetic nervous system that impedes intestinal motility. Hormonal factors, such as vasoactive intestinal peptide, substance P, and nitrous oxide released during the postoperative period, also have an inhibitory effect on gastrointestinal motility. In addition, increases in the levels of inflammatory mediators, such as interleukin-1 and interleukin-6, help to potentiate decreased motility.[3,13,14]

In the United States, the predominant risk factor for mechanical SBOs is previous abdominal surgeries, which causes intra-abdominal adhesions. Surgeries most frequently implicated with SBOs are colorectal and gynecologic surgeries. Other risk factors include abdominal wall or groin hernias, malignancies, inflammatory bowel disease (specifically Crohn disease), and prior radiation (**Fig. 1, Table 1**).[2,10]

Presentation and Diagnosis

Most patients with SBO typically have abdominal pain described as episodic and crampy, lasting seconds to minutes and located in the periumbilical area or diffusely.[1,2,15] If the patient begins to describe the pain as severe and constant, this may signal worsening intestinal ischemia.[2] Vomiting is also a common feature, with bilious vomitus present in proximal obstructions and more feculent vomitus in distal obstructions. Constipation and pain relief with vomiting have the highest specificity

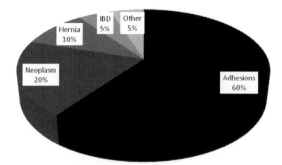

Fig. 1. Causes of mechanical SBOs. IBD, inflammatory bowel disease. (*Adapted from* Koch KL. Gastric neuromuscular function and neuromuscular disorders. In: Feldman M, Friedman LS, Brandt LJ, editors. Sleisenger and Fordtran's gastrointestinal and liver disease: pathophysiology/diagnosis/management. Philadelphia: Elsevier; 2010. p. 789–815.)

Table 1 Causes of mechanical SBO		
Intraluminal	**Intramural**	**Extramural**
Impaction	Congenital atresia	Adhesions
Foreign bodies/gallstones	Stricture	Hernia
Bezoars	Malignancy	Intussusception

with SBOs.[16] Partial SBOs allow the passing of stool and flatus, but patients with complete SBOs may cease to have bowel movements and flatus.

In SBO, abdominal distention is the most reliable sign and can be present even early in the presentation.[16] On percussion, the abdomen may be tympanic with high-pitched bowel sounds.[1] Depending on the length of time of obstruction, the bowel sounds may be decreased. Abnormal bowel sounds are the second most reliable indicator of SBOs.[16] Tenderness on abdominal examination may vary from minimal to severe and may not be localized. The presence of localized tenderness may be a sign of ischemia or perforation, indicating more severe disease. Examination of the abdomen for any surgical scars may help to aid in the diagnosis.

The patient may also have signs of dehydration because SBO may lead to profound volume loss. These signs include tachycardia, hypotension, dry mucous membranes, and decreased urine output. A fever may also be present because of ischemia and resulting infection. A rectal examination should be performed, because it may help reveal impaction or a mass. If the examination reveals a positive guaiac stool or hematochezia, it may indicate ischemia, malignancy, or inflammation of the intestinal mucosa.

Evaluation in the Emergency Department

Diagnostic strategies are needed to aid in the diagnoses, and computed tomography has become the most reliable imaging modality in the emergency department. **Table 2** describes the various imaging modalities that may be used in SBOs.[16,17]

Laboratory investigations should include a complete blood count and a basic metabolic profile. Leukocytosis may indicate translocation of bacteria, infection, or developing sepsis. If the levels are greater than $20,000/mm^3$ or the patient has significant left shift, bowel necrosis, intra-abdominal abscess, or peritonitis should be suspected.[1] As the patient becomes more dehydrated, blood urea nitrogen and creatinine levels may become increased. Patients may also have hypokalemia or hyponatremia and may show hypochloremic metabolic alkalosis. An increased lactate level may indicate bowel ischemia. One small study of 162 patients showed that increased procalcitonin levels were predictive of bowel ischemia.[18]

Treatment

Management of SBOs is 3-fold: correction of physiologic and electrolyte disturbances, bowel rest, and removing the source of the obstruction. First, resuscitation should be initiated to volume replete the patient. This resuscitation may require strict monitoring of urine output to assess the adequacy of resuscitation. Patients may need supplemental potassium because they may be significantly hypokalemic. If the patient shows fever or leukocytosis, antibiotics covering intra-abdominal flora and gram-negative and anaerobic bacteria are recommended.[2,8]

The second step to management involves bowel rest and conservative management. This step includes restricting the patient's oral intake in order to prevent further bowel distention. Gastrointestinal decompression with a nasogastric or orogastric tube may also be necessary but should be judged on a case-by-case basis. For

Table 2
Imaging modalities used to diagnose SBOs

	Pros and Cons	Imaging Findings
Abdominal radiograph	• Should be initial evaluation • Allows quick determination of perforation • Positive predictive value of 80% in high-grade obstruction • May be normal in early SBO • 75% sensitivity, 66% specificity	• Dilated loops of bowel (>2.5 cm) with distal bowel collapse • >2 air fluid levels • Stomach may also be dilated • Perforation may show free air
CT	• Most reliable test • Optimal information with oral and intravenous contrast • Can define cause and level of obstruction; ie, partial vs complete, strangulation or volvulus • Can show transition point • Slices 5–10 mm: 87% sensitivity, 81% specificity • Increasing sensitivity and specificity with thinner slices and higher grade obstructions	• Dilated loops of bowel with distal collapse • Air fluid levels • Absence of contrast material in rectum • Bowel wall thickening >3 mm • Pneumatosis intestinalis and mesenteric fat stranding suggest necrosis and perforation
Contrast fluoroscopy	• Rarely performed • Can help better delineate partial SBOs that are not clinically improving • Water-soluble contrast may also be therapeutic in partial SBO • Inferior to abdominal CT for closed-loop obstruction, ischemia, and determining cause • Contraindicated if there are signs of strangulation • If contrast reaches colon within 24 h, 96% sensitivity and 98% specificity in predicting resolution	• Dilated loops of proximal bowel highlighted with contrast material • Diameter change at transition point • No contrast distal to the obstruction
Ultrasonography	• Limited by poor visibility of gas-filled structures • May be useful in patients who cannot have CT scans • More sensitive and specific than radiographs, but cannot find grade, location, or cause • In trained individuals, 75%–97% sensitivity and 75%–90% specificity for high-grade SBO	• Dilated loops of bowel • Bowel wall thickening • Increased intestinal contents • Decreased peristalsis activity
MRI	• Limited by availability and time • Requires a cooperative patient • May be useful in patients who cannot have CT scans • May better identify strictures in cases of recurrent SBOs • Useful for low-grade bowel obstruction • 92% sensitivity, 89% specificity	• Dilated bowel loops • May show point of transition • Hyperintensity of injured bowel

Abbreviation: CT, computed tomography.

patients with high-grade or complete SBOs, gastrointestinal decompression may help to relieve abdominal distention and pain. It also helps to prevent further air swallowing and increased distention. In patients with a functional SBO, a nasogastric tube may not be necessary, and bowel rest is often enough.[1,2,8]

The final step involves relieving the obstruction, which often involves a trial of conservative management and depends on the cause of the obstruction. If the obstruction is thought to be secondary to adhesions, a laparoscopy or laparotomy is needed. There has been no difference in recurrence rates of SBO between laparoscopy versus laparotomy.[19] However, it is important to remember that further surgical trauma is a significant risk factor for recurrent SBOs. For an incarcerated hernia, if manual reduction is not possible, surgical intervention is needed. For malignant tumors, resection may be required. In the case of SBOs secondary to inflammatory bowel disease, bowel rest combined with high-dose steroids may help reduce the inflammation. All patients with complicated SBOs should have operative management. Surgery may be needed if patients have fever, leukocytosis, tachycardia, sepsis, lactic and metabolic acidosis, or worsening abdominal pain and peritonitis.

Conservative management is more successful in stable patients with partial SBOs. The success rate ranges from 40% to 70%.[20] However, if symptoms do not improve within 24 to 48 hours, operative management may be necessary. In one study comparing conservative versus operative treatment, patients treated operatively experienced a longer length of stay but had a lower rate of recurrence and longer time interval to recurrence.[21]

Summary

SBOs remain a significant reason for emergency department visits and hospital admissions. Through early diagnosis and appropriate management, the morbidity and mortality associated with SBOs can be significantly reduced.

CYCLIC VOMITING
Introduction

Cyclic vomiting syndrome (CVS) has been described in children since 1882,[22] and is defined by recurrent, stereotypical episodes of vomiting with return to baseline health between episodes.[23] CVS has been increasingly recognized in adults as well,[24] and research interest accelerated with the 2004 description of cannabinoid hyperemesis (CH) as a cause of recurrent vomiting (**Fig. 2**).[25] Among children, the incidence of CVS has been estimated at 3.2 per 100,000 children per year,[26] with a prevalence of 1.9% reported in 2 separate studies.[27,28] The median age at onset is 4 to 7 years,[26–29] with an average delay in diagnosis of 3.1 years after symptom onset,[30] and a slight female predominance (55:45).[29] CVS of childhood persists into adulthood in about 30% of patients,[29,31,32] but may develop de novo in adults, with a mean age at diagnosis of 34.8 years after a delay in diagnosis of 7.9 years.[30]

Pathophysiology

It is important to recognize that cyclic vomiting is a syndrome in the truest sense, defined by frequent co-occurrence of signs and symptoms rather than by shared mechanism. There is evidence that some cases of both pediatric and adult CVS may be related to undiagnosed mitochondrial dysfunction,[33,34] whereas other investigators attribute CVS to abdominal migraine because some cases are associated with migraine headaches.[32,35,36]

In the absence of a unifying pathophysiologic understanding of CVS, various professional societies have developed operational definitions and diagnostic approaches.[23,37]

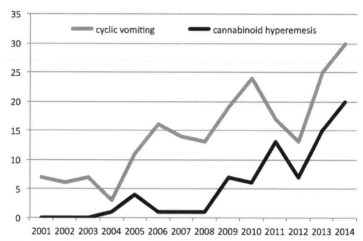

Fig. 2. PubMed search results by year for the terms "cyclic vomiting" and "cannabinoid hyperemesis."

Most prominently, the Rome process produced a definition and recommended management approach for CVS along with other functional gastrointestinal disorders (**Box 3**).[23] The North American Society for Pediatric Gastroenterology, Hepatology and Nutrition has published guidelines specific to the pediatric population that include recommendations concerning diagnosis, abortive and prophylactic therapies, and lifestyle modifications (**Box 4**).[37]

CH may represent a uniquely well-understood cause of adult CVS. CH is characterized by severe cyclic vomiting in the context of chronic heavy marijuana use and is associated with abdominal pain, compulsive hot water bathing behavior, and resolution of symptoms after cessation of use.[38] CH may be more common than was previously appreciated; an Internet survey of adult patients with CVS found that more than 80% used marijuana,[39] and cases have been reported in the pediatric population.[40] The prevalence of CH may increase with growing societal acceptance of cannabis use; diagnoses of CH doubled in Colorado following legalization of marijuana.[41]

Presentation and Diagnosis

The typical presentation of CVS in children involves between 8 and 12 attacks per year,[26,29] lasting between 20 and 48 hours,[26,28,30,33] with complete resolution of symptoms between episodes. Vomiting is typically severe, with at least 4 emeses per

---

Box 3
Rome III diagnostic criteria for cyclic vomiting syndrome

Must include all of the following:
1. Stereotypical episodes of vomiting regarding onset (acute) and duration (<1 week)
2. Three or more discrete episodes in the prior year
3. Absence of nausea and vomiting between episodes

Supportive criterion: personal or family history of migraine headaches.

Criteria fulfilled for the last 3 months with symptom onset at least 6 months before diagnosis.
   Data from Tack J, Talley NJ, Camilleri M, et al. Functional gastroduodenal disorders. Gastroenterology 2006;130:1466–79.

> **Box 4**
> **North American Society for Pediatric Gastroenterology, Hepatology and Nutrition (NASPGHAN) diagnostic criteria for cyclic vomiting syndrome in children**
>
> Must include all of the following:
>
> 1. At least 5 attacks in any interval or a minimum of 3 attacks during a 6-month period
> 2. Episodic attacks of intense nausea and vomiting lasting 1 hour to 10 days and occurring at least 1 week apart
> 3. Vomiting during attacks occur at least 4 times per hour for at least 1 hour
> 4. Return to baseline health between episodes
> 5. Not attributed to another disorder
>
> *Data from* Li BU, Lefevre F, Chelimsky GG, et al. North American Society for Pediatric Gastroenterology, Hepatology, and Nutrition consensus statement on the diagnosis and management of cyclic vomiting syndrome. J Pediatr Gastroenterol Nutr 2008;47:379–93.

hour,[33,42] and frequently commences in the early morning hours.[29] Concurrent abdominal pain is noted among 71% of patients.[26] Emotional stress and viral infections have been identified as precipitants.[29,33] Among adults the typical presentation is similar, except that episodes are of longer median duration (2.0 vs 3.8 days).[30]

CVS is a diagnosis of exclusion. The differential diagnosis of CVS is listed in **Box 5**.

> **Box 5**
> **Differential diagnosis of cyclic vomiting syndrome (CVS) among children and adults**
>
> Among children the differential diagnosis for CVS includes:
>
> 1. Primary gastrointestinal disorders (7%)
>   a. Delayed presentation of intermittent volvulus associated with malrotation
>   b. Gallbladder, liver, or pancreas disorders
>
> 2. Extra-abdominal disorders (5%)
>   a. Intermittent hydronephrosis
>   b. Diabetes mellitus
>   c. Acute intermittent porphyria
>   d. Intracranial neoplasms/masses/hydrocephalus
>   e. Metabolic conditions, including disorders of mitochondrial function, fatty acid oxidation, the urea cycle, or organic and amino acids
>
> These conditions may also exist in adults. Additional consideration should be given to:
>
> 1. Primary gastrointestinal disorders
>   a. Gastroparesis
>   b. Peptic ulcer disease
>   c. Intermittent SBO
>   d. Gallbladder disorder
>   e. Pancreatitis
>   f. Hepatitis
>
> 2. Extra-abdominal disorders
>   a. Nephrolithiasis
>   b. Intracranial neoplasms/masses/hydrocephalus
>   c. Adrenal insufficiency
>
> *Data from* Li BU, Lefevre F, Chelimsky GG, et al. North American Society for Pediatric Gastroenterology, Hepatology, and Nutrition consensus statement on the diagnosis and management of cyclic vomiting syndrome. J Pediatr Gastroenterol Nutr 2008;47:379–93; and Abell T, Adams K, Boles R, et al. Cyclic vomiting syndrome in adults. Neurogastroenterol Motil 2008;20:269–84.

Emergency Department Evaluation

As with all patients who present with abdominal pain, a careful history and physical examination are vital. Red flags include bilious emesis, abdominal tenderness, severe pain, or hematemesis. Additional testing in these patients may include urinalysis and abdominal ultrasonography to rule out ureteropelvic junction obstruction among children or nephrolithiasis in adults; acute abdominal series to rule out bowel obstruction; measurement of lipase levels, liver function tests, and gamma-glutamyl transferase levels to screen for pancreatitis, hepatitis, and gallbladder disease; with consideration of abdominal computed tomography scanning in lieu of or in addition to other imaging.

Among children, rare inborn errors of metabolism must be considered if fasting; if there is other illness or a high-protein meal is noted to provoke attacks; or if severe anion gap metabolic acidosis, altered mental status, or a peculiar odor are present.[37] Samples of blood and urine should be obtained during the attack before administration of carbohydrate-containing intravenous fluids. Serum ammonia level should be measured because urea cycle disorders are associated with increased serum ammonia levels while symptoms are present. Patients with possible delayed presentation of an inborn error of metabolism require hospitalization, because of the catastrophic outcome of these disorders if untreated.

Among children and adults, increased intracranial pressure secondary to obstructive hydrocephalus or intracranial mass may produce repetitive vomiting. Brain MRI is the test of choice given the limitations of computed tomography for evaluation of the posterior fossa. Rarely, temporal lobe epilepsy or other seizure disorders may cause cyclic vomiting, and thus electroencephalography and neurology consultation are appropriate in certain situations.

Treatment

Emergency department treatment of CVS and CH is directed at controlling symptoms of nausea and vomiting, addressing volume depletion and electrolyte abnormalities, and determining need for inpatient management or subspecialist consultation. Antianxiety and analgesic medications may also play a role depending on the severity of anxiety and pain.

Patients should be placed in a darkened, quiet room. Intravenous 5-hydroxytryptamine (5-HT$_3$ [serotonin]) receptor antagonists, such as ondansetron, are the cornerstone of symptomatic treatment during acute attacks.[37] Promethazine and prochlorperazine are less effective.[41,43] Other antiemetic agents have also been reported to be effective, including prokinetic agents such as metoclopramide and erythromycin,[44] although evidence is limited. Although ondansetron and prokinetic agents provide temporary relief, triptans (5-HT$_{1B/1D}$ agonists) have the potential to terminate an attack in migraine-associated cases.[37]

Initial resuscitation should be provided with isotonic crystalloid boluses until euvolemia is achieved and should be followed by dextrose-containing hypotonic maintenance fluids until the patient is able to tolerate oral intake. **Box 6** lists proposed indications for admission.[37] Some investigators advocate deep sedation and induced sleep with intravenous benzodiazepines,[45] although such an aggressive approach seems best reserved for refractory cases.

Acute kidney injury has been reported as a common complication of CH, perhaps in part caused by volume depletion associated with compulsive hot water bathing.[46] In addition to volume resuscitation and routine supportive care, haloperidol has been reported to improve symptoms among patients with CH who did not respond to

Box 6
Proposed indications for hospitalization for patients with CVS
Loss of greater than 5% of intravascular volume
Anuria for greater than 12 hours
Serum sodium level less than 130 mEq/L, anion gap greater than 18 mEq/L
Inability to control emesis
Data from Li BU, Lefevre F, Chelimsky GG, et al. North American Society for Pediatric Gastroenterology, Hepatology, and Nutrition consensus statement on the diagnosis and management of cyclic vomiting syndrome. J Pediatr Gastroenterol Nutr 2008;47:379–93.

ondansetron and other antiemetics.[47] Patients should be counseled to abstain from cannabis use.

Long-term therapy for CVS is directed at identifying and avoiding precipitating factors, pharmacologic prophylaxis, migraine-specific therapies for migraine-associated CVS, and psychological support.[45] Tricyclic antidepressants, amitriptyline in particular, are the mainstay of pharmacologic prophylaxis.[48] Among children, β-blockers, such as propranolol, have also been used.[45,49]

Summary

CVS is a condition of uncertain cause, defined by recurrent, stereotypical episodes of vomiting with return to baseline health between episodes. CH may account for a significant proportion of adult cases. Emergency department evaluation must be designed to identify red flags and rule out life-threatening alternative diagnoses. Treatment of acute episodes is primarily directed at symptom control, volume and electrolyte repletion, and arranging appropriate specialist follow-up.

GASTROPARESIS
Introduction

Gastroparesis is a chronic neuromuscular disorder of the upper gastrointestinal tract. It is characterized by chronic upper gastrointestinal symptoms, with objective evidence of delay in gastric emptying, in the absence of mechanical gastric outlet obstruction.[50] Characteristic symptoms of gastroparesis are described in **Table 3**.

Gastroparesis is estimated to affect up to 4% of the population and may produce mild, intermittent symptoms with little impairment of daily function to relentless vomiting with total disability and frequent hospitalizations.[51] A population-based study

Table 3	
Symptom profile of patients with gastroparesis	
Symptom	Percentage of Patients
Nausea	92
Vomiting	84
Bloating	75
Early satiety	60
Abdominal pain	46

Data from Parkman HP, Hasler WL, Fisher RS. American Gastroenterological Association technical review on the diagnosis and treatment of gastroparesis. Gastroenterology 2004;127:1592–622.

estimated that the age-adjusted incidence per 100,000 person-years for definite gastroparesis was 2.5 for men and 9.8 for women. The age-adjusted prevalence per 100,000 persons was 9.6 for men and 37.8 for women.[52] Hospitalizations with gastroparesis as a diagnosis more than doubled from 1995 to 2004, highlighting the importance of identifying and appropriately treating these patients when they present to the emergency department.[53]

Pathophysiology

Gastroparesis is a consequence of many systemic illnesses; it may complicate selected surgical procedures, or it may be idiopathic. In one case series, 29% of cases had underlying diabetes, 13% occurred after gastric surgery, and 36% were idiopathic (**Table 4**).[54] Of the idiopathic cases, postinfectious gastroparesis represented 21% of cases.[55]

Disruption of the normal physiology of gastric emptying (**Fig. 3**) caused by an abnormality in the smooth muscles, the enteric nervous system, the interstitial cells of Cajal, and the extrinsic innervation from the autonomic nervous system leads to delays in gastric emptying and the development of gastroparesis.[56]

Presentation and Diagnosis

Patients with suspected gastroparesis usually present with several nonspecific abdominal complaints. Symptoms typically include nausea, vomiting, bloating, early satiety, and abdominal pain.[54] The abdominal pain is often described as burning, vague, or crampy, with some patients localizing it to the epigastrium.[57] Sharp, well-localized pain is not characteristic, and other causes need to be ruled out in these situations.[58] Initial laboratory testing is not generally useful in diagnosing patients with gastroparesis. However, routine blood tests can help rule out other diagnoses. Diagnostic evaluation generally requires an esophagogastroduodenoscopy initially to rule out mechanical obstruction. If endoscopy is negative, patients require additional testing to assess their rate of gastric emptying.

Gastric emptying scintigraphy is currently the gold standard for measuring motility of the stomach.[52] Consensus standards for gastric emptying scintigraphy have been published by multiple societies.[59] Delayed gastric emptying is present if there is greater than 90% gastric retention at 1 hour, greater than 60% at 2 hours, and greater

Table 4
Causes of gastroparesis

Major Causes (%)	Less Common Causes
Diabetes mellitus (29)	Connective tissue disease
Post-surgical (13)	Ischemia
Idiopathic (36)	Cancer
	Neurologic disease (eg, Parkinson)
	Eating disorders
	Metabolic/endocrine conditions
	Medications (eg, anticholinergics, calcium channel blockers, and opiates)
	Critical illness

Data from Soykan I, Sivri B, Sarosiek I, et al. Demography, clinical characteristics, psychological and abuse profiles, treatment, and long-term follow-up of patients with gastroparesis. Dig Dis Sci 1998;43:2398–404; and Bityutskiy LP, Soykan I, McCallum RW. Viral gastroparesis: a subgroup of idiopathic gastroparesis–clinical characteristics and long-term outcomes. Am J Gastroenterol 1997;92:1501–4.

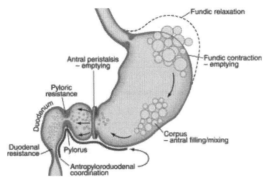

Fig. 3. Normal neuromuscular activity of the stomach in response to ingestion of food. (*Data from* Koch KL, Calles-Escandon J. Diabetic gastroparesis. Gastroenterol Clin North Am 2015;44:41; with permission.)

than 10% at 4 hours.[59,60] Other tests that measure delayed gastric emptying include wireless capsule motility, antroduodenal manometry, breath testing, transabdominal ultrasonography, and MRI.[61]

Emergency Department Evaluation

Although the diagnosis of gastroparesis is not typically made in the emergency department, an emergency department evaluation can help identify the severity of the disease and associated complications. Patients with mild gastroparesis often present with intermittent symptoms that worsen after a large solid meal. In severe cases, patients often complain of progressive nausea, distention, and pain that is relieved by vomiting old food residue. The history should also elicit existing comorbidities (eg, diabetes or scleroderma), prior gastric surgery, abdominal irradiation, or a recent viral illness.[51]

The physical examination in these patients can serve 2 purposes: to assess the severity of the presenting complaints and to facilitate diagnosis. Poor skin turgor, sunken eyes, dry mucous membranes, and orthostatic vital signs mandate prompt fluid resuscitation. Patients can also have abdominal distention and tympany on examination with or without abdominal tenderness. The clinician may also be able to elicit a succussion splash by gently rocking the patient from side to side.

Selected laboratory tests and radiologic studies may help direct further management of patients with presumed gastroparesis. Serum electrolyte levels can be used to assess for hypokalemia and contraction alkalosis. Tests for diabetes, uremia, and thyroid or parathyroid dysfunction are indicated in certain cases. Abdominal radiographs help rule out entities such as an SBO. If available, endoscopy may reveal mucosal lesions, such as reflux or candida esophagitis, which require treatments other than those typically used for treatment of gastroparesis.[62]

Treatment

Treatment of gastroparesis often includes dietary modifications, pharmacotherapy, and interventional therapy. Dietary modifications generally involve altering the meal content and frequency. Patients should be encouraged to eat more liquid-based meals, because they often have intact gastric emptying of liquids. Intake of fats and nondigestible fibers should be reduced, because they retard gastric emptying through various mechanisms.[63]

Management typically involves the use of pharmacotherapy. Nonetheless, treatment options should also include hydration with correction of electrolyte abnormalities and identification and treatment of the underlying disorder. However, the main aim of treatment is to alleviate the symptoms with medications (**Table 5**).

Metoclopramide
At present, metoclopramide is the only medication that is approved for the use of gastroparesis in the United States and should be considered the first-line treatment. Metoclopramide is a dopamine receptor antagonist, thereby stimulating the cholinergic receptors. This stimulation results in a reduction of esophageal sphincter and gastric tone, increased intragastric pressure, improved antroduodenal coordination, and accelerated gastric emptying.[64] Metoclopramide improved gastric emptying by 56% in patients with gastroparesis, compared with 37% in the placebo group.[65] However, multiple short-term studies generally showed a poor correlation of acceleration of gastric emptying with symptom improvement.[64,66-70] In addition, the US Food and Drug Administration has placed a black box warning on the use of metoclopramide. Acute dystonic reactions can occur with use of this medication, as well as irreversible tardive dyskinesia.[71]

Domperidone
Domperidone is approved only on an investigational basis in the United States. It is also a dopamine receptor antagonist. However, because it does not cross the blood-brain barrier, the central nervous system side effects are less evident. In addition, domperidone and metoclopramide have been shown to be equally efficacious in improving symptoms of gastroparesis.[67,72]

Erythromycin
Erythromycin, a macrolide antibiotic, acts as a motilin receptor agonist. It mimics the effects of motilin, a polypeptide involved in gastric smooth muscle contractions, and promotes gastric emptying.[73,74] Long-term use of erythromycin leads to tachyphylaxis and other complications of prolonged antibiotic use,[75,76] and thus there are an inadequate number of clinical trials evaluating the use of erythromycin for long-term treatment of gastroparesis.

Antiemetic agents
Given the lack of correlation between symptoms and gastric emptying, it is reasonable to propose that the primary goal of treating gastroparesis should focus on symptom relief. Because nausea and vomiting are the most common symptoms, medications targeted for symptomatic relief of these symptoms are often used. These medications work through a variety of peripheral and central pathways. **Box 7** lists these agents. To date, there have not been any controlled clinical studies formally evaluating nonprokinetic antiemetics in gastroparesis.[56]

Interventional therapy
Patients who fail medical therapy and are unable to meet their nutritional requirements should be considered for endoscopic and surgical options.[50] Endoscopic treatment involves onabotulinumtoxinA injections into the pyloric sphincter. Although earlier studies revealed a temporary improvement in symptoms, later studies have not been as promising.[77-80] Placement of a jejunostomy tube can be performed in patients with severe refractory gastroparesis. In a retrospective study, 39% of patients reported fewer symptoms, 52% reported fewer hospitalizations, 56% reported better nutritional status, and 83% reported overall improvement in their health.[81] The Food and Drug Administration approved gastric electrical stimulation as a surgical option

Table 5
Primary prokinetic agents used in the treatment of gastroparesis

Medication	Main Mechanism	Starting Oral Dose (mg)	Main Adverse Effects	Comments
Metoclopramide	Central and peripheral dopamine-2 receptor antagonist	10 TID and at bedtime	Extrapyramidal movement disorders (ie, tardive dyskinesia), hyperprolactinemia	Only FDA-approved drug for gastroparesis
Domperidone	Peripheral dopamine-2 receptor antagonist	10 TID and at bedtime	Hyperprolactinemia	Only available through investigational program in the United States
Erythromycin	Motilin receptor agonist	125 BID	Gastrointestinal upset, arrhythmias, and drug interactions	Macrolide antibiotic with antimicrobial properties

Abbreviations: BID, twice daily; FDA, US Food and Drug Administration; TID, 3 times daily.
Data from Tang DM, Friedenberg FK. Gastroparesis: approach, diagnostic evaluation, and management. Dis Mon 2011;57:74–101.

Box 7
Primary antiemetic agents used in gastroparesis

Phenothiazine derivatives

Prochlorperazine

Serotonin (5-hydroxytryptamine [5-HT₃]) receptor antagonists

Ondansetron

Dopamine receptor antagonists

Metoclopramide

Domperidone

Histamine H1 receptor antagonists

Diphenhydramine

Promethazine

Meclizine

Benzodiazepines

Lorazepam

Data from Tang DM, Friedenberg FK. Gastroparesis: approach, diagnostic evaluation, and management. Dis Mon 2011;57:74–101.

---

in 2000 for the treatment of refractory gastroparesis. It has been shown to significantly decrease gastrointestinal symptoms and improve quality of life, even over the long term.[82,83]

Summary

Gastroparesis is a chronic motility disorder. The most common causes include diabetes, postsurgical causes, and postinfectious causes. **Fig. 4** shows the general approach to these patients. They often present to the emergency department complaining of nausea, vomiting, bloating, early satiety, and abdominal pain. Evaluation should be designed to assess the severity of their symptoms. After restoration of fluid and electrolyte disturbances and glucose control, the mainstay of therapy is the use of the prokinetic agent metoclopramide. Treatment with domperidone, erythromycin, and antiemetics is also often used. Patients who have refractory gastroparesis should be considered for hospitalization to evaluate for interventional therapy.

SUMMARY: PEARLS AND PITFALLS
Small Bowel Obstruction

- Through early diagnosis and appropriate management, the morbidity and mortality associated with SBOs can be significantly reduced.
- Computed tomography has become the most reliable imaging modality in the emergency department.
- Management of SBOs is 3-fold: correction of physiologic and electrolyte disturbances, bowel rest, and removing the source of the obstruction.

Cyclic Vomiting

- CH may represent a uniquely well-understood cause of adult CVS.
- CVS is a diagnosis of exclusion, and emergency department evaluation must be designed to identify red flags and rule out life-threatening alternative diagnoses.

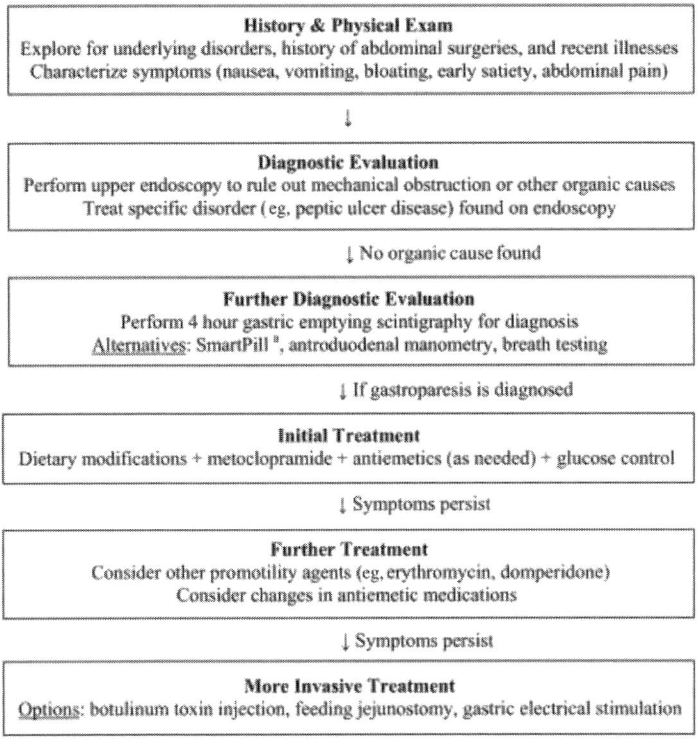

| **History & Physical Exam** |
| Explore for underlying disorders, history of abdominal surgeries, and recent illnesses |
| Characterize symptoms (nausea, vomiting, bloating, early satiety, abdominal pain) |

↓

| **Diagnostic Evaluation** |
| Perform upper endoscopy to rule out mechanical obstruction or other organic causes |
| Treat specific disorder (eg, peptic ulcer disease) found on endoscopy |

↓ No organic cause found

| **Further Diagnostic Evaluation** |
| Perform 4 hour gastric emptying scintigraphy for diagnosis |
| Alternatives: SmartPill [a], antroduodenal manometry, breath testing |

↓ If gastroparesis is diagnosed

| **Initial Treatment** |
| Dietary modifications + metoclopramide + antiemetics (as needed) + glucose control |

↓ Symptoms persist

| **Further Treatment** |
| Consider other promotility agents (eg, erythromycin, domperidone) |
| Consider changes in antiemetic medications |

↓ Symptoms persist

| **More Invasive Treatment** |
| Options: botulinum toxin injection, feeding jejunostomy, gastric electrical stimulation |

Fig. 4. General approach to gastroparesis. [a] SmartPill Corporation, Buffalo, NY. (*From* Tang DM, Friedenberg FK. Gastroparesis: approach, diagnostic evaluation, and management. Dis Mon 2011;57:86; with permission.)

- Treatment of acute episodes is primarily directed at symptom control, volume and electrolyte repletion, and arranging appropriate specialist follow-up.

Gastroparesis

- Gastroparesis is a chronic motility disorder, often associated with diabetic patients, postsurgical patients, and postinfectious patients.
- Evaluation should be designed to assess the severity of the patient's symptoms. After restoration of fluid and electrolyte disturbances and glucose control, the mainstay of therapy is the use of the prokinetic agent, metoclopramide.
- Patients with refractory gastroparesis should be considered for interventional therapy.

REFERENCES

1. Vicario SJ, Price TG. Bowel obstruction and volvulus. In: Tintinalli JE, Stapczynski JS, Ma JO, et al, editors. Tintinalli's emergency medicine: a comprehensive study guide. 7th edition. New York: McGraw-Hill; 2011. p. 581–3.
2. Torrey SP, Henneman PL. Disorders of the small intestine. In: Marx JA, Hockberger RS, Walls RM, editors. Rosen's emergency medicine. 7th edition. Philadelphia: Elsevier; 2010. p. 1184–8.
3. Carroll J, Alavi K. Pathogenesis and management of postoperative ileus. Clin Colon Rectal Surg 2009;22:47–50.

4. Scott FI, Osterman MT, Mahmoud NN, et al. Secular trends in small-bowel obstruction and adhesiolysis in the United States: 1988-2007. Am J Surg 2012; 204:315–20.

5. Maung AA, Johnson DC, Piper GL, et al. Evaluation and management of small-bowel obstruction: an Eastern Association for the Surgery of Trauma practice management guideline. J Trauma Acute Care Surg 2012;73:S362–9.

6. Duron J-J, Silva NJ-D, du Montcel ST, et al. Adhesive postoperative small bowel obstruction: incidence and risk factors of recurrence after surgical treatment. Ann Surg 2006;244:750–7.

7. Fevang BT, Fevang J, Lie SA, et al. Long-term prognosis after operation for adhesive small bowel obstruction. Ann Surg 2004;240:193–201.

8. Vallicelli C, Coccolini F, Catena F, et al. Small bowel emergency surgery: literature's review. World J Emerg Surg 2011;6:1.

9. Takeuchi K, Tsuzuki Y, Ando T, et al. Clinical studies of strangulating small bowel obstruction. Am Surg 2004;70:40–4.

10. Kulaylat MN, Doerr RJ. Small bowel obstruction. In: Holzheimer RG, Mannick JA, editors. Surgical treatment: evidence-based and problem-oriented. Munich (Germany): Zuckschwerdt; 2001. p. 102–13.

11. Sagar PM, MacFie J, Sedman P, et al. Intestinal obstruction promotes gut translocation of bacteria. Dis Colon Rectum 1995;38:640–4.

12. Rana SV, Bhardwaj SB. Small intestinal bacterial overgrowth. Scand J Gastroenterol 2008;43:1030–7.

13. Mattei P, Rombeau JL. Review of the pathophysiology and management of postoperative ileus. World J Surg 2006;30:1382–91.

14. Schwarz NT, Beer-Stolz D, Simmons RL, et al. Pathogenesis of paralytic ileus: intestinal manipulation opens a transient pathway between the intestinal lumen and the leukocytic infiltrate of the jejunal muscularis. Ann Surg 2002;235:31–40.

15. Jackson PG, Raiji MT. Evaluation and management of intestinal obstruction. Am Fam Physician 2011;83:159–65.

16. Taylor MR, Lalani N. Adult small bowel obstruction. Acad Emerg Med 2013;20: 528–44.

17. Maglinte DD, Heitkamp DE, Howard TJ, et al. Current concepts in imaging of small bowel obstruction. Radiol Clin North Am 2003;41:263–83.

18. Cosse C, Regimbeau JM, Fuks D, et al. Serum procalcitonin for predicting the failure of conservative management and the need for bowel resection in patients with small bowel obstruction. J Am Coll Surg 2013;216:997–1004.

19. Hill AG. The management of adhesive small bowel obstruction – An update. Int J Surg 2008;6:77–80.

20. Mosley JG, Shoaib A. Operative versus conservative management of adhesional intestinal obstruction. Br J Surg 2000;87:362–73.

21. Williams SB, Greenspon J, Young HA, et al. Small bowel obstruction: conservative vs. surgical management. Dis Colon Rectum 2005;48:1140–6.

22. Gee S. On fitful or recurrent vomiting. St Bartholomew Hosp Rev 1882;18:1–6.

23. Tack J, Talley NJ, Camilleri M, et al. Functional gastroduodenal disorders. Gastroenterology 2006;130:1466–79.

24. Prakash C, Clouse RE. Cyclic vomiting syndrome in adults: clinical features and response to tricyclic antidepressants. Am J Gastroenterol 1999;94:2855–60.

25. Allen JH, de Moore GM, Heddle R, et al. Cannabinoid hyperemesis: cyclical hyperemesis in association with chronic cannabis abuse. Gut 2004;53:1566–70.

26. Fitzpatrick E, Bourke B, Drumm B, et al. The incidence of cyclic vomiting syndrome in children: population-based study. Am J Gastroenterol 2008;103:991–5.

27. Ertekin V, Selimoglu MA, Altnkaynak S. Prevalence of cyclic vomiting syndrome in a sample of Turkish school children in an urban area. J Clin Gastroenterol 2006; 40:896–8.
28. Abu-Arafeh I, Russell G. Cyclical vomiting syndrome in children: a population-based study. J Pediatr Gastroenterol Nutr 1995;21:454–8.
29. Fleisher DR, Matar M. The cyclic vomiting syndrome: a report of 71 cases and literature review. J Pediatr Gastroenterol Nutr 1993;17:361–9.
30. Prakash C, Staiano A, Rothbaum RJ, et al. Similarities in cyclic vomiting syndrome across age groups. Am J Gastroenterol 2001;96:684–8.
31. Fitzpatrick E, Bourke B, Drumm B, et al. Outcome for children with cyclical vomiting syndrome. Arch Dis Child 2007;92:1001–4.
32. Dignan F, Symon DN, AbuArafeh I, et al. The prognosis of cyclical vomiting syndrome. Arch Dis Child 2001;84:55–7.
33. Moses J, Keilman A, Worley S, et al. Approach to the diagnosis and treatment of cyclic vomiting syndrome: a large single-center experience with 106 patients. Pediatr Neurol 2014;50:569–73.
34. Boles RG, Zaki EA, Lavenbarg T, et al. Are pediatric and adult-onset cyclic vomiting syndrome (CVS) biologically different conditions? Relationship of adult-onset CVS with the migraine and pediatric CVS-associated common mtDNA polymorphisms 16519T and 3010A. Neurogastroenterol Motil 2009;21:936-e72.
35. Li BU, Murray RD, Heitlinger LA, et al. Is cyclic vomiting syndrome related to migraine? J Pediatr 1999;134:567–72.
36. Abell TL, Kim CH, Malagelada JR. Idiopathic cyclic nausea and vomiting–a disorder of gastrointestinal motility? Mayo Clin Proc 1988;63:1169–75.
37. Li BU, Lefevre F, Chelimsky GG, et al. North American Society for Pediatric Gastroenterology, Hepatology, and Nutrition consensus statement on the diagnosis and management of cyclic vomiting syndrome. J Pediatr Gastroenterol Nutr 2008;47:379–93.
38. Simonetto DA, Oxentenko AS, Herman ML, et al. Cannabinoid hyperemesis: a case series of 98 patients. Mayo Clin Proc 2012;87:114–9.
39. Venkatesan T, Sengupta J, Lodhi A, et al. An Internet survey of marijuana and hot shower use in adults with cyclic vomiting syndrome (CVS). Exp Brain Res 2014; 232:2563–70.
40. Miller JB, Walsh M, Patel PA, et al. Pediatric cannabinoid hyperemesis: two cases. Pediatr Emerg Care 2010;26:919–20.
41. Kim HS, Anderson JD, Saghafi O, et al. Cyclic vomiting presentations following marijuana liberalization in Colorado. Acad Emerg Med 2015;22:694–9.
42. Abell T, Adams K, Boles R, et al. Cyclic vomiting syndrome in adults. Neurogastroenterol Motil 2008;20:269–84.
43. Li BU, Balint JP. Cyclic vomiting syndrome: evolution in our understanding of a brain-gut disorder. Adv Pediatr 2000;47:117–60.
44. Vanderhoof JA, Young R, Kaufman SS, et al. Treatment of cyclic vomiting in childhood with erythromycin. J Pediatr Gastroenterol Nutr 1995;21(Suppl 1):S60–2.
45. Hejazi RA, McCallum RW. Cyclic vomiting syndrome: treatment options. Exp Brain Res 2014;232:2549–52.
46. Habboushe J, Sedor J. Cannabinoid hyperemesis acute renal failure: a common sequela of cannabinoid hyperemesis syndrome. Am J Emerg Med 2014;32: 690.e1–2.
47. Witsil JC, Mycyk MB. Haloperidol, a novel treatment for cannabinoid hyperemesis syndrome. Am J Ther 2014. [Epub ahead of print].

48. Lee LY, Abbott L, Mahlangu B, et al. The management of cyclic vomiting syndrome: a systematic review. Eur J Gastroenterol Hepatol 2012;24:1001–6.
49. Haghighat M, Rafie SM, Dehghani SM, et al. Cyclic vomiting syndrome in children: experience with 181 cases from southern Iran. World J Gastroenterol 2007;13:1833–6.
50. Parkman HP, Hasler WL, Fisher RS. American Gastroenterological Association technical review on the diagnosis and treatment of gastroparesis. Gastroenterology 2004;127:1592–622.
51. Hasler WL. Gastroparesis: symptoms, evaluation, and treatment. Gastroenterol Clin North Am 2007;36:619–47.
52. Jung HK, Choung RS, Locke GR 3rd, et al. The incidence, prevalence, and outcomes of patients with gastroparesis in Olmsted County, Minnesota, from 1996 to 2006. Gastroenterology 2009;136:1225–33.
53. Wang YR, Fisher RS, Parkman HP. Gastroparesis-related hospitalizations in the United States: trends, characteristics, and outcomes, 1995-2004. Am J Gastroenterol 2008;103:313–22.
54. Soykan I, Sivri B, Sarosiek I, et al. Demography, clinical characteristics, psychological and abuse profiles, treatment, and long-term follow-up of patients with gastroparesis. Dig Dis Sci 1998;43:2398–404.
55. Bityutskiy LP, Soykan I, McCallum RW. Viral gastroparesis: a subgroup of idiopathic gastroparesis–clinical characteristics and long-term outcomes. Am J Gastroenterol 1997;92:1501–4.
56. Stein B, Everhart KK, Lacy BE. Gastroparesis: a review of current diagnosis and treatment options. J Clin Gastroenterol 2015;49:550–8.
57. Hoogerwerf WA, Pasricha PJ, Kalloo AN, et al. Pain: the overlooked symptom in gastroparesis. Am J Gastroenterol 1999;94:1029–33.
58. Friedenberg FK, Parkman HP. Advances in the management of gastroparesis. Curr Treat Options Gastroenterol 2007;10:283–93.
59. Abell TL, Camilleri M, Donohoe K, et al. Consensus recommendations for gastric emptying scintigraphy: a joint report of the American Neurogastroenterology and Motility Society and the Society of Nuclear Medicine. Am J Gastroenterol 2008; 103:753–63.
60. Tougas G, Eaker EY, Abell TL, et al. Assessment of gastric emptying using a low fat meal: establishment of international control values. Am J Gastroenterol 2000; 95:1456–62.
61. Koch KL, Calles-Escandon J. Diabetic gastroparesis. Gastroenterol Clin North Am 2015;44:39–57.
62. Parkman HP, Schwartz SS. Esophagitis and gastroduodenal disorders associated with diabetic gastroparesis. Arch Intern Med 1987;147:1477–80.
63. Tang DM, Friedenberg FK. Gastroparesis: approach, diagnostic evaluation, and management. Dis Mon 2011;57:74–101.
64. McCallum RW, Ricci DA, Rakatansky H, et al. A multicenter placebo-controlled clinical trial of oral metoclopramide in diabetic gastroparesis. Diabetes Care 1983;6:463–7.
65. Snape WJ, Battle WM, Schwartz SS, et al. Metoclopramide to treat gastroparesis due to diabetes mellitus. Ann Intern Med 1982;96:444.
66. Erbas T, Varoglu E, Erbas B, et al. Comparison of metoclopramide and erythromycin in the treatment of diabetic gastroparesis. Diabetes Care 1993;16:1511–4.
67. Patterson D, Abell T, Rothstein R, et al. A double-blind multicenter comparison of domperidone and metoclopramide in the treatment of diabetic patients with symptoms of gastroparesis. Am J Gastroenterol 1999;94:1230–4.

68. Perkel MS, Hersh T, Moore C, et al. Metoclopramide therapy in fifty-five patients with delayed gastric emptying. Am J Gastroenterol 1980;74:231–6.
69. Perkel MS, Moore C, Hersh T, et al. Metoclopramide therapy in patients with delayed gastric emptying: a randomized, double-blind study. Dig Dis Sci 1979;24: 662–6.
70. Ricci DA, Saltzman MB, Meyer C, et al. Effect of metoclopramide in diabetic gastroparesis. J Clin Gastroenterol 1985;7:25–32.
71. Ganzini L, Casey DE, Hoffman WF, et al. The prevalence of metoclopramide-induced tardive dyskinesia and acute extrapyramidal movement disorders. Arch Intern Med 1993;153:1469–75.
72. Sugumar A, Singh A, Pasricha PJ. A systematic review of the efficacy of domperidone for the treatment of diabetic gastroparesis. Clin Gastroenterol Hepatol 2008;6:726–33.
73. Hasler WL, Heldsinger A, Chung OY. Erythromycin contracts rabbit colon myocytes via occupation of motilin receptors. Am J Physiol 1992;262:G50–5.
74. Peeters T, Matthijs G, Depoortere I, et al. Erythromycin is a motilin receptor agonist. Am J Physiol 1989;257:G470–4.
75. O'Donovan D, Feinle-Bisset C, Jones K, et al. Idiopathic and diabetic gastroparesis. Curr Treat Options Gastroenterol 2003;6:299–309.
76. Richards RD, Davenport K, McCallum RW. The treatment of idiopathic and diabetic gastroparesis with acute intravenous and chronic oral erythromycin. Am J Gastroenterol 1993;88:203–7.
77. Miller LS, Szych GA, Kantor SB, et al. Treatment of idiopathic gastroparesis with injection of botulinum toxin into the pyloric sphincter muscle. Am J Gastroenterol 2002;97:1653–60.
78. Reddymasu SC, Singh S, Sankula R, et al. Endoscopic pyloric injection of botulinum toxin-A for the treatment of postvagotomy gastroparesis. Am J Med Sci 2009;337:161–4.
79. Arts J, Holvoet L, Caenepeel P, et al. Clinical trial: a randomized-controlled cross-over study of intrapyloric injection of botulinum toxin in gastroparesis. Aliment Pharmacol Ther 2007;26:1251–8.
80. Friedenberg FK, Palit A, Parkman HP, et al. Botulinum toxin A for the treatment of delayed gastric emptying. Am J Gastroenterol 2008;103:416–23.
81. Fontana RJ, Barnett JL. Jejunostomy tube placement in refractory diabetic gastroparesis: a retrospective review. Am J Gastroenterol 1996;91:2174–8.
82. McCallum RW, Snape W, Brody F, et al. Gastric electrical stimulation with Enterra therapy improves symptoms from diabetic gastroparesis in a prospective study. Clin Gastroenterol Hepatol 2010;8:947–54.
83. Cutts TF, Luo J, Starkebaum W, et al. Is gastric electrical stimulation superior to standard pharmacologic therapy in improving GI symptoms, healthcare resources, and long-term health care benefits? Neurogastroenterol Motil 2005;17: 35–43.

Diarrhea

Initial Evaluation and Treatment in the Emergency Department

Alexa R. Gale, MD*, Matthew Wilson, MD

KEYWORDS

- Diarrhea • Diagnosis • Management • Emergency department • Gastroenteritis

KEY POINTS

- A thorough history and examination to evaluate for dehydration or risk for treatment failure should drive the initial management of a diarrheal illness.
- Practitioners can provide valuable education for patients and caregivers regarding symptomatic care and expected course of their illness.
- Antibiotics are associated with hemolytic–uremic syndrome and should be used cautiously in patients presenting with bloody diarrhea and no fever.
- Notification of public health authorities is recommended if diarrheal illness is suspected from cholera, enterohemorrhagic *Escherichia coli*, *listeria*, *salmonella*, *shigella*, or norovirus.
- The initial emergency evaluation of chronic diarrhea should focus on stabilization with further testing coordinated with the patient's ongoing care provider.

INTRODUCTION

As a chief complaint, diarrhea generates a wide range of diagnostic considerations, ranging from benign, temporary alterations of intestinal motility to severe life-threatening disease. Diarrhea has profound individual and public health significance. The setting and circumstances under which a patient presents with diarrhea drastically influences the concern that is brought to the patient encounter. In the United States nausea, vomiting, and diarrhea are often provisionally labeled "gastroenteritis" with appropriate expectant management. However, it can carry significant morbidity/mortality in patients that are immunocompromised, at the extremes of age, or have an altered gastrointestinal system. There are 211 million to 375 million episodes of acute diarrhea each year in the United States (1.4 episodes per person per year), resulting in 900,000 hospitalizations and 6000 deaths. In resource-poor countries, the significance of diarrhea is even greater, where as many as 2 million deaths occur annually from diarrheal illness and survivors can be left with physical and cognitive impairment.[1]

ª Department of Emergency Medicine, Medstar Washington Hospital Center, 110 Irving Street NW, Washington, DC 20010, USA
* Corresponding author.
E-mail address: Alexa.R.Gale@medstar.net

Emerg Med Clin N Am 34 (2016) 293–308
http://dx.doi.org/10.1016/j.emc.2015.12.006   emed.theclinics.com

This review focuses on diarrhea and its initial evaluation and management in the emergency department (ED). Diarrhea accompanies many types of illnesses and practitioners need to maintain a wide differential to avoid labeling a severe systemic illness or abdominal surgical emergency as "gastroenteritis." Taking these pathologies into consideration, this article focuses on general diagnostics and management of diarrheal illness, as well as specific acute infectious etiologies and chronic diarrheas of importance to the ED practitioner.

GENERAL DIAGNOSTICS AND MANAGEMENT

Acute diarrhea is defined as increased stool frequency, up to 3 or more times per day or greater than 200 g of stool per day lasting less than 14 days.[1] The classification of *persistent diarrhea* is used for symptoms lasting longer than 14 days and symptoms lasting more than 30 days is termed *chronic diarrhea*.[2] Epidemiology data from the Centers for Disease Control and Prevention shows that bacterial etiologies for acute diarrhea are uncommon. Stool cultures grow *salmonella* (16.1 cases per 100,000 population), *campylobacter* (13.4 cases per 100,000 population), *shigella* (10.3 cases per 100,000 population), *Escherichia coli* O157:H7 (1.7 cases per 100,000 population), and *cryptosporidium* (1.4 cases per 100,000 population). *Vibrio, Yersinia, listeria,* and *Cyclospora* are reported in less than 1 person per 100,000. Infectious diarrhea agents for which clinical diagnostic testing is not routinely available include enterotoxigenic, enteropathogenic, enteroaggregative, and enteroinvasive strains of *E coli*, toxin-producing *Clostridium perfringens, Staphylococcus aureus, Bacillus cereus*, and noroviruses.[1]

The normal small bowel surface is designed for maximal nutrient absorption via villous tips, generating a tremendous surface area of intestinal epithelium for liquid, exocrine, and nutrient reabsorption (**Fig. 1**). This functional process is altered fundamentally during an acute diarrheal episode by microbial induced inflammation and toxins. This results in decreased absorption at the brush border, secretory losses, and an ongoing inflammatory response. The critical transporter that carries glucose and galactose into the enterocyte is the sodium-dependent hexose transporter-1. As a cotransporter, it requires both sodium and glucose for absorption to occur across

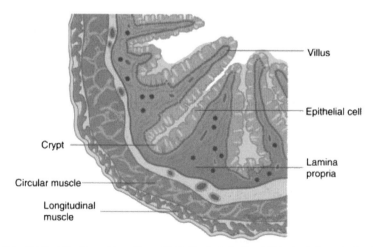

Fig. 1. Intestinal epithelium. (*From* Barrett KE. Gastrointestinal (GI) physiology. In: Caplan MJ, editor. Reference module in biomedical sciences. Philadelphia: Elsevier; 2014; with permission.)

the intestinal epithelium. Delivery of one, without the other, to the intestine results in suboptimal absorption and a persistent osmotic load that contributes to the ongoing volume losses during illness.

In acute diarrheal illness, the Infectious Disease Society of America emphasizes the importance of the history and physical examination for evaluation and diagnostic considerations. Although most acute diarrheal illnesses are self-resolving, it is also important to asses for high risk symptoms, exposures or stool characteristics to predict which patients will have a more severe course (**Table 1**). For example, a pregnant woman who is exposed to *listeria* may need long-term follow-up and care with multiple specialties, such as obstetrics and infectious disease. A travel history may prompt consideration of a treatable bacterial illness from traveler's diarrhea. High-risk food ingestions should prompt consideration of invasive bacterial illness and some exposures may clue the practitioner in to a more persistent atypical infectious illness that requires specific antimicrobials (high-risk sexual contacts, recent antibiotic use, untreated water exposure).

The history and physical examination is also of importance for public health as a pattern of exposure may become clear, for example, food exposures. Food service workers with inadequate hygiene or incomplete resolution of illness can further spread a gastrointestinal illness and should receive appropriate precautions.[2] The Centers for Disease Control and Prevention recommends notification of public health authorities for the following bacterial diarrheal illnesses when strongly suspected or definitively diagnosed: *cholera*, enterohemorrhagic *E coli*, *listeria*, *salmonella*, and *shigella*. Local health authorities should also be notified of suspected *norovirus* outbreaks. Even severe systemic illnesses can begin with an episode of diarrhea and appropriate isolation and contact precautions should be in place for patients with high-risk travel histories (eg, West Africa and the Ebola virus).

Laboratory tests are not required in the evaluation of low-risk patients who present with an acute diarrheal illness. Selected fecal studies can be considered in the ED; however, they take time to receive results, do not allow for rapid disposition, and need to be done in conjunction with ongoing follow-up. Local practice patterns may dictate when and how often these tests are ordered out of the ED as opposed to with a primary care provider. Another reason to consider performing these tests in selected patients with high-risk exposures is the public health significance of certain organisms causing invasive bacterial illness (**Table 2**).

Table 1	
High-risk symptoms and exposures in acute diarrheal disease	
Symptoms	**Exposures**
Profuse dehydration	Illness in extremes of age
Symptoms of hypovolemia	Illness in immunocompromised patients
Febrile	Travel/occupation history
Bloody diarrhea	Day care
Increased frequency	Raw/undercooked meat/seafood/dairy
Increased quantity	Sick contacts
	Drinking untreated fresh water
	Recent or regular medications
	Sexual contacts
	Pregnancy

Data from Guerrant RL, Van Gilder T, Steiner TS, et al. Practice guidelines for the management of infectious diarrhea. Clin Infect Dis 2001;32:331–50.

Table 2 Recommended stool studies		
Community-Acquired and Traveler's Diarrhea (When/ If Fever or Blood in Stool)	Hospital-Acquired or Recent Antibiotics/ Chemotherapy	Persistent Diarrhea
Culture/test for: *Salmonella*, *Shigella*, *Campylobacter*, *E coli* O157:H7, *C difficile* toxin	*C difficile* toxin	Test for parasites: giardia, cryptosporidium, cyclospora, isospora belli If HIV+: microsporidia, *M avium* complex

Data from Guerrant RL, Van Gilder T, Steiner TS, et al. Practice guidelines for the management of infectious diarrhea. Clin Infect Dis 2001;32:331–50.

The ordering of blood testing, urinalysis, and radiography should be dictated by clinical concern for severe disease or an acute surgical illness. These tests do not affect management or disposition in uncomplicated acute diarrheal illness. Although urine specific gravity and blood urea nitrogen have low sensitivities and specificities for dehydration, a normal serum bicarbonate level is reassuring that a child is not currently dehydrated, with a likelihood ratio between 0.18 (95% CI, 0.08–0.37) and 0.22 (95% CI, 0.12–0.43),[3,4] whereas a serum bicarbonate level of less than 13 mEq/L may reflect dehydration that is severe enough to fail an outpatient rehydration trial.[5]

The management of diarrheal illness is dictated by a patient's level of dehydration using a constellation of clinical signs and symptoms to identify those patients who are severely dehydrated who would benefit from aggressive initial management. In a study by Steiner and colleagues,[5] the authors noted that prolonged capillary refill, abnormal respiratory pattern, and decreased skin turgor were the most accurate clinical signs for dehydration. Abnormal vitals, fever, orthostatic hypotension, abdominal tenderness, or signs of an altered level of consciousness can point to a more severe illness, requiring aggressive resuscitation.

Patients with severe dehydration require attention to their airway, and respiratory and circulatory status to ensure that they are stable for further management and delineation of the acute etiology. The prudent practitioner can simultaneously manage volume resuscitation while evaluating for a correctable surgical or medical etiology that may have been masquerading as a diarrheal illness. For instance, an abdominal computed tomography scan may be required to identify an underlying surgical emergency such as appendicitis or obstruction, and/or laboratory work and fecal occult blood testing may be needed to identify a critical gastrointestinal bleed. Ongoing fluid management, either intravenously or with oral rehydration therapy (ORT), should be performed in conjunction with close monitoring of electrolytes, renal function, and for signs of end-organ failure such as a lactic acidosis. Supportive care should be continued to transition the patient to an appropriate level of care within the institution. Early empiric antimicrobial therapy, as presented in **Table 5**, should be considered for patients with severe dehydration because they are more likely to have an invasive bacterial illness and may even be presenting in septic shock.

For mild to moderate dehydration, general treatment focuses on replenishing fluids and electrolytes in a safe, cost-effective manner. ORT was developed in the 1970s to treat dehydration resulting from severe diarrhea and overcome the need for sterile intravenous hydration to overwhelming numbers of patients affected by diarrhea outbreaks (eg, cholera) in developing countries. ORS is an isoosmolar, glucose–electrolyte solution with a base added to treat dehydration and metabolic acidosis resulting from severe diarrhea.[6] The solution is designed to optimize the absorption of the sodium-dependent hexose transporter-1 co-transporter along the intestinal epithelium. It is of particular efficacy in diarrhea resulting from *Vibrio cholera* as the cholera enterotoxin results in increased secretion of cyclic adenosine monophosphate causing active Cl⁻ secretion and inhibition of NaCl reabsorption but the enterotoxin does not inhibit Na^+ and glucose reabsorption, which allows fluid absorption with oral rehydration solution (ORS) despite ongoing secretory losses. The value of ORT was demonstrated during the Bangladeshi war of independence in the early 1970s and its ongoing value has led to the conclusion by many "that ORS was the major therapeutic advance of the last (ie, twentieth) century."[6]

ORT is now the preferred method of rehydration in mild to moderate dehydration for children as confirmed in a metaanalysis of 16 studies looking at ORT showing it has fewer side effects and shorter durations of hospital stay compared with intravenous hydration.[7] An ORS is composed of sodium, dextrose, and bicarbonate in a ratio that does not overwhelm the hyperactive bowels with a hyperosmolar solution, but that is strong enough to replace the electrolyte loss.[3] The best options for rehydrating children at home are Pedialyte, Gatorade, Infalyte, or the World Health Organization (WHO) ORS. Parents should not use high sugar content drinks such as sodas and fruit juices, because they worsen diarrhea and dehydration.[8] Also, clear liquids (water, sodas, chicken broth, and apple juice) should not be substituted for ORS because they are hypoosmolar and do not adequately replace potassium, bicarbonate, and sodium, and can result in hyponatremia.[3] General principles for the use of ORT are presented in **Box 1**.

Ancillary medications can be considered for symptomatic therapy in diarrheal illness. Loperamide, an antimotility agent, has been shown to decrease the number of liquid bowel movements in the treatment of diarrheal illness without affecting the host's ability to eliminate diarrheal pathogens.[9] The median duration of diarrhea reduced to 19 hours (25th to 75th percentiles, 6–42 hours) for those receiving loperamide plus ciprofloxacin compared with 42 hours (21–46 hours) for those receiving ciprofloxacin alone ($P = .028$). However, antimotility agents may facilitate hemolytic uremic syndrome in enterohemorrhagic *E coli* as initially reported by Cimolai and colleagues[10] in their retrospective review of *E coli* cases from 1990, so they are not appropriate in bloody diarrhea or in patients with exposures or risk factors that generate concern for invasive illness.

Bismuth subsalicylate has also been investigated in the treatment of traveler's diarrhea specifically and it significantly reduced the number of unformed stools and increased the proportion of symptom resolution with only minor adverse effects noted.[11]

Box 1
Treating children with gastroenteritis and mild dehydration

Use oral rehydration with an over-the-counter oral rehydration solution

Begin rapid oral rehydration within 4 hours of symptom onset

Continue breastfeeding during the illness

Never dilute formula

Maintain a regular diet once rehydrated

Ongoing losses need to be replaced with additional rehydration solution

Avoid medications and unnecessary laboratory tests

Adapted from Churgay CA, Zahra A. Gastroenteritis in children: part I. Diagnosis. Am Fam Physician 2012;85:11.

There is also evidence supporting zinc supplementation in shortening the duration of diarrhea in children younger than 5 years of age. A systematic review encompassing 89 Chinese and 15 non-Chinese studies analyzing a total of 18,822 diarrhea cases found an overall 26% (95% CI, 20%-32%) reduction in the estimated relative risk of diarrhea lasting longer than 3 days among zinc-treated children. Studies conducted in and outside China report reductions in morbidity as a result of oral therapeutic zinc supplementation for acute diarrhea among children younger than 5 years of age. Lamberti and colleagues[12] subsequently conclude that the "WHO recommendation for zinc treatment of diarrhea episodes should be supported in all low- and middle-income countries" to ensure an adequate supply of zinc in patients at risk for deficiency.

A common question after the diagnosis of a diarrheal illness is regarding what foods are best to eat while recovering. General advice should include emphasizing the importance of a healthy diet to promote enterocyte recovery; however, patients do not have to be strictly limited to only bananas, rice, applesauce, and toast, as has been promoted in the past. Avoiding high-fat content and high lactose content foods while enterocytes are recovering can minimize the effects of any transient secondary lactose intolerance that developed. Probiotics have also been shown to be safe and beneficial in shortening an episode of acute diarrheal illness. A recent Cochrane review[13] looked at 63 studies with a total of 8014 participants showing no adverse events from probiotic intervention and a reduction in the duration of diarrhea (mean difference, 24.76 hours; 95% CI, 15.9–33.6 hours; n = 4555 patients; trials = 35).

Anticipatory guidance should be provided for patients and/or parents in the ED covering the expected course of their illness. Precautions for return should be discussed because many patients do not know what distinguishes a normal course of diarrhea from a more severe or progressive illness. This discussion should emphasize that diarrhea may persist, even for 3 days, but it is usually a self-limited illness. Return precautions should include fever, bloody diarrhea, or signs of severe dehydration such as decreased urine output, lightheadedness, or lethargy. Patients should also be instructed to limit spread of the illness through good hand hygiene with clean soap and water, food hygiene with strict separation of contaminated feces from food preparation, and even feces management in general with dedicated locations for stool separated from the food and water supply.

ACUTE INFECTIOUS ETIOLOGIES
Viral

The majority of acute infectious diarrhea cases are the result of a virus. Bacteria cultures are only positive in 1% to 5% of cases.[2] As seen in **Table 3**, the usual etiology in developed countries is norovirus, which has been implicated commonly in cruise ship outbreaks. Rotavirus is also identified as a common viral cause of acute diarrhea, but its frequency and the observed severity of seasonal outbreaks has decreased with the adoption of the Rotavirus vaccine.[14] Although viral cases of gastroenteritis do not have a specific antimicrobial agent of benefit for therapy, screening for dehydration and institution of symptomatic treatments are of importance in the ED setting.

Selected Bacterial Etiologies

There are numerous bacterial causes of acute diarrhea, as seen in **Table 3**. For the ED practitioner, the specific causal agent is usually not available for acute decision making and management. Therefore, empiric treatment can be instituted per the recommendations of the Infectious Disease Society of America provided in **Table 4**. The serious side effects of antibacterial agents in diarrhea should be

Table 3
Weighted average prevalence of enteric pathogen detection rate in adults older than 12 years

Pathogens	Middle East/North Africa Detection Rate (%)	Developed Countries Detection Rate (%)	Sub-Saharan Africa Detection Rate (%)
Bacteria			
Campylobacter	1.4	3.3	0.3
ETEC	N/R	0.1	1.0
Other E coli	37	0.1	3.6
Salmonella	0.7	1.9	4.0
Shigella	4.1	0.2	2.2
V cholerae	0.7	0.1	N/R
Viruses			
Adenovirus	6.8	1.0	0.3
Norovirus	0.7	10.5	0.3
Rotavirus	1.4	3.6	0.3
Parasites			
Ascaris	0.7	0.1	0.3
Cryptosporidium	0.7	0.3	9.4
Entamoeba	1.4	0.2	2.5
Giardia	0.7	0.3	1.4

Abbreviation: ETEC, enterotoxigenic E coli.
Data from Fletcher SM, McLaws ML, Ellis JT. Prevalence of gastrointestinal pathogens in developed and developing countries: systematic review and meta-analysis. J Public Health Res 2013;2:e9.

Table 4
Empiric antimicrobial considerations in acute infectious diarrhea

Clinical Scenario	Causative Etiology	Treatment
Traveler's diarrhea: international travel with acute diarrhea and often abdominal cramping, tenesmus, nausea, vomiting	ETEC, Norovirus, Rotavirus, Salmonella, Campylobacter, Shigella, Aeromonas, Bacteroides, and Vibrio	Fluoroquinolone or bactrim for 3 d shown to reduce duration by 2–3 d
Febrile/invasive: severe dysentery with fever/bloody diarrhea; very contagious	Campylobacter, Salmonella, Shigella, and Yersinia	Fluoroquinolone or bactrim for 3 d can be considered to reduce duration of shedding
Persistent diarrhea after untreated water exposure	Giardia	Metronidazole (500 mg TID for 7–10 d)
Bloody diarrhea, pain, lack of fever	Suspected STEC	No antimotility or antimicrobial agents as they may worsen the risk of hemolytic–uremic syndrome and do not ameliorate O157 illness

Abbreviations: ETEC, enterotoxigenic E coli; STEC, Shiga toxin-producing E coli; TID, 3 times a day.
Data from Guerrant RL, Van Gilder T, Steiner TS, et al. Practice guidelines for the management of infectious diarrhea. Clin Infect Dis 2001;32:344.

considered, including the development of antimicrobial resistance, medication cost, eradication of normal intestinal flora, and the induction of the shiga-toxin phage by quinolones.[2] Shiga-toxin phage induction by quinolones is of particular concern to practitioners because of the risk of the hemolytic–uremic syndrome after antibiotic treatment of *E coli* O157:H7 infections. Hemolytic–uremic syndrome results in microangiopathic hemolytic anemia, acute kidney injury, and thrombocytopenia after infection with *shigella*, *E coli*, or even *campylobacter*. The O157:H7 phage causes vascular endothelial damage and can be fatal or result in chronic kidney disease. In a prospective evaluation of risk factors, antibiotics were associated independently with the development of hemolytic–uremic syndrome.[15] Although polymerase chain reaction testing has been used in the research setting for rapid diagnosis of Shiga-toxin phage, it is not yet widely available to emergency practitioners and caution will continue to have to be used with any antimicrobial prescription in suspected or known Shiga toxin-producing *E coli* (also referred to as enterohemorrhagic *E coli*). Specific antimicrobial agents as well as key historical clues to the diagnosis of specific bacterial causes of acute infectious diarrhea are presented in **Table 5**.

Table 5
Selected bacterial causes of acute infectious diarrhea and their treatment

Clinical Scenario	Causative Etiology	Treatment
"Rice-water diarrhea"; Severely dehydrating secretory diarrhea from cholera enterotoxin; Only endemic in the United States along Gulf Coast	Cholera	Doxycycline 300 mg once or bactrim BID for 3 d or single dose fluoroquinolone
Severe dysentery with fever/bloody diarrhea; very contagious	*Shigella*	Bactrim or fluoroquinolone BID for 3 d
Acute watery diarrhea; associated with "pseudoappendicitis"	*Yersinia*	Antibiotics usually only needed in immunocompromised
Acute watery diarrhea; poultry reservoir; associated with Guillain-Barre, reactive arthritis and IBD	*Campylobacter*	Azithromycin 500 mg daily × 3 d
Food-borne, travelers or childhood diarrhea in developing countries; multiple strains	*E coli*	ETEC: bactrim or fluoroquinolone BID for 3 d
Systemic (fever, body aches, neck stiffness); transmitted from human to human (typhoid type)	*Salmonella*	Not routinely recommended unless immunocompromised, extremes of age, valvular heart disease or persistent; bactrim or fluoroquinolone BID for 5–7 d
Mild systemic symptoms (fever, body aches); severe invasive disease in pregnancy or immunocompromised	*Listeria*	Not routinely recommended unless immunocompromised or pregnant in which case ampicillin should be used

Abbreviations: BID, twice a day; ETEC, enterotoxigenic *E coli*; IBD, inflammatory bowel disease; TID, 3 times a day.
Adapted from Guerrant RL, Van Gilder T, Steiner TS, et al. Practice guidelines for the management of infectious diarrhea. Clin Infect Dis 2001;32:344; and Thielman NM, Guerrant RL. Acute infectious diarrhea. N Engl J Med 2004;350:38–47.

Bacterial Traveler's Diarrhea

With increased international travel, traveler's diarrhea is encountered commonly in the ED. It is seen in patients from high-income countries who travel to low- or moderate-income countries. Symptoms usually occur within the first 2 weeks of stay and decrease as more time is spent in the country. Although it affects men and women equally, infants and toddlers may experience more severe symptoms and require hospitalization.[16]

Many environmental factors have been linked to increased rates of traveler's diarrhea. Patients who obtain food from street vendors or partake in all-inclusive vacations are at greater risk. In addition to bacterial etiologies, cruise ships have high rates of Norovirus, resulting in outbreaks on the ship. The occurrence of traveler's diarrhea decreases in the winter months, when there is less rainfall and heat. Owing to the consumption of fecally contaminated food and beverages, the most common pathogens are enterotoxigenic E coli, enteroaggregative E coli, diffusely adherent E coli, Norovirus, Rotavirus, Salmonella species, Campylobacter jejuni, Shigella, Aeromonas species, Bacteroides fragilis, and Vibrio species[16] (**Box 2**).

Box 2
Symptoms of traveler's diarrhea

- Passage of 3 or more unformed stools in a 24-hour period plus any of the following symptoms: abdominal cramping, tenesmus, nausea, vomiting, fever, or fecal urgency.[16]
- Four- to 5-day duration.
- Patients may have nonspecific symptoms of a viral illness.
- Usually patients do not have symptoms of bloody diarrhea or purulent discharge mixed with stool.
- May cause longer symptoms in patients with inflammatory bowel disease.[17]

Travelers should be informed of the old adage: "Boil it, cook it, peel, it or forget it." Bismuth subsalicylate may provide moderate protection if given 4 times per day.[16,18,19] Prophylactic use of rifaximin has been shown in 4 trials to reduce the rates of noninvasive diarrhea.[16,20,21] Fluoroquinolone prophylaxis can prevent traveler's diarrhea. Studies have shown that it can reduce episodes of traveler's diarrhea by 90%; however, the risks of fluoroquinolone antibiotics should limit its prophylactic use to only travelers prone to complications.[16,18,22]

The treatment of traveler's diarrhea can proceed as outlined in the introduction for patients with mild to moderate dehydration. Antibiotics can be considered in patients with nonbloody diarrhea. A short 3-day course of ciprofloxacin or levofloxacin has been shown to decrease symptom duration by 1 to 3 days.[16,23,24] Practitioners should consider prescribing azithromycin to patients who have recently traveled from South East Asia to cover a species of Campylobacter that is resistant to fluoroquinolone antibiotics.[16,23,25,26]

Clostridium difficile

Clostridium difficile is one of the most serious causes of diarrhea affecting patients in the United States. It was first identified in 1978 as the cause of the majority of cases of antibiotic associated diarrhea. The earliest cases of C difficile were attributed to the use of clindamycin,[27] but most antibiotics have now been found to create an environment in the colon that allows colonization by *C difficile*. Data from the Centers for Disease Control and Prevention showed that, in 2011, approximately 500,000 patients sustained infections from *C difficile* and 83,000 of those patients had at least one recurrence. In that same year, 29,000 patients died within 30 days of their initial diagnosis.[28] The antibiotics that are often recognized to be at fault include, but are not limited to fluoroquinolones, clindamycin, cephalosporins, and penicillins. By altering gut flora, antibiotics allow for a perfect environment for *C difficile* to flourish. Increased duration, higher dose, and multiple antibiotics can increase the patient's risk for *C difficile*.

The most common manifestation of *C difficile* is diarrhea. It is a severe diarrhea, with 10 to 15 bowel movements a day with associated abdominal pain and cramping. Most patients have an associated systemic reaction, with a low-grade fever and leukocytosis on laboratory results. These symptoms generally occur approximately 7 to 10 days after starting antibiotic therapy; however, symptoms may develop up to 3 months after cessation of antibiotics.[29] On colonoscopy, patients with *C difficile* may have pseudomembranous colitis, which are yellow plaques concentrated in the right colon.[30] Severe cases of *C difficile* may develop toxic megacolon, which is an abnormal dilation of the colon observed on radiologic imaging.[31] Patients who do not respond to medical management require a surgical consultation owing to their high risk of perforation.[30] Recommended antibiotic choices for the treatment of *C difficile* infection are presented in **Box 3**. Please note that intravenous vancomycin has no effect on *C difficile*, because it is not excreted into the colon (**Table 6**).

Table 6 Recommended antibiotic choices for *Clostridium difficile*		
Timing	Mild Disease	Severe Disease
Initial episode	Metronidazole 500 mg orally 3 times daily for 10–14 d	Vancomycin 125 mg orally 4 times daily for 10–14 d
First relapse	May try as above or add fidaxomicin 200 mg orally for 10 d	May try as above or add fidaxomicin 200 mg orally for 10 d
Second relapse	—	Pulsed dose of vancomycin 125 mg orally 4 times a day for 7–14 d 125 mg orally twice a day for 7 d 125 mg orally once a day for 7 d 125 mg orally every other day for 7 d 125 mg orally every 3 d for 14 d
Additional relapse	—	Fidaxomicin 200 mg orally twice daily for 10 d

Data from Refs.[30,32,33]

PERSISTENT AND CHRONIC ETIOLOGIES

Persistent diarrhea is defined as diarrhea occurring for more than 14 days and chronic diarrhea as more than 30 days (Infectious Disease Society of America). The ED may be the first point of contact for patients with chronic diarrhea and their initial management should take consideration of subsequent follow-up testing and initiate tests or therapies with an eye toward their expected course. In addition, patients with chronic diarrhea may present to the ED because they are systemically ill, requiring rapid diagnosis and aggressive resuscitation. Chronic diarrheas for consideration in ED patients are presented in **Box 3** with selected topics discussed in additional detail.

Box 3
Chronic diarrheas for consideration in the emergency department

Surgical: ischemic bowel, partial obstruction, fecal impaction, malabsorption from resection or gastric bypass, cancer

Endocrine: chronic secretory diarrhea results from Addison disease, carcinoid tumors, Verner Morrison syndrome, gastrinoma (Zollinger–Ellison syndrome), mastocytosis, hyperthyroidism

Bacterial: *Tropheryma whippelei* (systemic antimicrobials for treatment); tropical sprue (presumed from enteric bacteria; requires a combination of antibiotics and folic acid supplementation for 3–6 months); small intestine bacterial overgrowth (occurs with postoperative motility disorders or immune deficiency or reduced gastric acid secretion requires prolonged management)

Parasitic: see below

Human immunodeficiency virus and diarrhea: see below

Other: irritable bowel syndrome (see below), inflammatory bowel disease, food sensitivities, carbohydrate malabsorption, celiac disease (see below), hepatobiliary or pancreatic disorder, diverticulitis, radiation colitis

Medications: laxative use and abuse, antibiotics, antineoplastics, colchicine, nonsteroidal anti-inflammatory drugs, acarbose, and others

Data from Murray JA, Rubio-Tapia A. Diarrhoea due to small bowel diseases. Best Pract Res Clin Gastroenterol 2012;26(5):581–600.

Parasitic

There are numerous parasitic causes of chronic diarrhea (*Cryptosporidium, Cyclospora, Entamoeba, Microsporidia, Strongyloides*) as seen in **Table 3**. The American College of Gastroenterology recommends consideration of the following cases for stool studies to look for ova and parasites: persistent diarrhea after travel to Russia, Nepal, mountainous regions, or in association with a day care center; diarrhea in patients with human immunodeficiency virus (HIV)/AIDS (see below); known outbreaks of *Giardia/Cryptosporidium*; and bloody diarrhea without a clear bacterial etiology because it may be the result of intestinal amebiasis. Specimens should be collected on 3 consecutive days to be complete so this testing needs to be instituted in the inpatient or outpatient setting.[34]

Giardia lamblia is the most common parasite among patients with chronic diarrhea.[35] It is a flagellated protozoan resulting in 280 million infections annually and is considered a neglected tropical disease by the WHO because of its disproportionate effect on children in developing countries.[36] The cyst form of the parasite is resistant and can be transmitted through contaminated food and water sources and is highly infectious. The giardiasis syndrome presents classically with severe abdominal cramping, bloating, and steatorrhea severe enough to result in weight loss.[36] It is thought that the parasite's products result in inflammation at the epithelial border causing the severe malabsorptive diarrhea.[37] *Giardia* may be treated presumptively with high dose metronidazole (500 mg 3 times a day for 7–10 days) with a suspected exposure and persistent diarrhea.[2] *Entamoeba histolytica* is another protozoan parasite transmitted through contaminated food and water that results in amebiasis (35–50 million cases annual cases predominantly in developing countries and particularly affecting children). The parasite is cytotoxic and, like giardia, should also be treated with metronidazole.[38]

Human Immunodeficiency Virus, AIDS, and Diarrhea

HIV and AIDS affects 33 million people worldwide.[39] Owing to the destruction of CD4 T lymphocytes, patients are at high risk of opportunistic infections, especially with CD4 counts of less than 350. Approximately 50% to 60% of these cases are owing to an identifiable infection source and the rest are owing to antiretroviral therapy, malabsorption states, and malignancies.[39–44] **Box 4** presents the most common identifiable causes of diarrhea in HIV patients and their recommended management.

Box 4
Common identifiable causes of diarrhea in HIV patients

Clostridium difficile

A patient on multiple antibiotics for PCP pneumonia presents to the ED with severe diarrhea, with multiple bowel movements. Cramping abdominal pain and clinical signs of dehydration. Patient has a low CD4 count and is cachectic looking in appearance.

Associated with antibiotic use and prophylactic treatment of PCP pneumonia[44]

Most common causes of diarrhea in patients with advanced AIDS[46]

Please see section on *C difficile* for more information

Cytomegalovirus

A patient with clinically documented AIDS presents to the ED with severe diarrhea. The patient also complains of increased weight loss, fever and severe abdominal pain with the diarrhea. The diarrhea is also associated with rectal bleeding. The patient looks dehydrated.

Most common viral GI infection in people with AIDS[46,47]

Symptoms include rectal bleeding, abdominal pain, fever and weight loss[46,48]

Treatment includes ganciclovir, foscarnet, and valganciclovir[49]

Cryptosporidium

A patient with HIV presents to the ED after a documented exposure to contaminated water source near a cattle farm. He states many of his friends with HIV have the same symptoms of watery diarrhea. He has lost weight and presents with tachycardia and hypotension.

Protozoa infection that causes 60,000 cases per year in the United States[46,50]

Increased risk in areas of poor sanitation[51–53]

Symptoms include watery diarrhea, malabsorptive state, severe dehydration, and electrolyte abnormalities[46,48,50]

Treatment includes supportive measures and treatment with nitazoxanide or rifampin[49]

Microsporidium

Protozoa that affects the small intestine[46]

Causes a malabsorptive state in immunocompetent patients[46]

Albendazole has seen treatment failure; other agents that have been used include metronidazole, azithromycin, and doxycycline

Entamoeba Histolytica

A patient with HIV presents with bright red blood per rectum, abdominal pain, and distention. The patient drank untreated water from a contaminated water source.

May cause colitis, ulceration, hematochezia, and toxic megacolon[46]

Treat with metronidazole

Mycobacterium avium Complex

A Patient with a CD4 count of less than 50 presents to the ED with cough, fever, weight loss, and diarrhea. Denies travel or known exposures to contaminated water or soil.

Found throughout the environment

Most infections occur through inhalation or ingestion

Can cause fever and weight loss[46]

Additional medications, such as amikacin or streptomycin, should be considered in severely immunocompromised patients (CD4 < 50)

Treatment includes a combination of clarithromycin and azithromcyin[49]

Protease Inhibitors

There is no change in the incidence of patients with chronic diarrhea with CD4 counts of less than 200[45]

There has been a decline in infectious diarrhea from 53% to 13%[45,46]

Although there has been a decrease in infectious causes, there has been an increase in noninfectious causes of diarrhea[45]

Treatment includes rehydration and repletion with electrolytes

Antidiarrheal agents, antimotility agents, and antisecretory agents have been used with success in limiting symptoms

Abbreviations: ED, emergency department; GI, gastrointestinal; HIV, human immunodeficiency virus; PCP, *Pneumocystis carinii* pneumonia.

Celiac Disease

Celiac disease, the most common inflammatory disorder of the small intestine in the Western world, may present as chronic diarrhea with weight loss, vitamin deficiency (iron, folic acid, B_{12}, and fat-soluble vitamins) and steatorrhea.[54] In the United States, more than 2 million persons have celiac disease, or about 1 in 133 persons, and this increases to as many as 1 in 22 persons if a first-degree relative is affected.[35] The inflammation results from an immune reaction against gluten that is present in wheat, barley, and rye and can be detected initially by tissue transglutaminase or endomysial antibodies and will ultimately require gastroenterological referral for biopsy (gold standard for diagnosis). Management focuses on a lifelong gluten-free diet.[54]

Pearls and pitfalls

- A thorough history and examination to evaluate for dehydration or risk for treatment failure should drive the initial management of a diarrheal illness.
- Practitioners can provide valuable education for patients and caregivers regarding symptomatic care and expected course of their illness.
- Antibiotics are associated with hemolytic uremic syndrome and should be avoided in patients presenting with bloody diarrhea and no fever.
- Notification of public health authorities is recommended if diarrheal illness is suspected from cholera, enterohemorrhagic *E coli*, *listeria*, *salmonella*, *shigella*, or norovirus.
- The initial emergency evaluation of chronic diarrhea should focus on stabilization with further testing coordinated with the patient's ongoing care provider.

REFERENCES

1. Thielman NM, Guerrant RL. Acute infectious diarrhea. N Engl J Med 2004;350: 38–47.

2. Guerrant RL, Van Gilder T, Steiner TS, et al. Practice guidelines for the management of infectious diarrhea. Clin Infect Dis 2001;32:331–50.
3. Churgay CA, Zahra A. Gastroenteritis in children: Part I. diagnosis. Am Fam Physician 2012;85:11.
4. Teach SJ, Yates EW, Feld LG. Laboratory predictors of fluid deficit in acutely dehydrated children. Clin Pediatr (Phila) 1997;36(7):395–400.
5. Steiner MJ, DeWalt DA, Byerley JS. Is this child dehydrated? JAMA 2004;291(22):2746–54.
6. Binder HJ, Brown I, Ramakrishna BS, et al. Oral rehydration therapy in the second decade of the twenty-first century. Curr Gastroenterol Rep 2014;16:376.
7. Fonseca BK, Holdgate A, Craig JC. Enteral vs intravenous rehydration therapy for children with gastroenteritis: a meta-analysis of randomized controlled trials. Arch Pediatr Adolesc Med 2004;158(5):483–90.
8. Pillow MT, Porter E, Hostetler MA. ACEP now focus on: current management of gastroenteritis in children. ACEP News 2008.
9. Murphy GS, Bodhidatta L, Echeverria P, et al. Ciprofloxacin and loperamide in the treatment of bacillary dysentery. Intern Med 1993;118(8):582.
10. Cimolai N, Carter JE, Morrison BJ, et al. Risk factors for the progression of Escherichia coli O157:H7 enteritis to hemolytic-uremic syndrome. J Pediatr 1990;116(4):589.
11. Steffen R. Worldwide efficacy of bismuth subsalicylate in the treatment of travelers' diarrhea. Rev Infect Dis 1990;12(Suppl 1):S80.
12. Lamberti LM, Walker CL, Chan KY, et al. Oral zinc supplementation for the treatment of acute diarrhea in children: a systematic review and meta-analysis. Nutrients 2013;5(11):4715–40.
13. Allen SJ, Martinez EG, Gregorio GV, et al. Probiotics for treating acute infectious diarrhoea. Cochrane Database Syst Rev 2010;(11):CD003048.
14. Centers for Disease Control and Prevention (CDC). Reduction in rotavirus after vaccine introduction - United States, 2000-2009. MMWR Morb Mortal Wkly Rep 2009;58:1146–9.
15. Wong CS, Jelacic S, Habeeb RL, et al. The risk of the hemolytic-uremic syndrome after antibiotic treatment of Escherichia coli O157:H7 infections. N Engl J Med 2000;342(26):1930.
16. Steffen R, Hill DR, Dupont HL. Traveler's diarrhea. A clinical review. JAMA 2015;313(1):71–80.
17. Baaten GG, Geskus RB, Kint JA, et al. Symptoms of infectious diseases in immunocompromised travelers. J Travel Med 2011;18(5):318–26.
18. Dupont HL, Ericsson CD, Farthing MJ, et al. Expert review of the evidence base for prevention of travelers' diarrhea. J Travel Med 2009;16(3):149–60.
19. Rao G, Aliwalas MG, Slaymaker E, et al. Bismuth revisited; an effective way to prevent traveler's diarrhea. J Travel Med 2004;11(4):239–41.
20. Dupont HL, Jiang ZD, Okhuysen PC, et al. A randomized, double-blind, placebo-controlled trial of rifaximin to prevent travelers' diarrhea. Ann Intern Med 2005;142(10):805–12.
21. Hu Y, Ren J, Zhan M, et al. Efficacy of rifaximin in prevention of travelers' diarrhea: a meta-analysis of randomized, double-blind, placebo-controlled trial. J Travel Med 2012;19(6):352–6.
22. Alajbegovic S, Sanders JW, Atherly DE, et al. Effectiveness of rifaximin and fluoroquinolones in preventing traveler's diarrhea (TD): a systematic review and meta-analysis. Syst Rev 2012;1:39.

23. Pandey P, Bodhidatta L, Lewis M, et al. Traveler's diarrhea in Nepal: an update on the pathogens and antibiotic resistance. J Travel Med 2011;18(2):102–8.

24. Ouyang-Latimer J, Jafri S, Van Tassel A, et al. In vitro antimicrobial susceptivility of bacterial enteropathogens isolated from international travelers to Mexico, Guatemala, and India from 2006-2008. Antimicrob Agents Chemother 2011; 55(2):874–8.

25. Tribble DR, Sanders JW, Pang LW, et al. Traveler's diarrhea in Thailand: randomized, double-blind trial comparing single-dose and 3-day azithromycin- based regimens with a 3-day levofloxacin regimen. Clin Infect Dis 2007;44(3):338–46.

26. Bottieau E, Clerinx J, Vilegehe E, et al. Epidemiology and outcome of Shigella, Salmonella and Campylobacter infections in travellers returning from the tropics with fever and diarrhoea. Acta Clin Belg 2011;66(3):191–5.

27. Bartlett JG. Narrative review: the new epidemic of clostridium difficile–associated enteric disease. Ann Intern Med 2006;145:758–64.

28. Bowen A, Hurd J, Hoover C, et al. Importation and domestic transmission of Shigella sonnei resistant to ciprofloxacin - United States, May 2014-February 2015. MMWR Morb Mortal Wkly Rep 2015;64(12):318–20.

29. Hensgens MP, Goorhuis A, Dekkers OM, et al. Time interval of increased risk for Clostridium difficile infection after exposure to antibiotics. J Antimicrob Chemother 2012;67(3):742–8.

30. Tintinalli JE, Stapczynski JS. Disorders presenting primarily with diarrhea. Tintinalli's emergency medicine: a comprehensive study guide. 7th edition. New York: McGraw-Hill; 2011. p. 531–40.

31. McDonald LC, Coignard B, Dubberke E, et al. Recommendations for surveillance of Clostridium difficile-associated disease. Infect Control Hosp Epidemiol 2007; 28(2):140–5.

32. Cornely OA, Miller MA, Louie TJ, et al. Treatment of first recurrence of Clostridium difficile infection: fidaxomicin versus vancomycin. Clin Infect Dis 2012;55(Suppl 2):S154–61.

33. Louie TJ, Miller MA, Mullane KM, et al. Fidaxomicin versus vancomycin for Clostridium difficile infection. N Engl J Med 2011;364(5):422–31.

34. DuPont AU. Guidelines on acute infectious diarrhea in adults. The Practice Parameters Committee of the American College of Gastroenterology. Am J Gastroenterol 1997;92(11):1962.

35. Juckett G, Trivedi R. Evaluation of chronic diarrhea. Am Fam Physician 2011; 84:10.

36. Bartelt LA, Sartor RB. Advances in understanding Giardia: determinants and mechanisms of chronic sequelae. F1000Prime Rep 2015;7:62.

37. Buret AG. Mechanisms of epithelial dysfunction in giardiasis. Gut 2007;56(3): 316–7.

38. Ralston KS, Petri WA. Tissue destruction and invasion by Entamoeba histolytica. Trends Parasitol 2011;27(6):254–63.

39. Nwachukwu CE, Okebe JU. Antimotility agents for chronic diarrhoea in people with HIV/AIDS. Cochrane Database Syst Rev 2008;(4):CD005644.

40. O'Brien ME, Clark RA, Besch CL, et al. Patterns and correlates of discontinuation of the initial HAART regimen in an urban outpatient cohort. J Acquir Immune Defic Syndr 2003;34(4):407–14.

41. Carcamo C, Hooton T, Wener MH, et al. Etiologies and manifestations of persistent diarrhoea in adults with HIV-1 infection: a case-control study in Lima, Peru. J Infect Dis 2005;191(1):11–9.

42. Silverberg MJ, Gore ME, French AL, et al. Prevalence of clinical symptoms associated with highly active antiretroviral therapy in the Women's Interagency HIV Study. Clin Infect Dis 2004;1(5):19–24.
43. Moyle GJ, Youle M, Higgs C, et al. Safety, pharmacokinetics and antiretroviral activity of the potent, specific human immunodeficiency virus protease inhibitor nelfinavir: results of a phase I/II trial and an extended follow-up in patients infected with human immunodeficiency virus. J Clin Pharmacol 1998;38:736–43.
44. Carr A, Cooper DA. Adverse effects of antiretroviral therapy. Lancet 2000;356: 1423–30.
45. Call SA, Heudebert G, Saag M, et al. The changing etiology of chronic diarrhea in HIV infected patients with CD4 cell counts less than 200 cells/mm3. Am J Gastroenterol 2000;95(11):3142–6.
46. Dikman AE, Schonfeld E, Srisarajivakul NC, et al. Human immunodeficiency virus-associated diarrhea: still an issue in the era of antiretroviral therapy. Dig Dis Sci 2015;60(8):2236–45.
47. Cello JP, Day LW. Idiopathic AID enteropathy and treatment of gastrointestinal opportunistic pathogens. Gastroenterology 2009;136:1952–65.
48. Lew EA, Poles MA, Dieterich DT. Diarrheal diseases associated with HIV infection. Gastroenterol Clin North Am 1997;26:259–90.
49. Thoden J, Potthoff A, Bogner JR, et al. Therapy and prophylaxis of opportunistic infections in HIV-infected patients: a guideline by the German and Austrian AIDS societies (DAIG/ÖAG) (AWMF 055/066). Infection 2013;41(Suppl 2):91–115.
50. Scallan E, Hoekstra RM, Angulo FJ, et al. Foodborne illness acquired in the United States—major pathogens. Emerg Infect Dis 2011;17(1):7–15.
51. Girma M, Teshome W, Petros B, et al. Cryptosporidiosis and Isosporiasis among HIV positive individuals in south Ethiopia: a cross sectional study. BMC Infect Dis 2014;14:100.
52. Mahmud MA, Bezabih AM, Gebru RB. Risk factors for intestinal parasitosis among antiretroviral-treated HIV/AIDS patients in Ethiopia. Int J STD AIDS 2014;25:778–84.
53. Baldursson S, Karanis P. Waterborne transmission of protozoan parasites: review of worldwide outbreaks- an update 2004-2010. Water Res 2011;45:6603–14.
54. Murray JA, Rubio-Tapia A. Diarrhoea due to small bowel diseases. Best Pract Res Clin Gastroenterol 2012;26(5):581–600.

Gastrointestinal Bleeding

Jose V. Nable, MD, MS, NRP[a],*, Autumn C. Graham, MD[b]

KEYWORDS

- Gastrointestinal bleeding • Hemorrhage • Upper gastrointestinal bleeding
- Lower gastrointestinal bleeding • Transfusion

KEY POINTS

- The emergency physician should have a structured approach to managing patients who present with acute gastrointestinal bleeding, directed toward preventing end-organ injury, limiting transfusion complications, averting rebleeding and managing comorbidities.
- Risk stratification is important to the management and disposition of patients with gastrointestinal bleeding, anticipating those who will need aggressive resuscitation and those who can be safely discharged home with outpatient management.
- Acute emergency department management may include localization of the bleed, appropriate volume and blood product resuscitation, vasoactive agents, antibiotics, reversal of anticoagulation, and specialty consultations.

INTRODUCTION

Gastrointestinal bleeding (GIB) is a serious, potentially life-threatening disease that leads to almost 1 million hospitalizations annually in the United States.[1,2] Because this is a commonly encountered chief complaint with high morbidity and mortality, the emergency physician is challenged to promptly diagnose, accurately risk assess, and aggressively resuscitate patients with gastrointestinal bleeding. Emergency medicine physicians are also tasked with identifying the subset of patients with GIB who can be safely discharged home with outpatient management. This article reviews risk stratification, diagnostic modalities, localization of bleeding, and management, including transfusion strategies and reversal of anticoagulation.

EPIDEMIOLOGY

GIB encompasses bleeding originating anywhere in the gastrointestinal tract, extending from the mouth to the anus. Most clinicians further delineate GIB by the location of

Disclosure Statement: The authors have nothing to disclose.
a Department of Emergency Medicine, MedStar Georgetown University Hospital, Georgetown University School of Medicine, 3800 Reservoir Road, Northwest, G-CCC, Washington, DC 20007, USA; b Department of Emergency Medicine, MedStar Georgetown University Hospital, MedStar Washington Hospital Center, 3800 Reservoir Road, Northwest, G-CCC, Washington, DC 20007, USA
* Corresponding author.
E-mail address: JoseVictor.L.Nable@medstar.net

bleeding. Upper gastrointestinal bleeding (UGIB), or bleeding from above the ligament of Treitz, and lower gastrointestinal bleeding (LGIB) each have unique etiologies (refer to **Box 1**), disease progression, and treatment.

The annual incidence of acute UGIB in the United States is estimated to be between 48 and 160 cases per 100,000.[3] The rates of UGIB are higher in men and the elderly.[3] The most common cause of UGIB remains peptic ulcer disease and accounts for up to 67% of UGIB fcases.[3,6] However, there has been a 23% decrease in admissions for UGIB from 2001 to 2009 and a corresponding 34% decrease in peptic ulcer disease admissions during that same time period.[7] Rebleeding rates with UGIB range from 25% to 30% in variceal bleeding and approximately 20% in peptic ulcer bleeding,[8] correlating with higher mortality rates ranging from 30% to 37%.[9] Risk factors for UGIB include *Helicobacter pylori* infection, nonsteroidal anti-inflammatory drugs (NSAIDs), antiplatelet medications, and anticoagulation. There is also a likely

---

Box 1
Etiologies of gastrointestinal bleeding

Upper Gastrointestinal Bleeding
- Peptic ulcer disease
- Gastritis
- Esophageal varices
- Gastric varices
- Vascular lesions
- Esophageal ulcer
- Malignancy
- Mallory-Weis tear
- Portal hypertensive gastropathy
- Aortoenteric fistula
- Crohn disease
- Pancreatic disease

Lower Gastrointestinal Bleeding
- Diverticular disease
- Gastrointestinal cancers
- Inflammatory bowel disease
- Colitis: ischemic, radiation, infectious
- Angiodysplasia
- Polyps
- Hemorrhoids
- Anal fissure
- Colonic ulcerations
- Rectal varices
- Upper gastrointestinal source

Data from Refs.[3–5]

association between selective serotonin reuptake inhibitors (SSRIs) and UGIBs. In a recent systematic review and meta-analysis of 22 studies with more than a million individuals, there was a twofold increase in risk of developing UGIB in those taking SSRIs.[10]

LGIB originates below the ligament of Treitz and has an estimated incidence of 20 patients per 100,000 annually.[11] The incidence increases with age and in one study, the average age of patients with LGIB was 75 years.[4] Risk factors for LGIBs include age, male sex, antiplatelet medications, NSAIDs, anticoagulation, and certain comorbid conditions such as human immunodeficiency virus.[11]

RISK STRATIFICATION OF GASTROINTESTINAL BLEEDING

GIB resolves spontaneously in up to 80% of patients and approximately 15% of patients will have continued bleeding that will require intervention.[12] Patients with GIB can be divided into 2 groups, high risk and low risk, with their emergency department evaluation and management customized to their anticipated course and disposition. High-risk patients are those whose continued bleeding will require interventions such as endoscopy, blood transfusion, or surgery, as well as those at risk for rebleeding, which is associated with higher morbidity and mortality rates. Low-risk patients are those who may need admission for a diagnostic workup or even those who may be safely discharged home with close outpatient follow-up but are unlikely to suffer poor outcomes.

Prognosis

The incidence of GIB increases with age and comorbidities, as does the mortality associated. Multiple studies have shown that most patients do not die from blood loss but rather end-organ injury, decompensation of comorbidities, and complications from subsequent blood transfusion. In one study of more than 10,000 patients with peptic ulcer disease, 80% of patients died of non–bleeding-related causes; mainly multiorgan failure, cardiopulmonary disease, and terminal malignancy.[13] Thus, prognosis correlates strongly with comorbidities. Identifying those patients at high risk for end-organ injury based on chronic medical conditions is imperative, specifically underlying pulmonary disease, coronary artery disease, cancer, liver disease, chronic alcoholism, and end-stage renal disease. Other historical features important for risk stratification include previous abdominal vascular surgery due to the risk of aortoenteric fistula development and the use of anticoagulants, including warfarin, novel anticoagulants, NSAIDs, and aspirin that independently are associated with worse outcomes. LGIB mortality also results from worsening comorbid conditions and nosocomial infection rather than severe bleeding.[14] In one study of LGIB patients, advanced age, intestinal ischemia, and comorbid illness were the strongest predictors of mortality.[5]

However, severe GIB, defined as documented GI blood loss with shock or a decrease in hematocrit level of 6%, does have a poor prognosis and is associated with mortality rates of 20% to 39%.[11,15] In massive GIB with hemodynamic instability, UGIB is the most likely source. Predictors of severe UGIB include nasogastric aspirate with red blood, tachycardia, and hemoglobin levels below 8 mg/L.[1] In LGIB, Strate and colleagues[5] identified 7 factors that correlated with severe bleeding; heart rate greater than 100 beats per minute, systolic blood pressure less than 115 mm Hg, syncope, nontender abdominal examination, rectal bleeding within first 4 hours of evaluation, use of aspirin and greater than 2 comorbid illnesses. In patients with more than 3 of the 7 factors, the likelihood of severe bleeding was 80%.

Historical Features and Physical Examination Findings

Initially, the patient's status can be determined by estimated blood volume loss and hemodynamic status. A patient's reported blood loss is often inaccurate. It is helpful to assess the degree of blood loss with a functional assessment. Dizziness, lightheadedness, syncope, confusion, and weakness may be indicative of hypovolemia. Chest pain and more often dyspnea or weakness can be symptoms of myocardial ischemia in the setting of GIB. Bright red hematemesis suggests recent or active bleeding from the esophagus, stomach, or duodenum, whereas coffee ground emesis suggests bleeding that has resolved. Melena is an important finding of significant blood loss but can be seen with as little as 50 mL of blood.[16]

Physical examination findings that correlate with low hemoglobin concentrations include color of the lower eyelid conjunctiva, nail bed rubor, nail bed blanching, and palmar crease rubor.[17] Abnormal vital signs should be followed closely in patients with suspected GIB. Supine tachycardia is one of the most sensitive, early vital sign abnormalities indicating clinically significant blood loss.[18] Orthostatics, in the setting of GIB, are recommended by multiple guidelines but its clinical value to identify hypovolemic patients remains controversial.[19]

Laboratory Studies

Laboratory data can be helpful in the risk stratification and resuscitation of patients with GIB. A low initial hemoglobin less than 10 g/dL has been associated with higher mortality rates.[20] However, a normal hemoglobin level can be falsely reassuring, as it can take up to 24 hours to accurately reflect the degree of blood loss. Coagulation profiles, platelet counts, and liver function tests can be helpful to assess for coagulopathy. As well, electrocardiogram and troponin should be liberally used to assess for coronary ischemia, as patients with GIB often experience ischemia without chest pain. In patients with known CAD, GIB is independently associated with higher mortality rates and ischemic complications.[21]

Lactate has been well validated in trauma literature to aid clinicians in the assessment of acute blood loss. In critically ill patients admitted for GIB, El-Kersh and colleagues[22] demonstrated that an admission lactate was predictive of outcome with a high sensitivity but low specificity. The median lactate level for nonsurvivors was 8.8 compared with 2.0 in survivors. Shah and colleagues[20] found that inpatient mortality was 6.4-fold higher in those patients with an ED lactate greater than 4 mmol/L. In hemodynamically stable patients, point of care lactate elevation greater than 2.5 mmol/L was associated with hypotension within 24 hours with a 90% specificity and 84% negative predictive value and with a lactate greater than 5 mmol/L the specificity increased to 98% with a negative predictive value of 87%.[23]

Prediction Scores

Multiple clinical prediction rules have been developed over the past couple of decades. In 1997, Kollef and colleagues[24] in the original BLEED study developed a prediction rule to risk stratify patients in the emergency department with UGIB or LGIB as high or low risk of developing in-hospital complications of rebleeding, surgery or mortality. Kollef and colleagues[24] found that visualized bleeding, hypotension, an elevated prothrombin time, "erratic" mental status, or unstable comorbid disease correlated with in-hospital complications and intensive care level care. Das and colleagues[25] performed a derivation and validation study testing the original BLEED criteria with a triage simulation model to determine high risk patients that should be admitted to the ICU versus low risk patients that would be stable for the floor. Das and colleagues[25] concluded that using the original BLEED criteria would result in unnecessary critical care admissions whereas a combination of visualized red blood by emesis or nasogastric aspirate and/or unstable comorbidities would more accurately assess which patients were at risk for decompensation in the first 24 hours of admission.

The 2 most commonly used clinical decision rules in the ED are the pre-endoscopic (Clinical) Rockall Score (CRS) and the Glasgow Blatchford Score (GBS). In 1996, Rockall and colleagues[26] identified independent risk factors to accurately predict mortality. The scoring system uses clinical criteria (increasing age, comorbidity, shock) but disregards the endoscopic components (diagnosis, stigmata of acute bleeding) included in the full Rockall Score. In 2000, Blatchford and colleagues[27] reported a prospective validation of a risk score based solely on clinical criteria that assesses the likelihood that a patient with an UGIB will need to have interventions, such as blood transfusion or endoscopy. Both GBS and CRS can accurately predict patients at risk for re-bleeding and mortality. However, GBS has been shown to be superior to the Rockall Score for predicting the need for admission, blood transfusion, or surgery.[28,29] Furthermore, in one controlled study, a low-risk subset of patients with a GBS of 0 accounting for 16% of the study group were found to have no deaths or require interventions. The investigators concluded that these patients could be safely managed in an outpatient setting and subsequent studies extending the low-risk group to a GBS less than 1 concurs.[30,31]

The AIMS65 score was developed and validated from a large database to predict inpatient mortality.[32] AIMS65 is easy to use with a simple score calculation and well adapted for use in the emergency department. However, in a comparison study of AIMS65 to the Glasgow Blatchford Score, GBS was superior or equal to AIMS65 for all clinically relevant outcomes, including rebleeding, endoscopy, surgery, intensive care admission, and 30-day mortality.[33] GBS was also superior to AIMS65 in identifying the lowest risk patients who might be appropriate for discharge.[34]

See **Table 1** for risk stratification scores.

Summary

Early identification of high-risk patients allows appropriate and timely interventions that may improve morbidity and mortality. Clinical predictors of increased risk for rebleeding or mortality include age older than 65 years, shock, poor overall health, comorbid illnesses, low initial hemoglobin levels, tachycardia, hypotension, melena, transfusion requirement, fresh red blood on rectal examination or in the emesis, blood on nasogastric aspirate, sepsis, elevated blood urea nitrogen (BUN), or elevated prothrombin time.[1] Other factors predictive of poor outcomes include chronic alcoholism, active cancer, or poor social support conditions.[45]

LOCALIZATION OF THE BLEED

Following initial stabilization, the emergency department evaluation and treatment of patients with a suspected upper GI bleed differs from those with a lower GI bleed. Thus, the emergency physician is first tasked with attempting to differentiate the suspected location of bleeding. Patients presenting with hematemesis are nearly always found to have an upper GI source of bleeding.[3] It is the patients with a GIB without hematemesis who are diagnostically challenging in determining their source of bleeding. Several factors, however, can be useful at assisting the emergency physician in differentiating an LGIB from an UGIB.

Table 1
Clinical decision rules for upper gastrointestinal bleeding

Rockall Score		Glasgow Blatchford Score		AIMS65	
Variable	Value	Variable	Value	Variable	Value
Age		*BUN mmol/L*			
<60	0	6.5–8.0	2	Albumin <3 mg/dL	1
60–79	1	8.0–10.0	3		
>80	2	10.0–25.0	4	INR >1.5	1
Shock		>25	6		
No Shock	0	*Hemoglobin (men)*		Altered Mental Status	1
Pulse >100 With SBP >100	1	12–12.9	1		
SBP <100	2	10.0–11.9	3	Systolic blood pressure >90 mm Hg	1
Comorbidity		<10.0	6		
None	0	*Hemoglobin (women)*		Age >65	1
CHF CAD Major morbidity	2	10.0–11.9	1		
Renal failure Liver failure Metastatic caner	3	<10.0	6		
Criteria for full Rockall below		*SBP mm Hg*			
		100–109	1		
Diagnosis		90–99	2		
Mallory Weiss	0	<90	3		
All other diagnoses	1	*Other Markers*			
GI malignancy	2	Pulse >100 (per min)	1		
		Presentation with melena	1		
Evidence of Bleeding		Presentation with syncope	2		
None	0	Hepatic disease	2		
Blood, adherent clot, spurting vessel	2	Cardiac failure	2		
Interpretation					
Score <3 good prognosis, Score >8 high risk of mortality		Score >6 associated with 50% risk of requiring intervention in UGIB patients		Risk factor correlation with mortality rate 0 = 0.3% 1 = 1% 2 = 3% 4 = 15% 5 = 25%	

Abbreviations: BUN, blood urea nitrogen; CAD, coronary artery disease; CHF, congestive heart failure; INR, international normalized ratio; SBP, systolic blood pressure; UGIB, upper gastrointestinal bleeding.
Data from Refs.[26,27,32,33]

Examination of Stool

A close examination of the patient's stool is naturally required for any patient with a suspected GIB. The presence of melena, for example, suggests an upper GI source of bleeding. With a demonstrated sensitivity of 80% in predicting an upper GI source,[46] and a likelihood ratio of up to 5.9,[1] the finding of melanotic stools is highly useful in localizing a GIB.

Although hemoccult-positive stool has often been used to detect LGIBs,[47] positive results of this test do not completely rule-out an upper GI source. A study by Lee and colleagues,[7] for example, found the guaiac-based test to be 17.9% sensitive at detecting an upper GI source.

Nasogastric Tube Aspiration

Controversy surrounds the placement of nasogastric tube (NGT) for aspiration in patients with suspected UGIBs, especially those without hematemesis.[48] One retrospective study found that in patients admitted for GIBs without hematemesis, bloody nasogastric aspiration (NGA) had a positive likelihood ratio of 11 in detecting a UGIB.[49] A negative NGA, however, had a likelihood ratio of 0.6, providing no useful diagnostic data. A recent systematic review also questioned the diagnostic utility for NGA, with sensitivity for upper GI bleeding ranging from 42% to 84%.[50] Nonetheless, a positive NGA has been demonstrated to predict the presence of high-risk lesions at risk for rebleeding, with a 75.8% specificity.[51]

Although a positive nasogastric aspiration is highly predictive of a UGIB,[1] emergency physicians cannot rely solely on placement of a nasogastric tube to determine the need for emergent endoscopy. The clinician should discuss with the gastroenterologist how placement of the NGT will affect the timing in performing an upper endoscopy given that NGT placement is an uncomfortable and painful procedure for patients.

Blood Urea Nitrogen:Creatinine Ratio

An increase in BUN in many patients with UGIB has long been documented in the literature.[52] More specifically, the ratio of BUN to creatinine (Cr) has been suggested as a means of differentiating UGIB from LGIB.[53] In addition to decreased perfusion of the kidneys, it has been hypothesized that this finding may be due to the absorption of digested blood.[54]

A systematic review found that a BUN:Cr ratio of greater than 30 is 93% specific for a UGIB, with a positive likelihood ratio of 7.5.[1] Although the sensitivity of this method is relatively low (39% in a study by Witting and colleagues[45]), a positive test is highly predictive of an upper GI source in the setting of GIB.

Age

The prevalence of LGIB is directly associated with age.[9] Indeed, a patient's relative youth has been demonstrated to be an independent predictor for UGIB. One study found that age younger than 50 years to be 92% specific for an upper GI source, with a positive likelihood ratio of 3.5.[22]

TREATMENT

The emergency physician must expeditiously evaluate and treat all patients with a suspected acute GIB. These patients are at risk for rapid deterioration. A minimum of 2 large-bore intravenous catheters should be placed. Those with significant UGIB may require intubation for airway protection. **Table 2** summarizes the following suggested treatment modalities for patients presenting with an acute GIB.

Table 2
Treatment of gastrointestinal bleeding

Treatment	
RBC transfusion	UGIB: • Indicated for exsanguinating hemorrhage. • Less than massive hemorrhage: Consider restrictive transfusion strategy to goal hemoglobin of 9.[35] LGIB: • Patient-specific, taking into account hemodynamic status.[36]
Platelet transfusion	Insufficient data for clear guidelines.[37]
Anticoagulation reversal	Vitamin K • IV vitamin K for patients on VKA with hemodynamic instability or large bleed.[38] • Oral vitamin K for patients on VKA with minor bleeding and INR >5.[39] PCC • Indicated for patients on VKA with unstable active bleeding.[39] • Consider FFP if PCC unavailable.
Proton pump inhibitor	Consider for all suspected UGIB.[40]
Somatostatin or octreotide	Consider for UGIB, especially suspected variceal-related bleeding.[41]
Vasopressin	Not recommended.[42]
Antibiotics	Consider for UGIB ceftriaxone 1 g IV.[43]
Tranexamic acid	Insufficient data for clear guidelines.[44]

Abbreviations: FFP, fresh frozen plasma; INR, international normalized ratio; IV, intravenous; LGIB, lower gastrointestinal bleeding; PCC, prothrombin complex concentrate; RBC, red blood cell; UGIB, upper gastrointestinal bleeding; VKA, vitamin K antagonist.

Red Blood Cell Transfusion

Patients with massive hemorrhage should emergently receive red blood cell transfusions. Rapid bleeding can result in significant loss of oxygen-binding capacity, leading to ischemia. A transfusion strategy, however, is more challenging in patients without exsanguinating hemorrhage, as transfusions carry significant risks to patients.[55–57] In euvolemic UGIB patients without a history of coronary artery disease, guidelines recommend transfusing red blood cells to a goal hemoglobin of 7 g/dL.[58] One study demonstrated that a restrictive transfusion strategy (goal hemoglobin 7 g/dL) in patients with UGIB had higher rates of 6-week survival when compared with a liberal transfusion strategy (goal hemoglobin 9 g/dL).[35]

Villaneuva and colleagues[35] found that the rates of further bleeding and transfusion-related adverse reactions were also less in the restrictive strategy group for patients with UGIB. Restitution of blood volume has been shown to be associated with portal hypertensive-related bleeding.[59] It is possible that transfusing too aggressively may exacerbate portal hypertension, leading to increased bleeding.

For patients with acute LGIB, the decision to provide red blood cell transfusions must be tailored to the individual patient. No specific target hemoglobin has been identified.[36] Instead, the clinician should evaluate the patient's hemodynamic status and assess the risks of infection, coagulopathies, and other transfusion-related adverse reactions.

Platelet Transfusion

Although the use of antiplatelet drugs, such as aspirin, has been shown to increase the risk of gastrointestinal hemorrhage,[60] the role of platelet transfusions during acute bleeds remains unclear. There are insufficient data in the literature to support a target transfusion goal for platelets.[37] Although a target of 50,000/μL has been suggested, this is based solely on expert opinion.[61]

Anticoagulation Reversal

Patients on anticoagulation therapies are at increased risk for an acute GIB.[62] The emergency physician must be prepared to reverse the effects of these medications in patients with ongoing GI bleeding. For patients on vitamin K antagonists (VKA), such as warfarin, presenting with active bleeding and hemodynamic compromise, intravenous vitamin K should be administered.[38] The clinician should recognize that it takes up to 12 hours to fully reverse VKA with vitamin K. Rapid reversal of coagulopathy is recommended with prothrombin complex concentrate (PCC), or fresh frozen plasma (FFP) if PCC is unavailable, in unstable actively bleeding patients.[39,51]

For actively bleeding patients without hemodynamic instability, intravenous vitamin K should still be administered.[51] The concomitant use of PCC or FFP may be considered in patients with a supratherapeutic international normalized ratio (INR), particularly those undergoing endoscopy within 6 to 12 hours.[51] For patients with minor GIB on VKA, oral vitamin K can be administered to those with an INR greater than 5.[51]

Because of the relative novelty of direct oral anticoagulants, such as dabigatran or rivaroxaban, the ideal strategy for managing acute GIB in these patients remains unclear.[63] In general, fluid resuscitation can promote renal metabolism of these drugs.[53] The off-label use of PCC may be considered in patients with significant bleeding.[64] Recombinant Factor VIIa has also been suggested in these situations, although data are limited to in vitro studies and healthy human volunteers.[65]

Idarucizumab has recently been shown to be effective at reversing dabigatran in an interim analysis of a prospective cohort study of patients with serious bleeding.[66] The final results of this study, however, are still pending.

Proton Pump Inhibitor

Intravenous proton pump inhibitor (PPI) therapy is recommended in patients with acute UGIB.[34] When given before endoscopy, PPIs have been shown to reduce stigmata of recent hemorrhage seen during endoscopy and the need for endoscopic intervention.[40,67] For ulcer-related UGIB, the use of PPIs is associated with decreased rates of rebleeding and need for surgery.[68] As the exact location of an UGIB may not be clearly known before endoscopy, the emergency physician should consider giving a PPI to all patients with a suspected upper GI source.

Somatostatin/Octreotide

Somatostatin and longer-acting octreotide reduce splanchnic blood flow and acid production.[69] Both these drugs can reduce the risks for continued bleeding in UGIB, regardless of the presence or absence of bleeding varices.[41,59] Although a Cochrane review found no effect on mortality, the rates of continued bleeding and need for transfusions are decreased when giving somatostatin for variceal-related UGIB.[70]

Vasopressin

Vasopressin has been used for variceal bleeds, as it reduces splanchic blood flow and decreases portal blood pressure.[71] However, significant systemic side effects, such as cardiac and bowel ischemia, are associated with vasopressin.[72] These deleterious effects have greatly limited the use of this vasoactive agent.[42]

Antibiotics

Patients with liver cirrhosis presenting with UGIB are at an increased risk for bacterial infection, with one study finding 36% of such patients developing an infection within 7 days of admission.[73] Rebleeding is also more likely in patients who develop bacterial infections.[38] Short-term prophylactic antibiotics in patients with cirrhosis patients presenting with acute GIB have been shown to improve survival.[74,75] Although oral norfloxacin has previously been a mainstay of prophylactic therapy,[76] 1 g intravenous ceftriaxone has been demonstrated to be more effective at preventing serious bacterial infections.[43]

Tranexamic Acid

The antifibrinolytic properties of tranexamic acid (TXA) have been shown to be beneficial in critically ill trauma patients, significantly reducing the risk of death.[77] Its role in acute GIB, however, remains unclear. Although a recent Cochrane review suggests a potential mortality benefit associated with TXA in patients with GIB, there are relatively few studies from which to draw a more definitive conclusion.[44] A large study examining the potential benefit of TXA with plans to enroll 8000 patients is currently under way.[78]

Balloon Tamponade

Balloon tamponade may be considered in an exsanguinating patient with UGIB as a temporizing measure until endoscopy is performed. The Sengstaken-Blakemore and Minnesota tubes are available, with both tubes consisting of esophageal and gastric balloons.[63] Significant complications, however, are associated with these tubes, including esophageal rupture, pressure necrosis, and aspiration pneumonia.[63,79,80] As balloon tamponade is a temporizing measure until definitive endoscopy, it should therefore be reserved for unstable patients with ongoing life-threatening bleeding refractory to all other treatments in whom endoscopy cannot be immediately performed.

IMAGING AND ENDOSCOPY
Upper Endoscopy

For patients with acute UGIB, upper endoscopy both confirms the source and allows potential control of bleeding. Early endoscopy (variably defined as endoscopy within 2–24 hours of presentation) has been shown to be safe and effective in all risk groups.[81] The emergency physician, however, may find it useful to discuss appropriate timing of an endoscopy for each patient with the gastroenterologist. Higher-risk patients, such as those with tachycardia, hypotension, bloody emesis, or nasogastric aspirate, have been shown to have a mortality benefit when endoscopy is performed within 12 hours of presentation.[34,82]

Hematochezia may be indicative of a brisk UGIB.[83] It is therefore reasonable to perform an upper endoscopy before colonoscopy in unstable patients with hematochezia.[36]

Video capsule endoscopy may emerge as an alternative to traditional endoscopy for patients with suspected UGIB. One study demonstrated the ability of emergency physicians to accurately detect GIB via this modality.[84] Further studies examining this modality are necessary, especially because the typical emergency physician is not trained to interpret video endoscopy.

Colonoscopy

Colonoscopy potentially allows for localization of the source of an LGIB. Colonoscopy may also allow for treatment of some cases of LGIB, possibly avoiding a colectomy.[85] Epinephrine injection and endoscopic band ligation are available therapies via colonoscopy, and are particularly useful for acute diverticular bleeds.[71,86] In patients with acute hematochezia, urgent colonoscopy without bowel preparation has been shown to safe and useful, localizing bleeding in 89% of cases in one study.[87]

Angiography

For patients with brisk LGIB, angiography potentially allows for localization and therapeutic intervention. Angiography also may be useful if endoscopy is unsuccessful at locating the source of bleeding.[88] Although it has traditionally been taught that a bleeding rate of 0.5 to 1.0 mL per minute is needed to detect via angiogram, digital subtraction angiography has been shown to be much more sensitive.[89] Angiography offers the ability to perform transcatheter embolization, which is particularly effective for LGIB.[90] Angiography, however, is not without possible complications. In particular, patients are at risk of acute kidney injury, contrast reactions, and bowel ischemia.[91] Angiography is therefore typically reserved for those with massive, ongoing bleeding in whom endoscopy is not possible or when colonoscopy is unable to locate the source of bleeding.[47]

Nuclear Scan

A nuclear scan with technetium Tc 99m–labeled red blood cells offers a noninvasive technique of detecting a bleed. Nuclear scans are more sensitive, but less specific, than angiography at hemorrhage localization, requiring a bleeding rate of at least 0.1 mL per minute.[92,93] Although nuclear scans are by themselves not therapeutic, their results can be used to guide treatment modalities, such as endoscopy, surgery, or angiography.

VARICEAL BLEEDING

By the time liver cirrhosis is diagnosed, varices are present in 30% of patients who are stable and 60% of those who are unstable.[90] Bleeding from varices is a medical emergency with a high mortality rate. However, with increased recognition and advances in care, the mortality rate for variceal bleeding has decreased from 43% in 1980 to 15% in 2000, representing a decrease in rebleeding and bacterial infections. On multivariable analysis, endoscopic therapy and antibiotic prophylaxis were independent predictors of survival.[94]

Because acute variceal bleeds can result in significant hemorrhaging, the emergency physician must ensure that at least 2 large-bore intravenous (IV) catheters are placed in these patients. Excessive volume resuscitation, however, may be harmful by deleteriously raising portal pressures.[63] Transfusions of red blood cells may be targeted to a goal hemoglobin of 9 g/dL to avoid transfusion-related adverse reactions.[45] Advanced airway management may be required, especially those who present with altered mental status or massive bleeding. Portal pressures should be reduced using vasoactive agents such as octreotide and somatostatin. Additionally, empiric antibiotic therapy with ceftriaxone can improve survival.[65] Finally, the emergency physician should consult with gastroenterology to potentially perform endoscopy, ligating sources of variceal bleeding.

PEARLS AND PITFALLS

- The emergency physician should have a structured approach to managing patients who present with acute GIB, directed toward preventing end-organ injury, limiting transfusion complications, averting rebleeding, and managing comorbidities.
- Risk stratification is important to the management and disposition of patients with GIB, anticipating those who will need aggressive resuscitation and those who can be safely discharged home with outpatient management.
  - Patients with UGIB can be effectively risk stratified by using the Glasgow Blatchford Score (GBS).
  - Patients with a GBS of 0 can likely be discharged with close outpatient follow-up established.
- Acute emergency department management may include localization of the bleed, appropriate volume and blood product resuscitation, vasoactive agents, antibiotics, reversal of anticoagulation, and specialty consultations.
  - A restrictive transfusion protocol (hemoglobin <7) should be followed in clinically stable patients.
  - A BUN:Cr ratio greater than 30 in patients without kidney injury suggests a UGIB, whereas advancing age suggests an LGIB.
  - PPIs are recommended for suspected UGIB; octreotide and ceftriaxone are recommended for variceal bleeding.

REFERENCES

1. Srygley FD, Gerardo CJ, Tran T, et al. Does this patient have a severe upper gastrointestinal bleed? JAMA 2012;307(10):1072–9.
2. Lewis JD, Bilker WB, Brensinger C, et al. Hospitalization and mortality rates from peptic ulcer disease and GI bleeding in the 1990s: Relationship to sales of nonsteroidal anti-inflammatory drugs and acid suppression medications. Am J Gastroenterol 2002;97:2540–9.
3. Rotondano G. Epidemiology and diagnosis of acute nonvariceal upper gastrointestinal bleeding. Gastroenterol Clin North Am 2014;43(4):643–63.
4. Das A, Ben-Menachem T, Cooper GS, et al. Prediction of outcome in acute lower gastrointestinal haemorrhage based on an artificial neural network: internal and external validation of a predictive model. Lancet 2003;362:1261–6.
5. Strate L, Ayanian J, Kotler G, et al. Risk factors for mortality in lower intestinal bleeding. Clin Gastroenterol Hepatol 2008;6(9):1004–10.
6. Khamaysi I, Gralnek IM. Acute upper gastrointestinal bleeding (UGIB)–initial evaluation and management. Best Pract Res Clin Gastroenterol 2013;27(5):633–8.
7. Lee YC, Chiu HM, Chiang TH, et al. Accuracy of faecal occult blood test and *Helicobacter pylori* stool antigen test for detection of upper gastrointestinal lesions. BMJ Open 2013;3(10):e003989.
8. van Leerdam ME. Epidemiology of acute upper gastrointestinal bleeding. Best Pract Res Clin Gastroenterol 2008;22(2):209–24.
9. Blatchford O, Davidson LA, Murray WR, et al. Acute upper gastrointestinal haemorrhage in east of Scotland; case ascertainment study. BMJ 1997;315(7107):510–4.
10. Jiang HY, Chen HZ, Hu X, et al. Use of selective serotonin reuptake inhibitors and risk of upper gastrointestinal bleeding: a systematic review and meta-analysis. Clin Gastroenterol Hepatol 2015;13:42–50.

11. Hussain H, Lapin S, Cappell MS. Clinical scoring systems for determining the prognosis of gastrointestinal bleeding. Gastroenterol Clin North Am 2000;29(2): 445–64.
12. Peura DA, Lanza FL, Gostout CJ, et al. The American College of Gastroenterology bleeding registry: preliminary findings. Am J Gastroenterol 1997;92(6): 924–8.
13. Sung J, Tsoi KE, Ma T, et al. Causes of mortality in patients with peptic ulcer bleeding: a prospective cohort study of 10,428 cases. Am J Gastroenterol 2010;105:84–9.
14. Longstreth GF. Epidemiology and outcome of patients hospitalized with acute lower gastrointestinal hemorrhage: a population-based study. Am J Gastroenterol 1997;92(3):419–24.
15. Afessa B. Triage of patients with acute gastrointestinal bleeding for intensive care unit admission based on risk factors for poor outcome. J Clin Gastroenterol 2000; 30(3):281–5.
16. Schiff L, Stevens R, Shaprio N, et al. Observations on the oral administration of citrated blood in man. Am J Med Sci 1942;203:409–12.
17. Strobach RS, Anderson SK, Doll DC, et al. The value of the physical examination in the diagnosis of anemia: correlation of the physical findings and the hemoglobin concentration. Arch Intern Med 1988;148(4):831–2.
18. Chappell MS, Friedel D. Initial management of acute upper gastrointestinal bleeding: from initial evaluation to gastrointestinal endoscopy. Med Clin North Am 2008;92:491–509.
19. McGee S, Abernethy WB 3rd, Simel DL. The rational clinical examination. Is this patient hypovolemic? JAMA 1999;281(11):1022–9.
20. Shah A, Chisolm-Straker M, Alexander A, et al. Prognostic use of lactate to predict inpatient mortality in acute gastrointestinal hemorrhage. Am J Emerg Med 2014;32:752–5.
21. Nikolsky E, Stone GW, Kirtane AJ, et al. Gastrointestinal bleeding in patients with acute coronary syndromes: incidence, predictors, and clinical implications: analysis from the ACUITY (Acute Catheterization and Urgent Intervention Triage Strategy) trial. J Am Coll Cardiol 2009;54(14):1293–302.
22. El-Kersh K, Chaddha U, Siddhartha R, et al. Predictive role of admission lactate level in critically ill patients with acute upper gastrointestinal bleeding. J Emerg Med 2015;49(3):318–25.
23. Ko B, Kim W, Ryoo S, et al. Predicting the occurrence of hypotension in stable patients with nonvariceal upper gastrointestinal bleeding: point of care lactate testing. Crit Care Med 2015;43:2409–15.
24. Kollef MF, O'Brien JD, Zuckerman GR, et al. BLEED: a classification tool to predict outcomes in patients with acute upper and lower gastrointestinal hemorrhage. Crit Care Med 1997;25:1125–32.
25. Das AM, Sood N, Hodgin K, et al. Development of a triage protocol for patients presenting with gastrointestinal hemorrhage: a prospective cohort study. Crit Care 2008;12:R57.
26. Rockall TA, Logan RF, Devlin HB, et al. Risk assessment after acute upper gastrointestinal bleeding. Gut 1996;38(3):316–21.
27. Blatchford O, Murray WR, Blatchford M. A risk score to predict need for treatment for upper gastrointestinal haemorrhage. Lancet 2000;356(9238):1318–21.
28. Bryant RV, Kuo P, Williamson K, et al. Performance of the Glasgow-Blatchford score in predicting clinical outcomes and intervention in hospitalized patients with upper GI bleeding. Gastrointest Endosc 2013;78(4):576–8.

29. Srirajaskanthan R, Conn R, Bulwer C, et al. The Glasgow Blatchford scoring system enables accurate risk stratification of patients with upper gastrointestinal haemorrhage. Int J Clin Pract 2010;64:868–74.

30. Stanley AJ, Ashley D, Dalton HR, et al. Outpatient management of patients with low-risk upper gastrointestinal haemorrhage: multicentre validation and prospective evaluation. Lancet 2009;373:42–7.

31. Mustafa Z, Cameron A, Clark E, et al. Outpatient management of low risk patients with upper gastrointestinal bleeding: can we safely extend the Glasgow Blatchford Score in clinical practice? Eur J Gastroenterol Hepatol 2015;27(5):512–5.

32. Saltzman JR, Tabak YP, Hyett BH, et al. A simple risk score accurately predicts in-hospital mortality, length of stay and cost in acute upper GI bleeding. Gastrointest Endosc 2011;74(6):1215.

33. Hyett BH, Abougergi MS, Charpentier JP, et al. The AIM65 score compared with the Glasgow-Blatchford score in predicting outcomes in upper GI bleeding. Gastrointest Endosc 2013;77(4):551.

34. Yaka E, Yilmaz S, Dogan N, et al. Comparison of the Glasgow-Blatchford and AIMS65 scoring systems for risk stratification in upper gastrointestinal bleeding in the emergency department. Acad Emerg Med 2015;22(1):23–30.

35. Villanueva C, Colomo A, Bosch A, et al. Transfusion strategies for acute upper gastrointestinal bleeding. N Engl J Med 2013;368(1):11–21.

36. Zuccaro G Jr. Management of the adult patient with acute lower gastrointestinal bleeding. American College of Gastroenterology. Practice Parameters Committee. Am J Gastroenterol 1998;93(8):1202–8.

37. Maltz GS, Siegel JE, Carson JL. Hematologic management of gastrointestinal bleeding. Gastroenterol Clin North Am 2000;29(1):169–87.

38. Radaelli F, Dentali F, Repici A, et al. Management of anticoagulation in patients with acute gastrointestinal bleeding. Dig Liver Dis 2015;47(8):621–7.

39. Holbrook A, Schulman S, Witt DM, et al. Evidence-based management of anticoagulant therapy: antithrombotic therapy and prevention of thrombosis, 9th ed: American College of chest physicians evidence-based clinical practice guidelines. Chest 2012;141(2 Suppl):e152S–84S.

40. Sreedharan A, Martin J, Leontiadis GI, et al. Proton pump inhibitor treatment initiated prior to endoscopic diagnosis in upper gastrointestinal bleeding. Cochrane Database Syst Rev 2010;(7):CD005415.

41. Jenkins SA, Shields R, Davies M, et al. A multicentre randomised trial comparing octreotide and injection sclerotherapy in the management and outcome of acute variceal haemorrhage. Gut 1997;41(4):526–33.

42. Dib N, Oberti F, Calès P. Current management of the complications of portal hypertension: variceal bleeding and ascites. CMAJ 2006;174(10):1433–43.

43. Fernández J, Ruiz del Arbol L, Gómez C, et al. Norfloxacin vs ceftriaxone in the prophylaxis of infections in patients with advanced cirrhosis and hemorrhage. Gastroenterology 2006;131(4):1049–56.

44. Bennett C, Klingenberg SL, Langholz E, et al. Tranexamic acid for upper gastrointestinal bleeding. Cochrane Database Syst Rev 2014;(11):CD006640.

45. Palmer ED. The vigorous diagnostic approach to upper-gastrointestinal tract hemorrhage. A 23 year prospective study of 1400 patients. JAMA 1969;207:1477.

46. Witting MD, Magder L, Heins AE, et al. ED predictors of upper gastrointestinal tract bleeding in patients without hematemesis. Am J Emerg Med 2006;24(3):280–5.

47. Rockey DC, Auslander A, Greenberg PD. Detection of upper gastrointestinal blood with fecal occult blood tests. Am J Gastroenterol 1999;94(2):344–50.

48. Pallin DJ, Saltzman JR. Is nasogastric tube lavage in patients with acute upper GI bleeding indicated or antiquated? Gastrointest Endosc 2011;74(5):981–4.

49. Witting MD, Magder L, Heins AE, et al. Usefulness and validity of diagnostic nasogastric aspiration in patients without hematemesis. Ann Emerg Med 2004; 43(4):525–32.

50. Palamidessi N, Sinert R, Falzon L, et al. Nasogastric aspiration and lavage in emergency department patients with hematochezia or melena without hematemesis. Acad Emerg Med 2010;17(2):126–32.

51. Aljebreen AM, Fallone CA, Barkun AN. Nasogastric aspirate predicts high-risk endoscopic lesions in patients with acute upper-GI bleeding. Gastrointest Endosc 2004;59(2):172–8.

52. Black DAK. Critical review. Azotemia in gastro-duodenal hemorrhage. Q J Med 1942;11:77–104.

53. Richards RJ, Donica MB, Grayer D. Can the blood urea nitrogen/creatinine ratio distinguish upper from lower gastrointestinal bleeding? J Clin Gastroenterol 1990; 12(5):500–4.

54. Ernst AA, Haynes ML, Nick TG, et al. Usefulness of the blood urea nitrogen/creatinine ratio in gastrointestinal bleeding. Am J Emerg Med 1999;17(1):70–2.

55. Hébert PC, Wells G, Blajchman MA, et al. A multicenter, randomized, controlled clinical trial of transfusion requirements in critical care. Transfusion requirements in critical care investigators, Canadian critical care trials group. N Engl J Med 1999;340(6):409–17.

56. Malone DL, Dunne J, Tracy JK, et al. Blood transfusion, independent of shock severity, is associated with worse outcome in trauma. J Trauma 2003;54(5): 898–905.

57. Rohde JM, Dimcheff DE, Blumberg N, et al. Health care-associated infection after red blood cell transfusion: a systematic review and meta-analysis. JAMA 2014; 311(13):1317–26.

58. Laine L, Jensen DM. Management of patients with ulcer bleeding. Am J Gastroenterol 2012;107(3):345–60.

59. Castañeda B, Morales J, Lionetti R, et al. Effects of blood volume restitution following a portal hypertensive-related bleeding in anesthetized cirrhotic rats. Hepatology 2001;33(4):821–5.

60. Lanas Á, Carrera-Lasfuentes P, Arguedas Y, et al. Risk of upper and lower gastrointestinal bleeding in patients taking nonsteroidal anti-inflammatory drugs, antiplatelet agents, or anticoagulants. Clin Gastroenterol Hepatol 2015;13(5): 906–12.e2.

61. Razzaghi A, Barkun AN. Platelet transfusion threshold in patients with upper gastrointestinal bleeding: a systematic review. J Clin Gastroenterol 2012;46(6): 482–6.

62. Hippisley-Cox J, Coupland C. Predicting risk of upper gastrointestinal bleed and intracranial bleed with anticoagulants: cohort study to derive and validate the QBleed scores. BMJ 2014;349:g4606.

63. Abraham NS, Castillo DL. Novel anticoagulants: bleeding risk and management strategies. Curr Opin Gastroenterol 2013;29(6):676–83.

64. Heidbuchel H, Verhamme P, Alings M, et al. European Heart Rhythm Association Practical Guide on the use of new oral anticoagulants in patients with non-valvular atrial fibrillation. Europace 2013;15(5):625–51.

65. Siegal DM, Cuker A. Reversal of novel oral anticoagulants in patients with major bleeding. J Thromb Thrombolysis 2013;35(3):391–8.
66. Pollack CV Jr, Reilly PA, Eikelboom J, et al. Idarucizumab for dabigatran reversal. N Engl J Med 2015;373(6):511–20.
67. Andrews CN, Levy A, Fishman M, et al. Intravenous proton pump inhibitors before endoscopy in bleeding peptic ulcer with high-risk stigmata: a multicentre comparative study. Can J Gastroenterol 2005;19(11):667–71.
68. Leontiadis GI, Sharma VK, Howden CW. Proton pump inhibitor therapy for peptic ulcer bleeding: Cochrane collaboration meta-analysis of randomized controlled trials. Mayo Clin Proc 2007;82(3):286–96.
69. Imperiale TF, Birgisson S. Somatostatin or octreotide compared with H2 antagonists and placebo in the management of acute nonvariceal upper gastrointestinal hemorrhage: a meta-analysis. Ann Intern Med 1997;127(12):1062–71.
70. Gøtzsche PC. Somatostatin analogues for acute bleeding oesophageal varices. Cochrane Database Syst Rev 2002;(1):CD000193.
71. Stump DL, Hardin TC. The use of vasopressin in the treatment of upper gastrointestinal haemorrhage. Drugs 1990;39(1):38–53.
72. Groszmann RJ, Kravetz D, Bosch J, et al. Nitroglycerin improves the hemodynamic response to vasopressin in portal hypertension. Hepatology 1982;2(6):757–62.
73. Bernard B, Cadranel JF, Valla D, et al. Prognostic significance of bacterial infection in bleeding cirrhotic patients: a prospective study. Gastroenterology 1995;108(6):1828–34.
74. Bernard B, Grangé JD, Khac EN, et al. Antibiotic prophylaxis for the prevention of bacterial infections in cirrhotic patients with gastrointestinal bleeding: a meta-analysis. Hepatology 1999;29(6):1655–61.
75. Herrera JL. Management of acute variceal bleeding. Clin Liver Dis 2014;18(2):347–57.
76. Rimola A, Bory F, Teres J, et al. Oral, nonabsorbable antibiotics prevent infection in cirrhotics with gastrointestinal hemorrhage. Hepatology 1985;5(3):463–7.
77. Roberts I, Shakur H, Coats T, et al. The CRASH-2 trial: a randomised controlled trial and economic evaluation of the effects of tranexamic acid on death, vascular occlusive events and transfusion requirement in bleeding trauma patients. Health Technol Assess 2013;17(10):1–79.
78. Roberts I, Coats T, Edwards P, et al. HALT-IT–tranexamic acid for the treatment of gastrointestinal bleeding: study protocol for a randomised controlled trial. Trials 2014;15:450.
79. Jayakumar S, Odulaja A, Patel S, et al. Surviving Sengstaken. J Pediatr Surg 2015;50(7):1142–6.
80. Nielsen TS, Charles AV. Lethal esophageal rupture following treatment with Sengstaken-Blakemore tube in management of variceal bleeding: a 10-year autopsy study. Forensic Sci Int 2012;222(1–3):e19–22.
81. Spiegel BM, Vakil NB, Ofman JJ. Endoscopy for acute nonvariceal upper gastrointestinal tract hemorrhage: is sooner better? A systematic review. Arch Intern Med 2001;161(11):1393–404.
82. Lim LG, Ho KY, Chan YH, et al. Urgent endoscopy is associated with lower mortality in high-risk but not low-risk nonvariceal upper gastrointestinal bleeding. Endoscopy 2011;43(4):300–6.
83. Jensen DM, Machicado GA. Diagnosis and treatment of severe hematochezia. The role of urgent colonoscopy after purge. Gastroenterology 1988;95(6):1569–74.

84. Meltzer AC, Ali MA, Kresiberg RB. Video capsule endoscopy in the emergency department: a prospective study of acute upper gastrointestinal hemorrhage. Ann Emerg Med 2013;61(4):438–43.e1.

85. Jensen DM, Machicado GA, Jutabha R, et al. Urgent colonoscopy for the diagnosis and treatment of severe diverticular hemorrhage. N Engl J Med 2000; 342(2):78–82.

86. Ishii N, Setoyama T, Deshpande GA, et al. Endoscopic band ligation for colonic diverticular hemorrhage. Gastrointest Endosc 2012;75(2):382–7.

87. Ohyama T, Sakurai Y, Ito M, et al. Analysis of urgent colonoscopy for lower gastrointestinal tract bleeding. Digestion 2000;61(3):189–92.

88. Walker TG, Salazar GM, Waltman AC. Angiographic evaluation and management of acute gastrointestinal hemorrhage. World J Gastroenterol 2012;18(11): 1191–201.

89. Krüger K, Heindel W, Dölken W, et al. Angiographic detection of gastrointestinal bleeding. An experimental comparison of conventional screen-film angiography and digital subtraction angiography. Invest Radiol 1996;31(7):451–7.

90. Defreyne L, Vanlangenhove P, De Vos M, et al. Embolization as a first approach with endoscopically unmanageable acute nonvariceal gastrointestinal hemorrhage. Radiology 2001;218(3):739–48.

91. Kumar R, Mills AM. Gastrointestinal bleeding. Emerg Med Clin North Am 2011; 29(2):239–52.

92. Suzman MS, Talmor M, Jennis R, et al. Accurate localization and surgical management of active lower gastrointestinal hemorrhage with technetium-labeled erythrocyte scintigraphy. Ann Surg 1996;224(1):29–36.

93. Smith R, Copely DJ, Bolen FH. 99mTc RBC scintigraphy: correlation of gastrointestinal bleeding rates with scintigraphic findings. AJR Am J Roentgenol 1987; 148(5):869–74.

94. Carbonell N, Pauwels A, Serfaty L, et al. Improved survival after variceal bleeding in patients with cirrhosis over the past two decades. Hepatology 2004;40:652–9.

Abdominal Vascular Catastrophes

Manpreet Singh, MD[a], Alex Koyfman, MD[b], Joseph P. Martinez, MD[c],*

KEYWORDS

- Mesenteric ischemia • Ruptured abdominal aortic aneurysm • Aorto-enteric fistula
- Gastrointestinal bleeding

KEY POINTS

- Mesenteric ischemia (MI) has a variety of causes, each with its own historical clues to assist in diagnosis.
- Early CT angiography without waiting for administration of oral contrast should be pursued in suspected cases of MI.
- Unexplained hypotension, syncope, or ecchymosis should prompt consideration of ruptured abdominal aortic aneurysm (AAA).
- Any amount of gastrointestinal (GI) bleeding in a patient with a history of AAA or AAA repair is an aortoenteric fistula (AEF) until proved otherwise.

INTRODUCTION

Abdominal vascular catastrophes are uncommon yet frequently fatal processes that are of great interest to emergency physicians because rapid recognition and initiation of definitive treatment are essential to prevent long-term morbidity and mortality. The list of abdominal vascular catastrophes is broad, but the focus of this article is on MI, AAA, and AEF.

MESENTERIC ISCHEMIA

Introduction

Acute MI continues to remain an elusive disease to diagnose despite clinicians being taught in medical school and residency about the classic pain out of proportion with examination presentation. Although a rare case of abdominal pain, with an annual incidence of 0.09% to 0.2% per year and approximately 1% of acute abdomen

Disclosure Statement: The authors have no financial relationships to disclose.
[a] Department of Emergency Medicine, Harbor-UCLA Medical Center, 1000 W. Carson Boulevard, Torrance, CA 90502, USA; [b] Department of Emergency Medicine, UT Southwestern Medical Center, 5323 Harry Hines Boulevard, Dallas, TX 75390, USA; [c] Department of Emergency Medicine, University of Maryland School of Medicine, 110 South Paca Street, Sixth Floor, Suite 200, Baltimore, MD 21201, USA
* Corresponding author.
E-mail address: jmartinez@som.umaryland.edu

Emerg Med Clin N Am 34 (2016) 327–339
http://dx.doi.org/10.1016/j.emc.2015.12.014
0733-8627/16/$ – see front matter © 2016 Elsevier Inc. All rights reserved.

hospitalizations,[1,2] this is offset with a 60% to 80% mortality within the first 24 hours.[3] It is imperative that there is no delay in diagnosis because delays in diagnosis lead to increased mortality and morbidity in terms of amount of bowel requiring resection. The presentation of patients with MI is usually nonspecific with a falsely reassuring objective abdominal examination, which can lead to a false sense of security because the late findings of this disease process (absent bowel sounds, positive fecal occult blood test, focal/generalized peritonitis from visceral ischemia, elevated lactate, hypotension, fever, and so forth) have not evolved. In general, a high degree of clinical suspicion should be based on a combination of history, examination, laboratory results, and imaging studies to arrive at the diagnosis of acute mesenteric ischemia.

Anatomy

The abdominal aorta gives off 3 major branches to the intestines (foregut, midgut, and hindgut), which are the celiac artery (CA), superior mesenteric artery (SMA), and inferior mesenteric artery (IMA).[4] The CA perfuses the foregut (distal esophagus to second portion of duodenum). Acute MI of the foregut is rare because the CA is a short, wide artery with good collateral flow. The SMA perfuses the midgut (duodenum to distal transverse colon), which encompasses nearly the entire small bowel and two-thirds of the large bowel. This is the most common embolic site of MI due to favorable takeoff angle (approximately 45°) from the aorta. The IMA perfuses the hindgut (transverse colon to rectum) and is rarely the sole vessel involved in MI. Collateral circulation from the CA or IMA generally allows sufficient perfusion in reduced SMA occlusion states.

Pathophysiology

In addition to the abdominal aortic anatomy, it is important to understand how the bowel layers are affected by MI, starting from the innermost to outermost layers (mucosa, submucosa, muscularis, and serosa). Early in the course of MI, the furthest layer from the blood supply (mucosa) is the first to become ischemic and is the reason for extreme pain, which is visceral in origin. Because the outer structures (muscle and serosa) have not become ischemic, however, there is minimal irritation of the parietal peritoneum when the examiner indents down against the serosa and the external layers of the bowel. Hence, there is pain out of proportion with the examination early on in the disease process. Over a period of hours, the muscularis and serosal layers become ischemic and infarct, leading to peritoneal irritation and guarding with rigidity. At this point, the pain is in proportion with the examination. It is also important to consider that between the early and late presentations (discussed previously), there is a deceptive pain-free interval of approximately 3 to 6 hours caused by a decline in intramural pain receptors from hypoperfusion.[5]

Etiology

MI can be classified as acute versus chronic or as occlusive versus nonocclusive. The following are the major 4 causes of acute MI[5]:

- Acute arterial emboli – the most frequent cause of MI, accounting for 40% to 50% of cases; the embolus usually lodges in the SMA.[3] The proximal branches of the SMA (jejunal and middle colic arteries) are usually preserved because the embolus lodges 3 cm to 10 cm distally from the SMA takeoff, where the artery tapers off and is just after the first major branch of the SMA (the middle colic artery). As a result, the proximal small and large bowels are usually spared.[6] Due to poorly developed collateral circulation, the onset of symptoms in cases of emboli is usually severe and dramatic pain.[4] When the bowel becomes ischemic, it has a propensity to empty itself, leading to vomiting or diarrhea, so-called gut emptying. This is one of the reasons that MI is often misdiagnosed as gastroenteritis. Common predisposing factors include atrial fibrillation, cardiomyopathy, recent angiography, and valvular disorders, such as rheumatic valve disease.[5] One-third of patients have had a previous embolic event, such as an embolic renal infarct, embolic stroke, or peripheral arterial embolus.

- Acute arterial thrombosis – patients with long-standing atherosclerosis may develop plaque build-up at the origin of the SMA, a site of turbulent blood flow. This subsequent stenosis may lead to long-standing postprandial pain (intestinal angina) and food fear with resultant weight loss. These symptoms of chronic MI can be seen in up to 80% of patients who develop arterial thrombosis. If the plaque acutely ruptures or the stenosis reaches a critical level, patients may present with acute pain, similar to those with arterial emboli.[3,6,7]
- Mesenteric venous thrombosis (MVT) – generally found in patients with an underlying hypercoagulable state; MVT accounts for 10% to 15% of cases. Patients typically present with less severe and more insidious pain than those with arterial occlusion.[5] A majority of patients present after more than 24 hours of symptoms. In 1 study, the mean symptom duration was 5 to 14 days, with many patients experiencing pain for 1 month prior to diagnosis.[3] Predisposing risk factors include malignancy, sepsis, liver disease or portal hypertension, sickle cell disease, and pancreatitis.[3,7] Many patients have heritable hematologic disorders, including protein C and protein S deficiency, antithrombin III deficiency, and factor V Leiden mutation. One-half of patients with MVT have a personal or family history of venous thromboembolism.
- Nonocclusive MI (NOMI) – this type of MI occurs in 20% of patients due to failure of autoregulation in low-flow states, such as hypovolemia, potent vasopressor use, heart failure, or sepsis.[3,6] The underlying ischemia from splanchnic vasoconstriction can further lead to hypotension from endogenous substances, perpetuating a vicious cycle.[4,5] This accounts for the extremely high mortality rate, usually due to the poor health of the affected population, with multiple comorbidities, combined with the difficulty in treating the primary cause of diminished intestinal blood flow. Patients who present with abdominal pain postdialysis may have NOMI secondary to intradialytic hypotension, leading to vasospasm.[8]

Clinical Findings

The presentation of MI is typically acute severe abdominal pain with a paucity of physical examination findings. There is a widely variable range of performance characteristics of the history and physical examination, which underlines the diagnostic challenge.[7] History and physical examination findings, such as acute abdominal pain, pain out of proportion, peritoneal signs, guaiac-positive stool, acute abdominal pain, heart failure, and atrial fibrillation, have a wide range of sensitivities and are frequently absent.[9] Therefore, clinicians should be vigilant in considering MI in the differential diagnosis of abdominal pain of unclear etiology. Assessing a patient's pretest probability for disease, actively searching for known risk factors, and adding in clues based on a patient's history and physical examination findings are an important process for wary clinicians. Early and aggressive imaging based on this process has been demonstrated to decrease overall mortality from MI.[10]

Laboratory Studies

Numerous laboratory abnormalities have been described in MI, including elevated amylase, lactate dehydrogenase, large base deficit, and metabolic acidosis. None of these findings is sensitive or specific for MI. Troponin I levels are often elevated. This finding is not specific for MI and has been shown to lead to delays in definitive care of these patients and inappropriate cardiology consultations.[11,12] Common laboratory abnormalities, such as hemoconcentration, leukocytosis, and high anion-gap metabolic acidosis with elevated lactate (specifically D-lactate), are neither sensitive nor specific enough to be diagnostic and usually late findings.

Diagnostic biomarkers are a tool that should bear a high sensitivity and specificity, especially in MI, where early symptoms are nonspecific and mortality rises with delayed or missed diagnosis. Many laboratory tests have been studied in AMI, including D-lactate, intestinal fatty acid–binding protein, glutathione S-transferase, ischemia-modified albumin, and D-dimer. Although some have shown promising early results, none is sufficiently well established to either make or exclude the diagnosis of AMI. The serum marker that practicing clinicians are most familiar with is lactate. Although MI mortality is associated with high lactate serum values, a normal serum lactate value does not exclude AMI.[13] Early in the disease process, lactate is generally normal as it travels through the portal venous system to the liver, where it is converted into glucose via the Cori cycle. As the ischemia load increases and the liver is not able to keep up with the demand, lactate spills over into the systemic circulation, where it eventually increases in late stages.

Imaging Studies

Various imaging methods have been studied and used in the diagnosis of MI, including lower GI endoscopy, radionuclide imaging, peritoneal fluid analysis, MRI, and peritoneoscopy. Imaging that is insensitive or low yield should be avoided, and any imaging that is performed should be pursued in as expeditious a manner as possible, given the time-sensitive nature of the disease. It has been shown that a multidisciplinary approach to suspected cases of AMI with streamlined protocols and early involvement of consultants can have an impact on overall mortality.[14] The following are common diagnostic modalities often described:

- Plain radiographs: the findings on a plain abdominal radiograph are usually nonspecific (ie, small bowel distention with air-fluid levels or ileus), and 25% of patients may have normal findings.[3] Patients with normal plain radiographs have a lower mortality rate, presumably because the findings that are visible on plain radiographs are late findings seen in more advanced disease. Characteristic findings, such as thumb printing or thickening of bowel loops, occur in less than 40% of patients.[3] Later findings, such as air in the bowel wall (pneumatosis intestinalis) and portal venous system, are ominous signs portending a poor prognosis.
- Ultrasound: the use of ultrasound to detect significant stenosis (>50%) in mesenteric vessels has been shown and has a role in chronic MI, but the role of ultrasound in making the diagnosis of acute ischemia is less well established. This likely is due to limited operator experience in AMI and the abnormality in patient bowel gas patterns that often accompanies AMI, which make visualization of the mesenteric vessels more difficult.
- CT scan: CT is the most commonly used diagnostic tool in suspected MI; the initial sensitivity was 64% but has now improved to 93% with the use of dynamic contrast-enhanced CT.[15,16] The addition of multidetector row CT (MDRCT) technology has further improved results (**Fig. 1**).[17,18] The use of MDRCT angiography does not require oral contrast,[16] which has been shown to increase time to image acquisition to 2 to 3 hours,[19] a potentially lethal delay in cases of suspected MI.

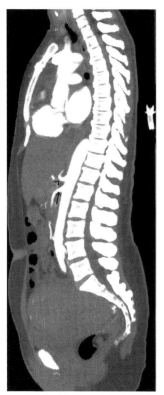

Fig. 1. Sagittal reconstruction of MDRCT angiography of normal celiac artery (*arrowhead*) and normal SMA (*arrow*).

- Angiography: angiography was once the diagnostic gold standard in work-up due to its high accuracy and therapeutic role; today it is used primarily as a confirmatory tool when noninvasive radiological studies do not produce conclusive results.[20,21] Catheter-based therapy and vasodilation still play a large role in management, especially in those patients who are deemed too risky for open surgical techniques. In addition, patients who undergo successful revascularization procedures may still require intra-arterial vasodilators to treat associated vasospasm.[22]
- Laparoscopy: depending on the institution, the availability of experienced radiologists to interpret CT angiograms and endovascular specialists to perform diagnostic and therapeutic angiography may be limited. In addition, acute renal failure from MI or those with known contrast allergy may prohibit obtaining a contrast study.[23,24] Furthermore, a CT scan may not show vascular/intestinal pathologies in patients with a high pretest probability of MI.[25,26] As a result, a diagnostic laparoscopy can fill this diagnostic gap. Studies have shown that the mean time between admission and diagnostic laparoscopy (10.2 h) was significantly shorter in patients who underwent successful revascularization and in those who survived with or without developing short bowel syndrome.[25]

Treatment

Treatment of AMI should be initiated while the diagnostic evaluation is commencing. Treatment often requires a multidisciplinary approach involving general and vascular surgeons as well as interventional radiologists. Aggressive fluid resuscitation should be started to correct fluid deficit and metabolic derangements. Broad-spectrum antibiotics are generally given as well. Early surgical consultation is warranted, even before definitive testing is performed, especially in cases of high pretest probability. The presence of peritoneal signs is usually an indicator of late stages of the disease requiring emergency laparotomy and may obviate any confirmatory imaging.

Once a diagnosis is established, surgical treatment of the underlying cause should be performed (ie, embolectomy, thrombectomy, endarterectomy, or bypass). Anticoagulation should be started, in consultation with the treating surgeon. An important part of the postsurgical care involves reducing the profound vasospasm that accompanies AMI. This is typically accomplished through intra-arterial papaverine infusion via an indwelling catheter in the SMA. A growing area of research involves minimizing ischemia-reperfusion injury.

Summary

MI is a vascular emergency, which all emergency physicians must consider early in their abdominal pain differential. It continues to remain a diagnostic challenge, and any delay in diagnosis can contribute to the increases in the already high mortality rate. Clues to the diagnosis should be sought for in the patient history (**Table 1**). Although the underlying cause varies, early diagnosis and prompt effective treatment can lead to improved clinical outcome. Time is bowel, so if there is a high clinical suspicion for MI, surgical and interventional radiology consultants should be involved early and in parallel with an expeditious diagnostic evaluation.

ABDOMINAL AORTIC ANEURYSM
Introduction

An AAA in itself is a hallmark emergency medicine presentation, where it is a ticking time bomb if not recognized because patients are asymptomatic until it becomes painful as it expands until it ruptures. Once ruptured, overall mortality is as high as 90%; even those with treatment have a 40% to 50% survival.[27] The classic presentation consists of abdominal/flank pain, hypotension, and a pulsatile abdominal mass, but this is only present in 50% of all cases at best.

Anatomy/Pathophysiology

A true aneurysm is a dilatation of all 3 arterial layers (intima, media, and adventitia) through a degenerative process that remains unclear but involves the degradation of the media, where elastin is normally found. As a result, the aortic wall becomes more susceptible to influences of high blood pressure. The aorta varies in size by

Table 1
Historical clues in suspected causes of mesenteric ischemia

Etiology	Historical Clue
SMA embolus	One-third have prior embolic event
SMA thrombosis	80% Have history of intestinal angina
MVT	One-half have personal or family history of deep vein thrombosis/pulmonary embolism
NOMI	More commonly seen in dialysis patients

age, gender, and body habitus, with the average diameter less than 2.0 cm, but, in general, anything above 3.0 cm is considered an aneurysm.[28] The risk of rupture increases with the size and rate of expansion.[29]

Most AAAs originate in the infrarenal aorta, below the takeoff of the renal vessels. In this area, the diameter of the aorta is decreasing and contains a lesser proportion of elastin. Although this is the most common location of AAAs, they may also occur in the suprarenal, pararenal, and juxtarenal areas. These anatomic variations are important when discussing patient candidates for endovascular aortic repair (EVAR), discussed later.

Causes/Risk Factors

Although the degenerative process remains unclear, the following are well-defined risk factors[30] that contribute to AAAs:

- Smoking
- Hypertension
- Male gender
- Connective tissue disorder (ie, Marfan syndrome and Ehlers-Danlos syndrome)
- Atherosclerosis
- Infection/arteritis

Clinical Findings

The clinical manifestation of an AAA varies considerably, depending on the location of rupture (**Box 1**). Intraperitoneal rupture typically manifests as sudden death and rarely survives to reach medical attention. Retroperitoneal bleeds may tamponade off temporarily, allowing a patient to present for medical care. In 75% of cases, acute severe pain is the most common presentation of rupture, where the location of pain varies based on the site of rupture.[31] Those close to renal vessels have flank pain leading to possible renal colic mimicry, whereas those anterior cause abdominal pain and posterior cause back pain. Once a rupture stabilizes, the pain may subside, leading to a false sense of security for both patient and physician. Other uncommon presentations of AAA rupture include radicular femoral/sciatic pain due to nerve compression from the hematoma, acute inguinal hernia from sudden increases in intraperitoneal pressure, and acute high-output heart failure or massive leg swelling from rupture into the inferior vena cava (aortocaval fistula). Unexplained hypotension or syncope, even transient, in a patient with risk factors for ruptured AAA should prompt consideration of the condition. This is evident because it is considered part of the differential of a hypotensive patient when performing the Rapid Ultrasound for Shock and Hypotension examination. Even without rupturing, AAAs can cause subacute flank,

---

Box 1
Location of rupture in abdominal aortic aneurysm (in decreasing frequency)

- Retroperitoneal
- Intraperitoneal
- Vena cava (aortocaval fistula)
- GI tract (AEF)

abdominal, or back pain due to rapid enlargement and compression of the surrounding structures.

The physical examination on these patients may be unrevealing but can offer clues to the diagnosis. Although insensitive, 50% of patients with an AAA have a pulsatile mass palpable in the epigastrium.[32] Besides an abdominal examination, a full vascular examination palpating major pulses (radial, carotid, femoral, and popliteal) should be done to look unequal pulses that can hint to acute aortic syndromes. Although ecchymotic signs, such as Grey Turner (flank), Cullen (periumbilical), Fox (inguinal ligament), and Bryant (scrotal) signs, are neither sensitive nor specific for an AAA, unexplained ecchymosis should always prompt consideration of this vascular emergency.

Imaging Studies

Bedside ultrasound has emerged as the test of choice when screening patients for AAA (**Fig. 2**). Ultrasound has a 98% sensitivity in fasted patients undergoing screening, and although bowel gas and body habitus can hinder the examination, this is less of an issue in imaging the larger aneurysms that are likely to present ruptured. If a patient with a known history of AAA arrives unstable with symptoms consistent with rupture, however, no confirmatory diagnostic tests are necessary and the patient should be transferred to an operating room expeditiously.

Abdominal CT imaging is generally advised for hemodynamically stable patients, although ultrasound should be performed immediately in patients with high clinical suspicion to aid in triage and to speed disposition. In addition to assessing for alternative conditions, CT provides important anatomic information about the AAA that may be important in surgical planning for open and closed (ie, endovascular) surgical approaches (**Fig. 3**). Although contrast is not required, its administration is helpful to obtain more aortic detail for preoperative planning and to ascertain whether the patient is a candidate for EVAR. Signs of rupture on CT include retroperitoneal hematoma, free intraperitoneal blood, an indistinct aortic wall, and loss of the normal fat plane around the aorta. Signs of impending rupture or an unstable aneurysm also may be seen and include layering of hematoma within the aorta (crescent sign), breaks in the calcification of the wall, and blebs or other irregularity within the wall.

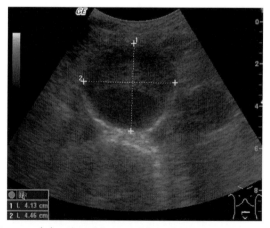

Fig. 2. Bedside ultrasound showing 4.1-cm × 4.5-cm AAA.

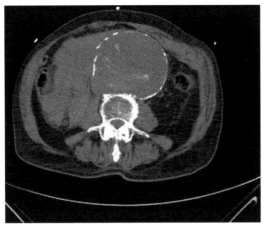

Fig. 3. CT of large AAA – axial slice of abdominal CT scan showing large, heavily calcified, and thrombosed AAA. The calcification exhibits significant discontinuity in the right posterolateral area and signs of retroperitoneal hematoma, suggestive of rupture.

Treatment

Those presenting in clinical shock require tandem resuscitation with bedside diagnosis if there is no known history of AAA. Initial misdiagnosis is common, occurring in approximately 40% of cases, where the most common incorrect diagnoses are renal colic, myocardial infarction, and diverticulitis.

Obtaining 2 large-bore intravenous (IV) lines with uncrossmatched type O blood immediately made available is key. Central access with a sheath introducer or multi-lumen access catheter should be weighed against possible delay in transport to an operating room. In anticipation for the operating room, 6 to 10 units of packed red blood cells, type and crossmatched, should be requested as well as fresh frozen plasma and platelets that may be required during resuscitation. Depending on the institution, implementing a massive transfusion protocol, as well as activating the patient as a trauma, may speed along the process of obtaining an OR room with a surgeon who is ready to go. Resuscitation effort should be focused on controlled volume resuscitation targeting a systolic blood pressure of 80 mm Hg to 90 mm Hg, analogous to patients with penetrating torso trauma.[33]

EVAR has become the mainstay for elective repair of AAAs, with 2 multicenter randomized controlled trials showing a 3-fold reduction in mortality.[19,34] Although randomized trials have not shown improved mortality rates for EVAR in the setting of acute rupture, it seems that perioperative morbidity is decreased and thus EVAR is favored for anatomically suitable patients.[35] The main criterion for EVAR is an adequately long aneurysm neck to allow seating of the graft without occlusion of the renal arteries, which is met in 70% of AAAs.[36] Although infrarenal aneurysms are preferred (especially in the emergent use), suprarenal and pararenal aneurysms are amenable to EVAR with custom grafts.

Summary

Ruptured or symptomatic AAA is a fatal and time-sensitive condition that emergency physicians should be familiar with and ready for, where timely diagnosis and appropriate resuscitation with operative team management can mean the difference between life and death.

AORTOENTERIC FISTULAS
Introduction

Development of an AEF is a life-threatening and devastating cause of upper GI bleed, which can be difficult to diagnose and treat. Although rare, it is most commonly seen as a delayed complication of aortic reconstruction.

Pathophysiology

The disease is divided into 2 types – primary AEF and secondary AEF. Although uncommon, primary AEF occurs when a large, previously untreated aneurysm erodes de novo into the adjacent bowel. This is often diagnosed unexpectedly during exploratory laparotomy. The third portion of the duodenum, fixed retroperitoneally and in proximity to the descending aorta, is the bowel segment most vulnerable to this. The nidus for this process starts with ischemia and subsequent necrosis of the intestinal wall as a consequence of repetitive traumatic pulsations of an adjacent aortic aneurysm. Subsequent rupture of an expanding aneurysm or perforation of the aorta as a result of contamination with GI contents results in the formation of a communication with the bowel and the potential for rapid exsanguination. Less commonly encountered conditions that may lead to primary AEFs include syphilis, tuberculosis, mycotic infection, and collagen vascular disease, where the chronic inflammation leads to aortitis, erosion, and formation of the fistula. In the absence of treatment, the mortality rate is almost 100%. With surgical intervention, survival ranges from 18% to 93%.

In contrast, secondary AEF occurs as a complication of aortic reconstructive surgery. An estimated 80% of secondary AEFs affect the duodenum, mostly the third and fourth parts (the horizontal and ascending duodenum). As a result of advanced perigraft infection from chronic low-grade infection and the repetitive pressure on the intestine from aortic pulsations, fistulas are formed.

Clinical Findings

The typical symptoms of AEFs include acute abdominal pain, GI hemorrhage (melena, hematemesis, and dark blood per rectum), and sepsis. The most common clinical features of primary AEFs are upper GI bleeding (64%), abdominal pain (32%), and a pulsatile abdominal mass (25%), where these 3 features are concomitantly present in only 10% to 23% of patients. Patients with a secondary AEF usually present with 1 or more of the following clinical signs and symptoms: GI bleeding (80%), sepsis (44%), abdominal pain (30%), back pain (15%), groin mass (12%), and abdominal pulsatile mass (6%). With both primary and secondary AEFs, transient, self-limited, intermittent bleeding episodes (herald bleeds) often precede a major hemorrhagic episode by hours, days, or weeks. This is a result of a small fistula tamponaded by thrombus formation and bowel contraction around it.

Imaging Studies

Three modalities are available to assist in diagnosis: abdominal CT scan with IV contrast, esophagogastroduodenoscopy (EGD), and arteriography. Of the 3, CT scan offers superiority because it is less invasive, more readily available, and more expedient than the latter 2. In addition, it offers the advantage of being unlikely to dislodge the aortic thrombus. The CT may show abnormal communication between the aorta and the bowel, may disclose loss of continuity of the aneurysmal wall, and may demonstrate air bubbles in the aneurysm wall that are pathognomonic for the existence of a fistula.

An EGD with a water-soluble contrast material is usually considered second line but should be performed only on a hemodynamically stable patient. An AEF is usually present when there is leakage of oral contrast material from the disrupted bowel wall into the perigraft space. In addition to evaluating the presence or absence of an AEF, an EGD assists in ruling out other causes of upper GI bleeding, including varices, bleeding masses, and ulcers. A normal EGD or the finding of other pathology without stigmata of recent bleeding does not exclude an AEF, especially if there is a high index of suspicion.

Arteriography is of some value but rarely used in critically ill patients for diagnosis. Its true value lies in embolization therapy and stent placement.

Treatment

AEF requires definitive and emergent operative management, where various surgical modalities exist (graft excision and extra-anatomic bypass, in situ graft replacement, and simple graft excision or endovascular repair). The role of emergency physicians, in the perioperative phase, includes optimally resuscitating the patient with fluids and blood products while initiating broad-spectrum IV antibiotics to cover gram-positive, gram-negative, and enteric pathogens as part of sepsis management.

Summary

AEF is a life-threatening entity that is challenging to diagnose and carries high morbidity and mortality. Any patient who presents with any degree of GI bleeding and has a prior history of aortic aneurysm repair should be considered as having an AEF until proved otherwise.

REFERENCES

1. Sise MJ. Acute mesenteric ischemia. Surg Clin North Am 2014;94(1):165–81.
2. van den Heijkant TC, Aerts BA, Teijink JA, et al. Diagnosis of mesenteric ischemia. World J Gastroenterol 2013;19(9):1338–41.
3. Lewiss RE, Egan DJ, Shreves A. Vascular abdominal emergencies. Emerg Med Clin North Am 2011;29:253–72.
4. Oldenburg WA, Lau LL, Rodenberg TJ, et al. Acute mesenteric ischemia: a clinical review. Arch Intern Med 2004;164(10):1054–62.
5. Martinez JP, Hogan GJ. Mesenteric ischemia. Emerg Med Clin North Am 2004; 22(4):909–28.
6. Lotterman S. Mesenteric Ischemia: A Power Review. 2014. Available at: http://www.emdocs.net/mesenteric-ischemia-power-review/. Accessed December, 2015.
7. McKinsey JF, Gewertz BL. Acute mesenteric ischemia. Surg Clin North Am 1997; 77:307–18.
8. Diamond S, Emmett M, Henrich WL. Bowel infarction as a cause of death in dialysis patients. JAMA 1986;256:2545.
9. Cudnik MT, Darbha S, Jones J, et al. The diagnosis of acute mesenteric ischemia: a systematic review and meta-analysis. Acad Emerg Med 2013;20:1087–100.
10. Boley SJ, Sprayregen S, Siegelman SJ, et al. Initial results from an aggressive roentgenologic and surgical approach to acute mesenteric ischemia. Surgery 1977;82:848.
11. Acosta S, Block T, Bjornsson S, et al. Diagnostic pitfalls at admission in patients with acute superior mesenteric artery occlusion. J Emerg Med 2012;42(6): 635–41.

12. Huynh LN, Coughlin BF, Wolfe J, et al. Patient encounter time intervals in the evaluation of emergency department patients requiring abdominopelvic CT: oral contrast versus no contrast. Emerg Radiol 2004;10:310–3.

13. Cohn B. Does this patient have acute mesenteric ischemia? Ann Emerg Med 2014;5(64):533–4.

14. Clark RA, Gallant TE. Acute mesenteric ischemia: angiographic spectrum. AJR Am J Roentgenol 1984;142:555.

15. Menke J. Diagnostic accuracy of multidetector CT in acute mesenteric ischemia: systematic review and meta-analysis. Radiology 2010;256:93–101.

16. Kirkpatrick ID, Kroeker MA, Greenberg HM. Biphasic CT with mesenteric CT angiography in the evaluation of acute mesenteric ischemia: initial experience. Radiology 2003;229:91–8.

17. Klar E, Rahmanian PB, Bücker A, et al. Acute mesenteric ischemia: a vascular emergency. Dtsch Arztebl Int 2012;109:249–56.

18. Horton KM, Fishman EK. CT angiography of the mesenteric circulation. Radiol Clin North Am 2010;48:331–45.

19. Prinssen M, Verhoeven ELG, Buth J, et al. A randomized trial comparing conventional and endovascular repair of abdominal aortic aneurysms. N Engl J Med 2004;351:1607–18.

20. Aschoff AJ, Stuber G, Becker BW, et al. Evaluation of acute mesenteric ischemia: accuracy of biphasic mesenteric multidetector CT angiography. Abdom Imaging 2009;34:345–57.

21. Ofer A, Abadi S, Nitecki S, et al. Multidetector CT angiography in the evaluation of acute mesenteric ischemia. Eur Radiol 2009;19:24–30.

22. Stone JR, Wilkins LR. Acute mesenteric ischemia. Tech Vasc Interv Radiol 2015; 18:24–30.

23. Gupta PK, Natarajan B, Gupta H, et al. Morbidity and mortality after bowel resection for acute mesenteric ischemia. Surgery 2011;150:779–87.

24. Kougias P, Lau D, El Sayed HF, et al. Determinants of mortality and treatment outcome following surgical interventions for acute mesenteric ischemia. J Vasc Surg 2007;46:467–74.

25. Gonenc M, Dural CA, Kocatas A, et al. The impact of early diagnostic laparoscopy on the prognosis of patients with suspected acute mesenteric ischemia. Eur J Trauma Emerg Surg 2013;39(2):185–9.

26. Smerud MJ, Johnson CD, Stephens DH. Diagnosis of bowel infarction: a comparison of plain films and CT scans in 23 cases. Roentgenol 1990;154:99–103.

27. Brown LC, Powell JT. Risk factors for aneurysm rupture in patients kept under ultrasound surveillance. Ann Surg 1999;230(3):289–96.

28. Johnston KW, Rutherford RB, Tilson MD, et al. Suggested standards for reporting on arterial aneurysms. Subcommittee on Reporting Standards for Arterial Aneurysms, Ad Hoc Committee on Reporting Standards, Society for Vascular Surgery and North American Chapter, International Society for Cardiovascular Surgery. J Vasc Surg 1991;13:452.

29. Chaikof EL, Brewster DC, Dalman RL, et al. SVS practice guidelines for the care of patients with an abdominal aortic aneurysm: executive summary. J Vasc Surg 2009;50:880.

30. Wilmink AB, Quick CG. Epidemiology and potential for prevention of abdominal aortic aneurysm. Br J Surg 1998;85:55–62.

31. Rinckenbach S, Albertini JN, Thaveau F, et al. Prehospital treatment of infrarenal ruptured abdominal aortic aneurysms: a multicentre analysis. Ann Vasc Surg 2010;24:308.

32. Azhar B, Patel SR, Holt PJ, et al. Misdiagnosis of ruptured abdominal aortic aneurysm: systematic review and meta-analysis. J Endovasc Ther 2014;21:568.
33. Dick F, Erdoes G, Opfermann P, et al. Delayed volume resuscitation during initial management of ruptured abdominal aortic aneurysm. J Vasc Surg 2013;57:943.
34. Greenhalgh RM, Brown LC, Kwong GPS, et al. Comparison of endovascular aneurysm repair with open repair in patients with abdominal aortic aneurysm (EVAR trial 1), 30-day operative mortality results: randomised controlled trial. Lancet 2004;364:843–8.
35. van Beek SC, Conijn AP, Koelemay MJ, et al. Editor's Choice – Endovascular aneurysm repair versus open repair for patients with a ruptured abdominal aortic aneurysm: a systematic review and meta-analysis of short-term survival. Eur J Vasc Endovasc Surg 2014;47:593.
36. Antoniou GA, Georgiadis GS, Antoniou SA, et al. Endovascular repair for ruptured abdominal aortic aneurysm confers an early survival benefit over open repair. J Vasc Surg 2013;58:1091.

Pediatric Abdominal Pain

An Emergency Medicine Perspective

Jeremiah Smith, MD[a],*, Sean M. Fox, MD[b]

KEYWORDS

- Functional constipation • Pyloric stenosis • Necrotizing enterocolitis • Appendicitis
- Incarcerated inguinal hernia • Gonadal torsion • Functional gastrointestinal disorder

KEY POINTS

- Avoid diagnostic momentum, especially when evaluating functional constipation and functional gastrointestinal disorders.
- Bilious vomiting in a neonate is a surgical emergency until proven otherwise.
- Always consider gonadal torsion in a child with lower abdominal pain.
- Do not overlook the potential for psychosocial causes of abdominal pain.
- Constipation is not an innocuous condition.

BACKGROUND

Pediatric abdominal pain is a common complaint evaluated in emergency departments (EDs). Although often due to benign causes, the varied and nonspecific presentations present a diagnostic challenge. Emergency care providers are tasked with the difficult job of remaining vigilant for the rare, yet devastating conditions while sorting through the much more common, benign causes of abdominal pain. This task is akin to finding the needle in the haystack. Diagnostic momentum can further threaten to divert the provider's attention from the true cause. Pediatric abdominal pain is a challenging complaint to evaluate and deserves specific attention.

EPIDEMIOLOGY

Overall, 5% to 10% of all ED visits by pediatric patients are for abdominal pain.[1,2] In the United States alone, up to 38% of school-aged children complain of abdominal

Disclosures: The authors have nothing to disclose.
[a] Department of Emergency Medicine, Carolinas Medical Center, 1000 Blythe Boulevard, MEB Floor 3, Charlotte, NC 28203, USA; [b] Emergency Medicine Residency Program, Department of Emergency Medicine, Carolinas Medical Center, 1000 Blythe Boulevard, MEB Floor 3, Charlotte, NC 28203, USA
* Corresponding author.
E-mail address: jeremiah.smith@carolinashealthcare.org

Emerg Med Clin N Am 34 (2016) 341–361
http://dx.doi.org/10.1016/j.emc.2015.12.010
0733-8627/16/$ – see front matter © 2016 Elsevier Inc. All rights reserved.
emed.theclinics.com

pain weekly and up to 24% of them have had that pain for greater than 8 weeks.[3,4] What makes finding the rare, but potentially life-threatening case of abdominal pain even more difficult is that *only 5% to 10% of children* with abdominal pain have underlying organic disease and that the causes vary substantially with the age of the patients (**Table 1**).[3]

HISTORY

The history of present illness and past medical history are the foundation on which appropriate medical decisions are built. A thorough history helps pare down the large differential for abdominal pain. Although daunting in a busy ED, it is possible to obtain a thorough but efficient history.

When taking the history, question both the caregiver and child themselves separately, if age appropriate. Sitting or kneeling may help minimize anxiety in both children and parents. Interview the child where he or she is most comfortable. For older children and adolescents, a history for sexual activity, drug use, possible abuse, and suicidal ideation is best obtained with the caregivers out of the room.

PHYSICAL EXAMINATION

A complete history should always be followed by an equally thorough physical examination. Although the abdominal examination is the centerpiece, significant information can be gleaned from a full examination (**Box 1**). The patients' general appearance and activity level are also helpful in sorting out the potential causes, especially if infants are lethargic or inconsolable. Focusing only on the abdomen may lead to missing simple clues to other causes.

Table 1
Common causes of abdominal pain by age

Age	<1 y	1–5 y	5–12 y	>12 y
Common or benign	Colic, GERD, milk protein allergy	UTI, constipation	UTI, constipation, FGID, GAS	UTI, constipation, FGID, GAS
Urgent	AGE, malrotation without volvulus	AGE, HSP, pneumonia, Meckel diverticulum	AGE, IBD, pneumonia	AGE, IBD, pneumonia, hepatitis, pancreatitis, nephrolithiasis, PID
Emergent	Trauma, NAT, midgut volvulus, NEC, omphalitis, incarcerated hernia, pyloric stenosis, intussusception	Trauma, appendicitis, asthma	Trauma, appendicitis, gonadal torsion, DKA, asthma	Trauma, appendicitis, gonadal torsion, ectopic pregnancy, DKA, asthma

Abbreviations: AGE, acute gastroenteritis; DKA, diabetic ketoacidosis; FGID, functional gastrointestinal disorders; GAS, group A strep; GERD, gastroesophageal reflux disease; HSP, Henoch-Schönlein purpura; IBD, inflammatory bowel disease; NAT, nonaccidental trauma; NEC, necrotizing enterocolitis; PID, pelvic inflammatory disease; UTI, urinary tract infection.

Box 1
Physical examination for a child with abdominal pain

General

- Play with the child and engage him or her in a fun activity before the examination.
- Use a stuffed animal to show what you will do and how easy it is.
- Attempt to perform as much of the examination as possible in the caregivers lap if possible.
- Use a distraction during the examination.
- Use child life if they are available at your institution.

Constitutional

- Observation of the child before entering the room can direct your examination.
- Check for the absence or presence of a fever.
- Check for any other vital sign abnormality (ie, tachycardia, tachypnea, hypoxia).

Abdominal examination

- Use visualization for distention, masses, visible peristalsis, or bruising.
- Use auscultation for bowel sounds.

Palpation

- Check for the location of maximal tenderness, masses, or guarding.
- Having patients bend their knees while lying will help relax abdominal muscles and improve your examination.
- It is sometimes helpful to push with the stethoscope during auscultation to evaluate for tenderness.

Percussion

- It is possible to percuss for abdominal fluid.
- It can be helpful in evaluating for rebound tenderness.
- Asking patients to jump and give you a high 5 is a great way to assess for rebound tenderness.

Rectal

- This examination is not always necessary and *should not be routine* in all examinations.
- Directed reasons for a rectal examination are as follows: evaluate for bloody stool, possible fecal impaction, and question of Hirschsprung disease.

Genitourinary examination

- A genital examination should be performed in all male patients with abdominal pain and, at least, externally in all female patients.
- A complete gynecologic examination is sometimes required in sexually active female patients.

Remaining examination

- The remaining physical examination should not be skipped over.
- Evaluate for other causes of abdominal pain, such as pneumonia or pharyngitis.

IMAGING

Judicious use of imaging is often integral to a complete evaluation of abdominal pain. It is important to know the benefit and potential limitations of each modality. **Box 2** highlights some of the important considerations of various imaging modalities.

PEDIATRIC CAUSES OF ABDOMINAL PAIN

Constipation is a ubiquitous problem with a worldwide prevalence of 3% to 5%[6,7] (**Box 3**). In the United States, retrospective studies have shown constipation to account for 19.3% of all ED visits for abdominal pain and 0.4% of all visits to the ED.[1,7]

Box 2
Judicious use of imaging

Abdominal radiograph

- It is rarely useful because of low sensitivity and specificity.
- An acute abdominal series may show signs of obstruction or perforation.
- A fecalith in the right lower quadrant of a patient with appendicitis may occasionally be seen.
- It *should not be routinely* ordered for patients with constipation.
- It may show a basilar pneumonia.

Ultrasound

- It is often the image modality of choice for many diseases because it has no radiation exposure.
- It can be performed at the bedside.
- It may be very user dependent and is best at institutions that use it often.
- It is the imaging modality of choice for hydronephrosis from possible nephrolithiasis, gallstones, gonadal torsion, intussusception, pyloric stenosis, appendicitis, and Focused Assessment with Sonography in Trauma examinations.

Computed tomography

- It has high sensitivity and specificity for many intra-abdominal diseases.
- Sensitivity and specificity are often maintained between community and academic facilities.
- It exposes children to ionizing radiation.
  - 25.8 to 33.9 cases of solid organ cancer per 10,000 abdomen/pelvis CTs in girls[5]
  - 13.1 to 14.8 cases of solid organ cancer per 10,000 abdomen/pelvis CTs in boys[5]
- Children are more radiosensitive to ionizing radiation.
- Children have longer expected lifetime to manifest latent injury.
- There is greater potential for radiation overdose from inappropriate CT protocols.
- Helical computed tomography is the most sensitive test for nephrolithiasis in children.

MRI

- It has high sensitivity and specificity for many intra-abdominal diseases.
- It is expensive.
- It is time intensive.
- It is not readily available at many EDs.
- It may require sedation in children.

Diagnosis and Workup

Functional constipation is a diagnosis of exclusion, and the evaluation begins with a thorough history and physical examination.

Abdominal radiographs are often ordered to evaluate for constipation, but they only have a reported sensitivity of 60% to 80% and *should not be routinely ordered*.[6] In fact, there is no evidence to support routine testing of any sort if the child does not have any concerning signs or symptoms (**Box 4**), yet it is important to remain vigilant for other concealed conditions, such as Hirschsprung disease in the neonate with constipation.

Management

The management of constipation can be broken up into 2 groups: *ED management* and *home management*. The cornerstone of ED management for constipation begins with setting reasonable expectations and explanation that this is a long-term process. An enema in the ED may be required, but daily osmotic laxatives (eg, polyethylene glycol 3350) or glycerin suppositories at home, behavioral modifications, and close follow-up with their primary care provider will keep them out of the ED.

PYLORIC STENOSIS

- The pylorus is a single unit of smooth muscle at the lower end of the stomach.
- It connects to the duodenum via the pyloric sphincter.
- Stenosis occurs with elongation and thickening of the pylorus.

Gastric outlet obstruction occurs when the pyloric sphincter is unable to open. Pyloric stenosis is the most common surgical cause of nonbilious emesis in infants less than 6 months of age and typically occurs around 4 to 6 weeks.[9–11] Up to 43% of patients with pyloric stenosis are firstborn, and it is 4 to 5 times more common in males.[10–12]

Diagnosis and Workup

Any infant with true vomiting is concerning and deserves a thorough evaluation. Most clinicians will easily recognize the classic presentation of pyloric stenosis; however, not every presentation is classic. The physical examination can heighten suspicion for pyloric stenosis as well as help sort through other causes of vomiting.

If the infant has worsening projectile vomiting or failure to thrive, diagnostic testing to evaluate for pyloric stenosis should be done.

- Laboratories
  - Classically, infants develop hypochloremic hypokalemic metabolic alkalosis.
  - With earlier diagnosis, less than 50% of infants will present with electrolyte abnormalities.[13,14]
  - Electrolyte changes often after vomiting for greater than 1 week.[13]
- Abdominal ultrasound
  - It is the imaging modality of choice with a sensitivity of 98% to 100% and specificity up to 100%.[9,15]
  - Findings are consistent with pyloric stenosis: pylorus length greater than 14 to 17 mm and a single-wall thickness greater than 3.0 to 4.5 mm[9,13,16] (**Fig. 1**).
  - ED physicians using point-of-care ultrasound had 100% sensitivity (95% confidence interval [CI] 66%–100%) and 100% specificity (95% CI 92%–100%) when able to identify the pylorus (wide CIs for sensitivity makes this a nonideal screening test).[9]
- Upper gastrointestinal (GI) study
  - It is the former gold standard, but rarely used now.[15]
  - It is useful if bilious vomiting is present as it also evaluates for malrotation and volvulus.[10,15]

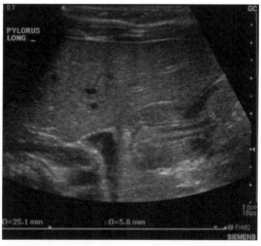

Fig. 1. Length 25.1 mm, thickness 5.8 mm. (*From* Shah S. An update on common gastrointestinal emergencies. Emerg Med Clin North Am 2013;31:775–93.)

○ Findings are as follows:
  ■ String sign: a string of contrast through the elongated pyloric channel
  ■ Double-track sign: several linear tracks of contrast separated by redundant mucosa
- Abdominal radiographs
  ○ It is rarely useful but may show gas in the stomach and a paucity distal to the pylorus.

Management

These infants may present ill appearing and may require stabilization with fluid resuscitation. It may be difficult to differentiate between sepsis and pyloric stenosis in a severely dehydrated infant, and a sepsis evaluation may be necessary as well. Once volume resuscitated and stable, surgical correction is required. Being mindful of the management will ideally help avoid potential pitfalls (**Box 5**).

INTUSSUSCEPTION

- Telescoping of one portion of intestines into itself
- Most common cause of GI obstruction in children
- Second most common abdominal surgical emergency in children

Intussusception is the most common cause of GI obstruction in children and is the second most common pediatric acute abdominal surgical emergency. Its peak incidence is at 5 to 10 months of age.[17–19]

Diagnosis and Workup

Often the need for evaluation will be predicated on the history and a high index of suspicion. The classic history of colicky abdominal pain interspersed with episodes of normal activity or lethargy is seen in only 7.5% to 50.0% of patients.[17,20,21] It may even be painless in up to 40% of patients less than 4 months of age.[22] Red currant jelly stools represents bowel ischemia. Up to 75% of children without these grossly bloody stools may still be hemoccult positive.[23]

- Using history and examination alone, physicians are better at determining patients who do not have intussusception rather than who do (specificity of 85% and an negative predictive value of 94%).[21]
- Laboratory evaluation is often unnecessary, although abnormalities like leukocytosis, elevated band count, and elevated lactate can be seen with bowel perforation.[24]

Abdominal radiographs

- A paucity of gas in the right lower quadrant, intracolonic mass, rim sign, or signs of small bowel obstruction may be seen.

Box 5
Pitfalls of pyloric stenosis

- Failing to perform a comprehensive history and physical in every vomiting infant
- Ruling out pyloric stenosis automatically in an infant with bilious vomiting
- Deciding an infant does not need a full diagnostic workup for pyloric stenosis because they do not have an olivelike mass or hypochloremic hypokalemic metabolic alkalosis
- Forgetting to check a glucose level in a child with severely altered oral intake

- Overall sensitivity for ileocolic intussusception is 74% to 90% and is 88% to 100% sensitive if there is air in the ascending colon in all images of a 3-view abdominal radiograph.[17,25]
- *Up to 24% of children with intussusception may have normal radiographs.*[26]

Abdominal ultrasound

- Evaluate for a target, donut, or pseudokidney sign (**Fig. 2**).
- In the radiology department, ultrasound has a 97.9% to 100% sensitivity.[25]
- One study showed ED physician point-of-care ultrasound to have a sensitivity of 85% and specificity of 97%.[19]

Abdominal computed tomography/MRI

- Rarely necessary and is not cost-effective
- May be necessary to identify a pathologic lead point in an older child or for recurrent intussusception

Fluoroscopy enema

- Diagnostic and therapeutic for intussusception
- Avoid if you have a concern for peritonitis, perforation, or necrosis

Management

Once diagnosed, the intussusception must be reduced. The largest controversy associated with intussusception management has to do with final disposition. It is common for most hospitals to admit and observe children after successful nonoperative reduction because of the 7.5% to 43.0% recurrence rate.[18,27] A recent meta-analysis showed that 2.2% to 5.3% of patients had a recurrence at 24 hours and 7.1% at 48 hours.[18,28] After 48 hours, recurrence was seen in 5.1% and there was rarely adverse events.[26] This finding, along with a growing body of supportive evidence,

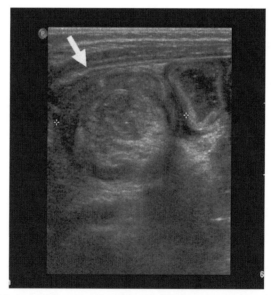

Fig. 2. Sonographic image showing the target or donut sign associated with intussusception. (*From* Marin J, Alpern E. Abdominal pain in children. Emerg Med Clin North Am 2011;29:401–28.)

has led many practitioners to begin observing patients for approximately 6 hours after successful nonoperative reduction and then discharging home with strict return precautions and close follow-up.[18,27,28] Naturally, disposition planning requires coordination with the pediatric surgical team to help avoid potential pitfalls (**Box 6**).

MALROTATION WITH OR WITHOUT MIDGUT VOLVULUS

- Malrotation refers to a spectrum of abnormal rotation of the duodenum around the superior mesenteric artery (SMA) axis.
- This abnormal rotation leads to a shortened mesenteric root and predisposes to midgut volvulus.
- Additionally, fibrous peritoneal bands (ie, Ladd bands) can lead to volvulus or obstruction themselves.

Midgut volvulus is abnormal rotation and fixation of the midgut around the SMA axis that impedes lymphatic drainage, venous outflow, and arterial blood flow leading to massive bowel infarction.

Although malrotation is traditionally thought of as a disease of infancy, up to 25% of patients may not be diagnosed until 5 years of age.[29] Sixty percent of patients with malrotation, however, will present by 1 month and *90% with volvulus present within the first year of life.*[22,30,31]

Diagnosis and Workup

Bilious vomiting is present in greater than 90% of neonates with volvulus and should always be considered a surgical emergency until proven otherwise.[32] Neonates with volvulus are typically irritable because of poor feeding with vomiting, abdominal pain and/or distention, and hematochezia. Older children with bilious vomiting have a larger differential diagnosis, but there should always be a high index of suspicion for malrotation with volvulus because 22% of children and 12% of adults with malrotation present with a volvulus.[32] They will often have a history of chronic abdominal pain or cyclic vomiting and present with abrupt worsening of abdominal pain, and 50% will have nonbilious vomiting.[30]

Naturally, any patient with signs of decompensation requires aggressive resuscitation before further diagnostic testing. Surgical consultation may be required based solely on clinical suspicion if the child remains unstable with findings concerning for abdominal catastrophe. Once the child is stable, imaging should be performed to evaluate for malrotation and volvulus.

- Abdominal radiograph
  - It is often the initial study of choice because it is quick and readily available.
  - Findings are as follows:
    - Double bubble sign signifying duodenal obstruction
    - Lack of bowel gas distal to the duodenum

Box 6
Pitfalls of intussusception

- Not considering and evaluating for a possible pathologic lead point in an older child with intussusception or in cases of recurrence
- Failing to recognize that intussusception can lead to somnolence and lethargy
- Missing the diagnosis because the infant had fever, anorexia, or diarrhea initially

- Bowel malposition
- Air fluid levels
- Pneumatosis
- The most common finding is "normal bowel gas pattern."[33]
- Upper GI with small bowel follow-through
  - It is considered the gold standard and defines size, shape, rotation, and presence of obstruction.
  - Malrotation with or without volvulus is suggested if the duodenal-jejunal junction (DJJ) is in low position, DJJ is not left of the vertebral body pedicle, the jejunum is on the right and coiled like a spring, there is duodenal redundancy, or there is a corkscrew appearance of the DJJ **(Fig. 3)**.
  - Sensitivity is 93% to 100%, but the false-positive rate is 15% and false-negative rate is 2% to 3%.[34]
  - Equivocal findings are seen in up to 37% of patients.[35]
- Ultrasound
  - Normally, the superior mesenteric vein (SMV) should be right of the SMA.
  - With malrotation, the SMV will be anterior or leftward or the duodenum will not be between the SMA and aorta.
  - If volvulus is present, a whirlpool sign, whereby the SMV wraps around the SMA on color-flow Doppler, may be seen.
  - There is a clinical spectrum of normal variant anatomy, and confirmatory testing is often still necessary.
- Other imaging modalities
  - *Barium enema* may show the cecum in the right upper quadrant or in the central abdomen but is not a reliable sign for malrotation.
  - *Abdominal CT* can evaluate the anatomic relationship between the SMA, SMV, and DJJ positioning with a sensitivity of 97.3% and specificity of 99.0%.[33]
  - *Abdominal MRI* can identify malrotation as well but is often time and cost prohibitive.

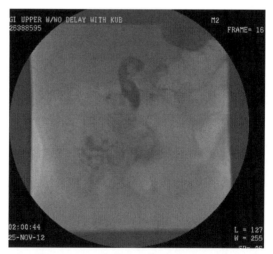

Fig. 3. Upper GI series demonstrates inferior displacement of the DJJ to the right. DJJ does not pass to the left of the spine and does not rise to the level of the duodenal bulb. Proximal small bowel appears on the right side of the abdomen. Likely corkscrew pattern of duodenum indicating volvulus. (*From* Shah S. An update on common gastrointestinal emergencies. Emerg Med Clin North Am 2013;31:775–93.)

Management

Management of malrotation depends on the presence of an associated midgut volvulus. Midgut volvulus is a true surgical emergency. Immediate surgical consultation and operative repair with a Ladd procedure is necessary. Aggressive resuscitation and correction of hypoglycemia is imperative. Additionally, gastric decompression and initiation of broad-spectrum antibiotics that cover gut flora are vitally important. Unfortunately, even with prompt resuscitation and emergent surgical correction, the mortality rate for a midgut volvulus is 3% to 9%. Asymptomatic pediatric patients with malrotation but no midgut volvulus can be managed electively by pediatric surgery (**Box 7**).

NECROTIZING ENTEROCOLITIS

- Classic triad of abdominal distention, GI bleeding, and pneumatosis on radiograph
- Modified Bells staging: stage I suspected necrotizing enterocolitis (NEC), stage II mild NEC, and stage III severe NEC

NEC is often thought of as a disease of prematurity, but nearly 10% to 13% of neonates with NEC are full term within the first 10 days of life.[36,37] Presentation can vary from being nonspecific with temperature instability and feeding intolerance to overt shock with grossly bloody stool. Often times, full-term NEC is associated with infection, hypoxic event at birth, congenital heart disease or cardiac surgery, and umbilical artery catherization.[37]

Diagnosis and Workup

Full-term NEC can often present in a nonspecific fashion, and the clinician needs to maintain a high index of suspicion while sorting through the other potential diagnoses.

Because these patients will often appear similar to a septic neonate, a full septic workup including glucose level, complete blood count, comprehensive metabolic panel, urinalysis, blood and urine cultures, and cerebrospinal fluid (CSF) studies is beneficial. An abdominal radiograph, with either a cross-table lateral or decubitus view, may show an abnormal gas pattern, pneumatosis, free air, or portal gas. Abdominal ultrasound may show a pseudokidney sign. Additional studies are often required to evaluate for uncommon causes of NEC in a full-term neonate.

Management

These patients can become critically ill rapidly and may require cardiopulmonary and fluid resuscitation. Twenty percent to 30% of neonates with NEC have bacteremia,

---

Box 7
Pitfalls of malrotation with or without volvulus

- Not appreciating that an infant with bilious vomiting is a surgical emergency until proven otherwise

- Delaying surgical consultation by obtaining time-intensive testing in an acutely ill neonate/child with a suggestive history of malrotation with volvulus

- Dismissing the idea of malrotation with volvulus in a worrisome child because imaging was negative

- Always be vigilant of patients with chronic abdominal pain and vomiting who have been labeled cyclic vomiting—avoid diagnostic momentum because they patients may be an older patient with undiagnosed malrotation.

and broad-spectrum antibiotics (eg, ampicillin + cefotaxime + metronidazole) that cover gut flora should be initiated promptly. The neonate should have nothing by mouth, and a nasogastric tube should be placed for gastric decompression. Early coordination with pediatric surgery is necessary. Neonates with pneumoperitoneum, an abdominal mass or stricture with obstruction, or signs of sepsis require operative intervention[37] (**Box 8**).

APPENDICITIS

- It is inflammation of the appendix.
- It can affect all age groups but is difficult to diagnosis in the very young.
- Children less than 3 years of age have the highest perforation risk.

Appendicitis is the most common pediatric surgical emergency, and 250,000 cases are seen annually with a lifetime risk of developing it of 8.6% for men and 6.7% in women.[38–40] The perforation rate is 80% to 100% in children younger than 3 years and up to 38% in older children.[24,41]

Diagnosis and Workup

The diagnosis of appendicitis may be quite clear or rather confounded but typically involves a combination of physical examination findings, laboratories, and imaging.

- History and physical examination
  - Studies have shown experienced practitioners in pediatric emergency medicine are able to accurately diagnose men with appendicitis at a rate of 78% to 92% and women at 58% to 85%.[42]
  - Unfortunately, physical examination alone leads to a false-negative rate of 9.8% when taken to the operating room (OR) directly based on examination as opposed to 4.5% with imaging.[43]
  - Overall, there is no single predictor highly indicating appendicitis; but rebound tenderness has a positive likelihood ratio (LR) of 2.3 to 3.9, and right lower quadrant (RLQ) pain to percussion has a positive LR of 2.56.[24,44]
  - As always, being mindful of the other potential causes of abdominal pain is necessary.
- Laboratory values
  - A complete blood count (CBC) with differential is often ordered but has relatively low diagnostic yield. If it is greater than 10,000 mm^3 it has a positive LR of 1.77 and a sensitivity and specificity for appendicitis of 65% to 85% and 32% to 83%, respectively.[44,45]
  - Increased polymorphonuclear cells and bandemia may provide diagnostic clues but are not indicative by themselves.
  - A C-reactive protein (CRP) greater than 10 mg/L is not sensitive or specific for appendicitis but may be a strong predictor of perforation.[46]

Box 8
Pitfalls of NEC

- Failing to consider NEC as a possible diagnosis for abdominal pain in a full-term neonate
- Not searching for uncommon causes associated with NEC in a full-term neonate, such as congenital heart disease (eg, coarctation or patent ductus arteriosus)
- Forgetting that sepsis may cause NEC and a full workup including CSF is needed
- Not stopping feeds and starting antibiotics when you suspect NEC

- ○ Pooled laboratory tests may increase the predictive power and generate a sensitivity of 98% to 99%, but they still have low specificity (only 6%–12%).[45]
- ○ Overall, laboratory test results may help determine which patients are at low risk for appendicitis, but they do not help determine who actually needs to go the OR for an appendectomy.
- ○ A pregnancy test in female patients should always be done.
- Imaging
  - ○ Abdominal radiographs are rarely useful, showing an appendicolith less than 5% of time.[42]
  - ○ Abdominal ultrasound is often used as the first imaging of choice when evaluating appendicitis (**Fig. 4**)
    - ▪ It has become the imaging modality of choice at many institutions and is recommended by the American College of Emergency Physicians to *diagnose but not exclude*.[47]
    - ▪ It has a sensitivity of 72.5% to 94.0% and specificity of 89% to 98% when the appendix is visualized (25%–73% of the time).[48,49]
    - ▪ False negatives can be seen with perforation or tip appendicitis.[50]
    - ▪ The diagnostic accuracy increases with the duration of symptoms.[49]
  - ○ Abdominal computed tomography (CT) may be used when abdominal ultrasound was non-diagnostic for appendicitis or other diagnoses are being considered concurrently.
    - ▪ It is the imaging modality of choice for many institutions because it has a sensitivity of 90% to 97% and specificity of 91% to 99%.[25,51]
    - ▪ This high accuracy is maintained between large academic hospitals and small rural community hospitals.[38]

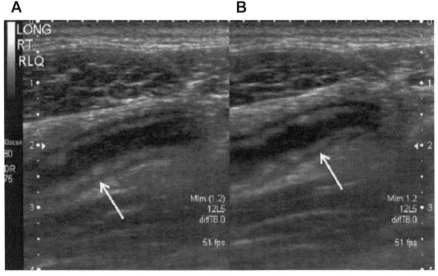

Fig. 4. Thickened wall, noncompressible. (*A*) Sonographic image of appendix without compression. (*B*) Sonographic image of appendix with compression showing noncompressible appendix. Sonographic image of the thickened wall of the appendix with appendicitis (*arrow*). (*From* Parks N, Schroeppel T. Update on imaging for acute appendicitis. Surg Clin North Am 2011;91:141–54.)

■ Unfortunately, children are much more sensitive to the ionizing radiation and have a lifetime radiation-induced cancer risk of 20.1 to 26.1 per 100,000.[52]
  ○ Abdominal MRI has 100% sensitivity and 96% specificity without radiation exposure but is not readily available in all EDs.
- Scoring systems
  ○ The Alvarado scoring system was initially designed to use in adults but only has a specificity of 59% to 100% in children.[53,54]
  ○ The Pediatric Appendicitis Score was designed specifically for children but again has a specificity range of 50% to 98%.[54,55]
  ○ The a priori judgment of experienced practitioners in emergency medicine has a specificity of 49.6% to 90.2% *and is equal* to these appendicitis scoring systems.[44]
  ○ Scoring systems seem to be most useful for trainees or as adjuncts to optimize and standardize patient management.[44]

Management

The primary challenge for the emergency care provider is in considering and diagnosing appendicitis. Its subsequent ED management is relatively straightforward as long as potential pitfalls are appreciated (**Box 9**).

INCARCERATED INGUINAL HERNIA

- It is entrapment of peritoneal contents in an inguinal hernia.
- Strangulation occurs when the hernia is tightly constricted and the vascular supply of the herniated contents becomes severely compromised.

Inguinal hernias are the *most common congenital abnormality that requires surgery* occurring in 0.8% to 4.4% of the general population but up to 6% to 31% in pediatric patients.[56,57] It is 6 times more common in males and typically occurs on the right side.[58]

Diagnosis and Workup

Incarcerated inguinal hernias are often diagnosable with history and physical examination alone, which has a sensitivity of 84%.[56] They typically present with an abrupt bulge in the groin area that increases in size when the child is upset and disappears when calm. The child is usually comfortable appearing unless it is incarcerated. If incarcerated, the hernia is not easily reduced and the child is inconsolable. Bloody stools and bilious emesis occur with bowel strangulation.

Bedside point-of-care ultrasound can augment the evaluation. If a hernia is present, peristalsis with air or fluid within the lumen of the inguinal mass will be seen.

Box 9
Pitfalls of appendicitis

- Assuming a child who has a concerning examination does not have appendicitis because of a negative or indeterminate ultrasound
- Not ensuring adequate follow-up within 24 hours for children discharged home with a worrisome history but reassuring laboratory test results/imaging
- Failing to consider gonadal torsion in any child with lower abdominal pain and concern for appendicitis
- Relying on only one sign or symptom to diagnose or exclude appendicitis

Ultrasound in the radiology department has a sensitivity of 97.9% and can help differentiate between indirect and direct hernias.[56] Formal sonographic evaluation should be considered in female patients to evaluate for ovarian contents.

Management

Nonoperative management of incarcerated hernias with bedside reduction requires adequate analgesia and possibly sedation (50% of children do not receive analgesia before this procedure).[59] If bedside reduction fails, pediatric surgical consultation with possible operative repair is necessary (**Box 10**).

GONADAL TORSION

- Ovarian torsion
  - It is a rotated ovary on its pedicle leading to obstruction of venous outflow, lymphatic drainage, and arterial blood flow once the ovary is engorged and edematous.
  - Adnexal torsion occurs with torsion of the ovary and/or fallopian tube.
- Testicular torsion
  - It is the rotation of spermatic cord resulting in compromise of testicular blood flow.

Ovarian torsion accounts for up to 2.7% of all cases of acute abdominal pain in female patients, but only 15% of those are in children.[60,61] Forty percent to 84% of cases of ovarian pathology have some abnormal features upon histologic examination but this is rarely malignancy.[62]

Testicular torsion occurs in 3.8 to 4.5 males per 100,000, but only 3% to 38% of males with acute scrotal pain have testicular torsion.[61–64] A bell-clapper deformity is a predisposing condition for torsion and occurs bilaterally in 12% of patients who develop testicular torsion.[62]

Diagnosis and Workup

Whether it is a female or male patient being evaluated, early diagnosis and a high clinical suspicion is important for gonadal salvage. There are obvious differences between their respective diagnostic evaluations.

Ovarian torsion

- Diagnosis is difficult because of the nonspecific symptoms often seen, and up to 38% are initially diagnosed with appendicitis.[65]
- Colicky RLQ pain is common with associated fever, nausea, vomiting, and dysuria.
- A previous history of torsion or ovarian mass is often seen.
- On average, girls wait 2.5 times as long for imaging and 2.7 times as long to go to the OR as males with testicular torsion.[66]

Box 10
Pitfalls of incarcerated inguinal hernia

- Failing to consider ovarian involvement in female patients
- Not providing adequate analgesia and sedation before nonoperative reduction
- Failing to evaluate for testes below the hernia, that is, not a retracted testicle

> **Box 11**
> **Pitfalls of gonadal torsion**
>
> - Only looking at the appendix in female patients with a concerning history—historically leads to ovarian salvage rates of 9% to 50%[67]
> - Not maintaining a high clinical suspicion for ovarian torsion in female patients with RLQ abdominal pain
> - Ruling out gonadal torsion based on there being normal blood flow on color Doppler
> - Not performing a testicular examination on all males with abdominal pain

- Laboratory values are nonspecific, but urinalysis and urine pregnancy tests should be performed.
- A pelvic ultrasound has a sensitivity of 100% and specificity of 98% for ovarian torsion and will often reveal an enlarged adnexal mass or ovary with a whirlpool sign.[60,67]
- Color Doppler sonography is useful, but up to two-thirds of cases will have arterial blood flow because the *ovary is fed by both the ovarian and uterine arteries* (**Box 11**).[60,61]
- The presence of pelvic mass or an ovarian cyst greater than 5 cm is 83% sensitive for ovarian torsion.[60]
- It is useful to ultrasound the appendix at the same time because they have similar presentations.
- It is important to note that nonsexually active and prepubescent girls require a transabdominal ultrasound with a full bladder, whereas older, sexually active females require a transvaginal ultrasound with an empty bladder.
- Abdominal/pelvic CT may see an adnexal mass or other abdominal pathology but does not rule in ovarian torsion.
- Overall, diagnosis takes a high index of suspicion, a consistent history and examination, and only sometimes an abnormal sonographic finding.

Testicular torsion

- High position of the testicle and abnormal cremasteric reflex have an odds ratio of 58.8 and 27.7, respectively, for testicular torsion.[63]
- Pain less than 24 hours with associated nausea/vomiting increase the likelihood of testicular torsion if they have an acute scrotum.[63]
- Testicular ultrasound is the most used imaging modality and has a sensitivity of 88% to 96% and specificity of 78% to 98%.[62,64]
- It may reveal a torsion knot in the spermatic cord, which has 96% to 99% sensitivity and specificity for testicular torsion.[62,68]
- If blood flow is present, the testis is more likely to be salvageable with emergent reduction and orchidopexy (**Box 12**).

> **Box 12**
> **Functional GI disorder**
>
> - Chronic abdominal pain in the absence of organic disease
> - Possibly related to dysregulation of the brain-gut axis expressed by visceral hypersensitivity
> - 3 major subsets: functional dyspepsia, functional abdominal pain, and irritable bowel syndrome

---

Box 13
Important aspects of the history for FGID

Functional abdominal pain

- Episodic or continuous periumbilical abdominal pain

IBS

- Diffuse abdominal pain
- Related to bowel movement frequency and improves after defecation

Functional dyspepsia

- Nausea
- Vomiting
- Symptoms consistent with gastroesophageal reflux disease

General

- Often have anxiety, depression, social isolation, and school absenteeism[71]
- Family history of celiac disease, IBD, peptic ulcers, FGID, and constipation

---

Functional GI disorder (FGID) is a common worldwide problem with a prevalence of 1.6% to 41.2%. Up to 45% of these children will be diagnosed with irritable bowel syndrome (IBS).[69,70] Seventy percent of diagnosed cases of IBS occur in females, but there is more sex variability with the other subsets of FGID.[69,71] It is no surprise that this entity is the most common disease leading to consultation with a pediatric gastroenterologist.[72]

Diagnosis and Workup

The American Academy of Pediatrics recommends that evaluation for FGID should take place in the primary care setting, but these children will often present to the ED.[3] When they do, a full history and physical examination (**Box 13**) should be performed to ensure that there are no red flags for organic disease, abuse, depression, or suicidal ideation (**Box 14**).

If they have a reassuring history and physical examination, diagnostic testing is often low yield.[3] If there are red flags on examination, laboratory values, such as CBC, CRP, liver function tests, lipase, erythrocyte sedimentation rate, celiac serologies, urinalysis, urine pregnancy test, and stool studies, may be indicated. Imaging though is not routinely recommended. Without a concerning red flag, less than 1%

Box 14
Red flags for organic cause of abdominal pain in children

- Weight loss
- Severe vomiting
- Chronic severe diarrhea
- GI bleeding
- Hematemesis
- Fever
- Family medical history of inflammatory bowel disease

Box 15
Pitfalls of FGID

- Not considering psychosocial conditions like depression, suicidal ideation, or child abuse in your differential—this may be how the child is reaching out for help
- Failing to recognize and workup worrisome red flags associated with FGID
- Failing to perform a thorough examination in child already labeled with chronic abdominal pain

---

of children will have an abnormality on ultrasound.[3] If further workup is needed, but children are stable and there is not concern for an emergent condition, the need for evaluation should be explained and then deferred to patients' primary care provider.

Management

The mainstay of management for children with FGID is thorough anticipatory guidance discussions and the setting of reasonable expectations (**Box 15**).

SUMMARY

Up to 10% of all visits to a pediatric ED are for abdominal pain.[48] The astute clinician needs to have a high index of suspicion while evaluating any child with abdominal pain. The challenge is to remain vigilant for the rare, yet significant pathologic condition, while not overtesting the more common, benign conditions.

REFERENCES

1. Caperell K, Pitetti R, Cross K. Race and acute abdominal pain in a pediatric emergency department. Pediatrics 2013;131:1098–106.
2. Pollack E. Pediatric abdominal surgical emergencies. Pediatr Ann 1996;25:448–57.
3. Romano C, Porcaro F. Currents issues in the management of pediatric functional abdominal pain. Rev Recent Clin Trials 2014;9:13–20.
4. Saps M, Seshadri R, Sztainberg M, et al. A prospective school-based study of abdominal pain and other common somatic complaints in children. J Pediatr 2009;154:322–36.
5. Miglioretti D, Johnson E, Williams A, et al. Pediatric computed tomography and associated radiation exposure and estimated cancer risk. JAMA Pediatr 2013;167:700–7.
6. Tabbers M, DiLorenzo C, Berger M, et al. Evaluation and treatment of functional constipation in infants and children: evidence-based recommendations from ESPGHAN and NASPGHAN. J Pediatr Gastroenterol Nutr 2014;58:258–74.
7. Diamanti A, Bracci F, Reale A, et al. Incidence, clinical presentation, and management of constipation in a pediatric ED. Am J Emerg Med 2010;28:189–94.
8. Fox S. Recurrent abdominal pain. Charlotte (NC): Pediatric EM Morsels; 2014.
9. Sivitz A, Tejani C, Cohen S. Evaluation of hypertrophic pyloric stenosis by pediatric emergency physician sonography. Acad Emerg Med 2013;20:646–51.
10. Taylor N, Cass D, Holland A. Infantile hypertrophic pyloric stenosis: has anything changed? J Paediatr Child Health 2013;49:33–7.

11. Eberly M, Eide M, Thompson J, et al. Azithromycin in early infancy and pyloric stenosis. Pediatrics 2015;135:483–8.
12. Piroutek M, Brown L, Thorp A. Bilious vomiting does not rule out infantile hypertrophic pyloric stenosis. Clin Pediatr 2012;51:214–8.
13. Glatstein M, Carbell G, Boddu S, et al. The changing clinical presentation of hypertrophic pyloric stenosis: the experience of a large, tertiary care pediatric hospital. Clin Pediatr 2011;50:192–5.
14. Tutay G, Capraro G, Spirko B, et al. Electrolyte profile of pediatric patients with hypertrophic pyloric stenosis. Pediatr Emerg Care 2013;29:465–8.
15. Askew N. An overview of infantile hypertrophic pyloric stenosis. Paediatr Nurs 2010;22:27–30.
16. Hernanz-Schulman M. Infantile hypertrophic pyloric stenosis. Radiology 2003; 227:319–31.
17. Mandeville K, Chien M, Willyerd F, et al. Intussusception: clinical presentation and imaging characteristics. Pediatr Emerg Care 2012;28:842–4.
18. Gray M, Li S, Hoffmann R, et al. Recurrence rates after intussusception enema reduction: a meta-analysis. Pediatrics 2014;134:110–9.
19. Riera A, Hsiao A, Langhan M, et al. Diagnosis of intussusception by physician novice sonographers in the emergency department. Ann Emerg Med 2012;60: 264–8.
20. Lam S, Wise A, Yenter C. Emergency bedside ultrasound for the diagnosis of pediatric intussusception: a retrospective review. World J Emerg Med 2014;5: 255–8.
21. Weihmiller S, Monuteaux M, Bachur R. Ability of pediatric physicians to judge the likelihood of intussusception. Pediatr Emerg Care 2012;28:136–40.
22. Shah S. An update on common gastrointestinal emergencies. Emerg Med Clin North Am 2013;31:775–93.
23. Fleisher G. Textbook of pediatric emergency medicine. 6th edition. Philadelphia: Lippincott Williams & Wilkins; 2010. Print.
24. Pepper V, Stanfill A, Pearl R. Diagnosis and management of pediatric appendicitis, intussusception, and Meckel diverticulum. Surg Clin North Am 2012;92: 505–26.
25. Henderson A, Anupindi S, Servaes S, et al. Comparison of 2-view abdominal radiographs with ultrasound in children with suspected intussusception. Pediatr Emerg Care 2013;29:145–50.
26. Hernandez J, Swischuk L, Angel C. Validity of plain films in intussusception. Emerg Radiol 2004;10:323–6.
27. Beres A, Baird R, Fung E, et al. Comparative outcome analysis of the management of pediatric intussusception with or without surgical admission. J Pediatr Surg 2014;49:750–2.
28. Chien M, Willyerd F, Mandeville K, et al. Management of the child after enema-reduced intussusception: hospital or home? J Emerg Med 2013;44:53–7.
29. Aboagye J, Goldstein S, Salazar J. Age at presentation of common pediatric surgical conditions: reexamining dogma. J Pediatr Surg 2014;49:995–9.
30. Millar A, Rode H, Cywe S. Malrotation and volvulus in infancy and childhood. Semin Pediatr Surg 2003;12:229–36.
31. Sivitz A, Lyons R. Mid-gut volvulus identified by pediatric emergency ultrasonography. J Emerg Med 2013;45:e173–4.
32. Nehra D, Goldstein A. Intestinal malrotation: varied clinical presentation from infancy through adulthood. Surgery 2011;149:386–93.

33. Tackett J, Muise E, Cowles R. Malrotation: current strategies navigating the radiologic diagnosis of a surgical emergency. World J Radiol 2014;6:730–6.

34. Applegate K, Anderson J, Klatte E. Intestinal malrotation in children: a problem-solving approach to the upper gastrointestinal series. Radiographics 2006;26: 1485–500.

35. Lodwik D, Minneci P, Deans K. Current surgical management of intestinal rotational abnormalities. Curr Opin Pediatr 2015;27:383–8.

36. Short S, Papillon S, Berel D, et al. Late onset of necrotizing enterocolitis in the full-term infant is associated with increased mortality: results from a two-center analysis. J Pediatr Surg 2014;49:950–3.

37. Sakellaris G, Partalis N, Dede O, et al. Gastrointestinal perforations in neonatal period: experience over 10 years. Pediatr Emerg Care 2012;28:886–8.

38. Parks N, Schroeppel T. Update on imaging for acute appendicitis. Surg Clin North Am 2011;91:141–54.

39. Paulson E, Kalady M, Pappas T. Clinical practice. Suspected appendicitis. N Engl J Med 2003;348:910–25.

40. Cole M, Maldonado N. Evidence-based management of suspected appendicitis in the emergency department. Emerg Med Pract 2011;13:1–32.

41. Lavine E, Saul T, Frasure S, et al. Point-of-care ultrasound in a patient with perforated appendicitis. Pediatr Emerg Care 2014;30:665–7.

42. Old J, Dusing R, Yap W, et al. Imaging for suspected appendicitis. Am Fam Physician 2005;71:71–8.

43. The SCOAP Collaborative, Cuschieri J, Florence M, Flum DR, et al. Negative appendectomy and imaging accuracy in the Washington State Surgical Care and Outcomes Assessment Program. Ann Surg 2008;248:557–63.

44. Fleischman R, Devine M, Yagapen M, et al. Evaluation of a novel pediatric appendicitis pathway using high- and low-risk scoring systems. Pediatr Emerg Care 2013;29:1060–5.

45. Shogilev D, Duus N, Odom S, et al. Diagnosing appendicitis: evidence-based review of the diagnostic approach in 2014. West J Emerg Med 2014;7:859–71.

46. Wu H, Lin C, Chang C, et al. Predictive value of C-reactive protein at different cutoff levels in acute appendicitis. Am J Emerg Med 2005;23:449–53.

47. Howell J, Eddy O, Lukens T, et al. Clinical policy: critical issues in the evaluation and management of emergency department patients with suspected appendicitis. Ann Emerg Med 2010;55:71–116.

48. Mittal M, Dayan P, Macias C, et al. Performance of ultrasound in the diagnosis of appendicitis in children in a multicenter cohort. Acad Emerg Med 2013;20: 697–702.

49. Ross M, Liu H, Netherton S, et al. Outcomes of children with suspected appendicitis and incompletely visualized appendix on ultrasound. Acad Emerg Med 2014;21:538–42.

50. Horn A, Ufberg J. Appendicitis, diverticulitis, and colitis. Emerg Med Clin North Am 2011;29:347–68.

51. Birnbaum B, Wilson S. Appendicitis at the millennium. Radiology 2000;215: 337–48.

52. Hall E. Lessons we have learned from our children: cancer risks from diagnostic radiology. Pediatr Radiol 2002;32:700–6.

53. Escriba A, Gamell A, Fernandez Y, et al. Prospective validation of two systems of classification for the diagnosis of acute appendicitis. Pediatr Emerg Care 2011; 27:165–9.

54. Pogorelic Z, Rak S, Mrklic I, et al. Prospective validation of Alvarado score and pediatric appendicitis score for the diagnosis of acute appendicitis in children. Pediatr Emerg Care 2015;31:164–8.
55. Goldman R, Carter S, Stephens D, et al. Prospective validation of the pediatric appendicitis score. J Pediatr 2008;153:278–82.
56. Till L, Kessler D. Rapid evaluation of an inguinal mass in a female infant using point-of-care ultrasound. Pediatr Emerg Care 2014;30:366–7.
57. Lau S, Lee Y, Caty M. Current management of hernias and hydroceles. Semin Pediatr Surg 2007;16:50–7.
58. Cascini V, Lisi G, Di Renzo D, et al. Irreducible indirect inguinal hernia containing uterus and bilateral adnexa in a premature female infant: report of an exceptional case and review of the literature. J Pediatr Surg 2013;48:E17–9.
59. Al-Ansari K, Sulowski C, Ratnapalan S. Analgesia and sedation practices for incarcerated inguinal hernias in children. Clin Pediatr 2008;47:766–9.
60. Appelbaum H, Abraham C, Choi-Rosen J, et al. Key clinical predictors in the early diagnosis of adnexal torsion in children. J Pediatr Adolesc Gynecol 2013;26: 167–70.
61. Schmitt E, Ngai S, Gausche-Hill M, et al. Twist and shout! Pediatric ovarian torsion clinical update and case discussion. Pediatr Emerg Care 2013;29:518–26.
62. Baldisserotto M. Scrotal emergencies. Pediatr Radiol 2009;39:516–21.
63. Beni-Israel T, Goldman M, Bar Chaim S, et al. Clinical predictors for testicular torsion as seen in the pediatric ED. Am J Emerg Med 2010;28:786–9.
64. Shah M, Caviness A, Mendez D. Prospective pilot derivation of a decision tool for children at low risk for testicular torsion. Acad Emerg Med 2013;20:271–8.
65. Ryan M, Desai B. Ovarian torsion in a 5-year old: a case report and review. Case Rep Emerg Med 2012;2012:679121.
66. Piper H, Oltmann S, Xu L, et al. Ovarian torsion: diagnosis of inclusion mandates earlier intervention. J Pediatr Surg 2012;47:2071–6.
67. Ochsner T, Roos J, Johnson A, et al. Ovarian torsion in a three-year-old girl. J Emerg Med 2010;38:e27–30.
68. Dajusta D, Granberg C, Villanueva C, et al. Contemporary review of testicular torsion: new concepts, emerging technologies and potential therapeutics. J Pediatr Urol 2013;9:723–30.
69. Korterink J, Rutten J, Venmans L, et al. Pharmacologic treatment in pediatric functional abdominal pain disorders: a systematic review. J Pediatr 2015;166: 424–31.
70. Korterink J, Diederen K, Benninga M, et al. Epidemiology of pediatric functional abdominal pain disorders: a meta-analysis. PLoS One 2015;10(5):1–17.
71. Varni J, Shulman R, Self M, et al. Symptom profiles in patients with irritable bowel syndrome or functional abdominal pain compared to healthy controls. J Pediatr Gastroenterol Nutr 2015;61(3):323–9.
72. Saps M, Biring H, Pusatcioglu C, et al. A comprehensive review of randomized placebo-controlled pharmacological clinical trials in children with functional abdominal pain disorders. J Pediatr Gastroenterol Nutr 2015;60:645–53.

Abdominal Pain in the Geriatric Patient

Amy Leuthauser, MD, MS[a],*, Benjamin McVane, MD[b]

KEYWORDS

- Abdominal pain in the elderly
- Atypical presentations of common abnormalities in the elderly • Approach • Geriatric

KEY POINTS

- Evaluation of the elderly patient with abdominal pain can be difficult, time-consuming, and fraught with potential missteps.
- Abdominal pain is the most common emergency department complaint and the fourth most common complaint among elderly patients.
- The physiologic, pharmacologic, and psychosocial aspects of elderly patients make evaluation of their abdominal pain different than in the general population.
- Having a lower index of suspicion for abnormality and ordering tests will help make diagnoses, and getting ancillary services like pharmacy involved in the patients' care, can be of innumerable benefit.

INTRODUCTION

Evaluation of the elderly patient with abdominal pain can be difficult, time-consuming, and fraught with potential missteps. Still, it will be an increasingly common task of the emergency physician as the population ages. The US population over the age of 65 continues to grow, and patients of this age group are the fastest growing group of emergency department (ED) users. Accordingly, the past few years have seen a dramatic increase in research and focus on the emergency care of elderly patients.[1]

Abdominal pain is the most common ED complaint and the fourth most common complaint among elderly patients. The physiologic, pharmacologic, and psychosocial aspects of elderly patients make evaluation of their abdominal pain different than in the general population. Consequently, this population is prone to worse outcomes, higher rates of admission and surgical interventions, and prolonged ED and hospital stays

---

Disclosures: Neither author has any disclosures to report.
^a Department of Emergency Medicine, Bay of Plenty District Health Board, Tauranga Hospital, Cameron Road, Private bag 12024, Tauranga 3142, New Zealand; ^b Department of Emergency Medicine, Icahn School of Medicine, Mount Sinai Hospital, 1 gustav levy place, New York, NY 10028, USA
* Corresponding author.
E-mail address: amyleuthauser@gmail.com

Emerg Med Clin N Am 34 (2016) 363–375
http://dx.doi.org/10.1016/j.emc.2015.12.009
0733-8627/16/$ – see front matter © 2016 Elsevier Inc. All rights reserved.

compared with younger patients.[2] Alarmingly, mortality in patients greater than age 80 with abdominal pain nearly doubles if initial diagnosis is delayed.[3] This article aims to address general aspects of approaching abdominal pain in elderly patients as well as specific commonly encountered abnormalities in this population.

GENERAL APPROACH
Limitations to History-Taking

Within the initial step of gathering a history of the presenting illness, a clinician should be aware of potential complexities unique to an elderly patient. Elderly patients often present later in their disease course with vaguer and broader symptoms than their younger counterparts.[4] Normal age-related decline in hearing and vision may impede the patient's ability to communicate effectively with a physician. Cognitive impairments may further limit communication or diminish a patient's effective recollection of their illness progression. Patients themselves may underreport symptoms because of assumptions that symptoms are a part of the normal aging process or for fear of loss of independence with increased health care needs.[5] Alternatively, a provider may need to rely on family members or home health assistants to supplement the clinical history.

Limitations to Physical Examination

Physiologic changes inherent in the aging process can diminish the usefulness of the physical examination for elderly patients. Changes in the gastrointestinal (GI) as well as neurologic, musculoskeletal, and immunologic system lead to much higher rates of atypical presentations of common disease. Only 17% of elderly patients with perforated appendicitis presented with "classic" complaints.[6] Atrophy of abdominal wall musculature diminishes rebound and guarding.[7] Changes in peripheral nerve functioning lead to later and subtler presentation of pain.[8] Medications commonly taken by elderly patients, including β-blockers, steroids, nonsteroidal anti-inflammatory drugs (NSAIDs), and opiates, may blunt or alter their response to disease. They may also impair their ability to demonstrate a fever or the expected tachycardic response seen in younger patients. Similarly, changes to T-cell functioning in the elderly patient lead to a higher susceptibility to infection and decreased rate of leukocytosis on laboratory results. One study showed that 30% of patients over the age of 80 with intra-abdominal abnormality requiring surgery developed neither fever nor leukocytosis.[9]

Imaging

The high pretest probability of surgical abnormality and the decreased reliability of physical examination should lead the ED physician to a low threshold for using advanced imaging in elderly patients with abdominal pain. In this population, disposition and management decision may be significantly altered by results of computed tomographic (CT) imaging, which should be the imaging test of choice in most cases of elderly abdominal pain. In one study, the diagnostic certainty of emergency physicians assessing elderly patients with abdominal pain was increased from 36% to 77% after obtaining a CT scan.[10]

Plain films are generally of limited diagnostic use, although they may be helpful for identifying features such as sigmoid or cecal volvulus, bowel obstruction, or the presence of free intraperitoneal air. Ultrasound is the imaging of choice for biliary and pelvic diseases as well as for early identification of abdominal aneurysms, although it may be limited by body habitus, bowel gas, and operator competence.

General Treatment and Disposition Considerations

Symptomatic and definitive treatment of elderly patients poses unique concerns that cannot be categorized into traditional teachings. Selecting and dosing appropriate analgesic medication may be complicated by comorbid renal and liver insufficiency, dementia and fall risk, patient tolerance or intolerance of opiates, and difficulties in obtaining vascular access. Both underdosing and overdosing of medications are relevant concerns in elderly patients, unsurprisingly leading to widespread discomfort of emergency physicians in managing elderly pain.[11] Consequently, elderly patients are less frequently screened for pain and often inadequately provided analgesia.[12] The Beers Criteria for potentially inappropriate medications (PIM) for use in older adults caution against several commonly used medication for the treatment of abdominal pain, most notably ketorolac and metoclopramide.[13]

In general, assessing the risk-benefit ratios of disposition options is multifactorial and more complicated than in younger cohorts. Nearly half of elderly patients with abdominal pain will require admission, and one-third will require surgical intervention.[2] Forty percent of abdominal surgeries in geriatric patients occur in an acute (urgent or emergent) time frame, with a corresponding 10- to 15-fold increase in morbidity and 3- to 5-fold increase in mortality compared with elective surgery and worse outcomes compared with younger cohorts.[14] Although the prevalence of multiple comorbidities makes many elderly patients less than ideal surgical candidates, it is not clear how to fully incorporate these into accurate prognoses.[15] Similarly, the iatrogenic risks of hospitalization, including falls, physical deconditioning, and nosocomial infection, increase with age, underscoring the potential harm of even conservative observation of undifferentiated abdominal pain.[16] Still, given the difficult and unreliable nature of evaluating elderly abdominal pain, a low threshold for observation or hospitalization should be used.

SPECIFIC ABNORMALITIES
Small-Bowel Obstruction

Small-bowel obstructions (SBOs) are a common cause of abdominal pain in the elderly and may present more subtly than in younger patients.[17] Although symptoms classically include diffuse abdominal pain, distention, vomiting, and constipation/obstipation, these symptoms may not manifest early in the presentation. Paradoxically, diarrhea may be present as a result of hyperperistalsis distal to the obstruction point. Previous studies have suggested concerning mortalities for SBO in geriatric patients up to 26%, although more recent studies suggest outcomes in geriatric patients similar to the general population.[18] For patients without indications for urgent surgery, initial conservative medical management should include intravenous fluid resuscitation, nasogastric decompression, and temporary NPO (nothing by mouth) status, with surgery following if not improved in 24 to 48 hours. Patients admitted to a surgical, rather than medical service, are noted to have less delay in progression to surgery when necessary, and corresponding improvements in outcomes.[18] As in younger patients, hernias or intra-abdominal adhesions cause most SBOs in the elderly. However, unique to elderly patients, gallstone disease may contribute to 25% of bowel obstructions compared with 2% in the general population.[19]

Large-Bowel Obstruction

Although still uncommon, large-bowel obstructions occur more frequently in elderly patients than in the general population. Most cases result from diverticulosis and malignancy, the rates of which increase with age. Accordingly, elderly patients presenting with large-bowel obstructions should be questioned regarding symptoms and risk factors for colorectal cancer. Similar to a SBO, patients classically present with abdominal pain, vomiting, and constipation/obstipation, although diarrhea is seen in one-fifth of patients, and only one-half will report constipation or vomiting.[20] Similar to SBOs in this age group, large-bowel obstructions are commonly only discovered late in their course and accordingly have a high mortality, ranging from 12% to 50%.[21]

Sigmoid and cecal volvulus account for a smaller subset of large-bowel obstructions, but more often requires emergent surgical intervention.[22] Reported symptoms can provide some differentiation between volvulus site. Sigmoid volvulus, causing close to 80% of volvuli, causes a more gradual onset of pain, whereas cecal volvulus presents more acutely. As would be expected anatomically, sigmoid volvulus can often be decompressed with a rectal tube, sigmoidoscope, or barium enema, whereas cecal volvulus requires surgical repair. Volvulus of either site is at risk for perforation and should be decompressed urgently.[23] Sigmoid volvulus has a high rate of recurrence and often requires definitive surgery, which may be performed electively if the volvulus can be decompressed nonoperatively.

Functional impairment and decreased motility of the GI tract can occur from medications and mimic symptoms of large- or small-bowel obstructions.[24] Given the increased rates of polypharmacy in older adults, this possibility should be noted when evaluating elderly patients. Medications with opioid or anticholinergic effects can cause ileus. In a more severe form, patients may develop acute colonic pseudo-obstruction, or Ogilvie syndrome. Ogilvie syndrome, a functional obstruction of the GI tract, occurs more commonly in elderly, debilitated patients, particularly those that are institutionalized or in prolonged hospital course.[25] Treatment is conservative medical management similar to SBOs. Alternatively, treatment with neostigmine has been offered as an acute therapy.[26] This treatment is highly effective in a short time period but requires careful monitoring because of the risk of bradycardia.

Biliary Tract Disease

The incidence of cholelithiasis increases with age to up to 33% by age 70, as does the severity of subsequent biliary tract disease in elderly patients.[27] Gallbladder perforation, gangrene, emphysematous cholecystitis, ascending cholangitis, gallstone ileus, choledocholiathisis, and gallstone-induced pancreatitis are all more prevalent in elderly patients than the general population.[28] As such, biliary disease constitutes the leading reason for acute abdominal surgery in elderly patients.[29]

Cholecystitis may be harder to detect in elderly patients than the general population. Although right upper quadrant or epigastric pain and tenderness are common, more than half of elderly patients with acute cholecystitis will lack nausea, vomiting, or fever.[30] Laboratory and imaging studies may be similarly unhelpful. Leukocytosis may be absent in 30% to 40% of those with acute cholecystitis.[31] Evaluation by ultrasound (**Fig. 1**) may be less helpful given the increased prevalence of acalculous cholecystitis as well as cholodocolithiasis. If available, HIDA (hepatobiliary) scan may be useful when a high clinical suspicion exists.

With the increased rate of complications of cholecystitis in older adults, broad-spectrum antibiotics and prompt surgical evaluation should be pursued once a diagnosis of cholecystitis is made. Delay in surgery may result in an increased mortality.[32]

Pancreatitis

The incidence of pancreatitis increases 200-fold after the age of 65, making it the most common nonsurgical emergent abdominal abnormality in the elderly.[33] The mortality for elderly patients exceeds that of the general population, approaching 40%.[34] Compared with the broader causes of pancreatitis seen in younger patients, nearly

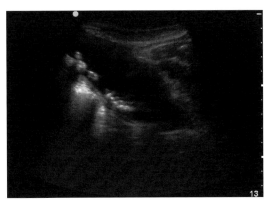

Fig. 1. Ultrasound of gallbladder, demonstrating stones with acoustic shadowing. (*Courtesy of* Nelson B, MD, New York City, NY.)

half of pancreatitis in elderly patients results from gallstones.[33] As with other abdominal processes, pancreatitis may present in elderly patients in a manner different than the classic upper abdominal pain radiating to the back with nausea and vomiting. Recent guidelines suggest that a diagnosis of pancreatitis should be made if at least 2 of 3 criteria are fulfilled: upper abdominal pain, elevated pancreatic enzymes, ultrasound/CT/MRI findings suggestive of pancreatitis, with CT being the preferred imaging modality.[35] The index of suspicion for pancreatitis should be low, prompting a low threshold for imaging in elderly patients. The rate of necrotizing pancreatitis in elderly patients is increased, underscoring the importance of imaging.[36]

Peptic Ulcer Disease

There is a high incidence of peptic ulcer disease (PUD) in the elderly population, due in part to the increasing use of NSAIDs in that age group. Users of NSAIDs are 5 to 10 times more likely to develop PUD.[37] Similarly, patients on corticosteroids are at increased risk, particularly when combined with NSAIDs. It is important to take a thorough drug history, because patients may not consider an over-the-counter medication as part of the list they provide to staff. There is a significant amount of patients who will not admit their use of aspirin, even on direct questioning, so it must always be considered.[38]

Helicobacter pylori colonization is greatly increased in the elderly, with some estimates of 53% to 73% of elderly being colonized,[39] leading to increased risk of PUD. The risk of bleeding from PUD is about 14 times higher in the population over the age of 70 than patients under the age of 40,[40] and the overall mortality from PUD is 100 times higher in the elderly population.[23] Elderly patients are more likely to bleed, rebleed, require blood transfusions, and require surgery to control bleeding than younger patients.

Diagnosing PUD in elderly patients can be difficult in the absence of typical pain. A common presentation may just be melena,[41] or even signs of long-term blood loss, like heart failure or chest pain. In elderly patients, visceral perforation is often painless, with no rigidity on examination. Free air may be absent on radiograph; thus, a low threshold for ordering a CT scan is indicated. In one study, up to 50% of patients with perforation did not show free air on the plain radiographs.[19]

Diverticular Disease

The formation of diverticula in the colon is related to chronic constipation, a lack of enough water, and physical inactivity, as well as increased bowel transit time. They are usually seen in patients older than 40 years and are present in approximately 50% to 80% of older patients.[42] Approximately 80% of patients with diverticulosis are asymptomatic.[43]

Acute diverticulitis occurs when the diverticula become obstructed by fecal matter, resulting in lymphatic obstruction, inflammation, and perforation. The usual presenting complaints are left lower quadrant abdominal pain, with or without bloody stools, nausea, and fever. Atypical presentations include lack of fever, leukocytosis, and absence of guaiac-positive stool. Nearly 30% of the geriatric presentations of acute diverticulitis do not have abdominal tenderness on examination.[44] It is important that endoscopy be performed to rule out carcinoma after an acute episode of diverticulitis. Neoplasms are found in about 15% of patients with diverticulitis.[45]

Most cases of diverticulitis in Western countries are located in the left colon; right colonic involvement is more common in Eastern nations. Right-sided diverticula are more often the case of bleeding than the left colon.[46] Most acute flares of diverticulitis, even those with small perforations, can be managed medically, with antibiotics covering gram-negative and anaerobes, intravenous fluids, and bowel rest. If there are larger perforations or abscess formation, surgery or percutaneous drainage may be indicated.

Unfortunately, in the elderly, acute diverticulitis tends to present in a more severe manner, most likely due to the use of antiplatelet medication in this age group. The operative risk in this group is high, approaching 5%.[47,48]

Diverticular bleeding is one of the most common causes of lower GI bleeds. The risk of bleeding increases with age, male gender, and the use of NSAIDs or anticoagulants.[49]

Appendicitis

Appendicitis is a very common surgical emergency. It is often a very difficult diagnosis to make in the elderly patient population and is missed in the elderly about 54% of the time.[50] As mentioned in the introduction of this section, studies show that only 17% of elderly patients with perforated appendicitis had a classic presentation.[6] The classic presentation is defined as right lower quadrant pain, fever, and elevated white blood cell count.

The widespread use of CT scanning has helped to minimize unnecessary surgery and is very sensitive in the elderly population, showing 91% to 99% sensitivity.[51] The rates of renal insufficiency in the elderly make the use of intravenous contrast dye for the study sometimes contraindicated. In recent years, literature has emerged supporting the use of noncontrast CT imaging for suspected appendicitis, and it seems to be appropriate for decision-making in the ED.[52,53] There is a growing body of literature regarding the use of ultrasound in diagnosing appendicitis. As with any ultrasonography study, it is operator-dependent and made more difficult by patients' body habitus and bowel gas patterns.

The prognosis of uncomplicated appendicitis in both young and old age groups is nearly equal. However, perforation worsens the condition, dramatically resulting in higher rates of morbidity and mortality.[54] In this same article, the investigators concluded that although the rate of perforation is similar in age ranges, the elderly often have a delay in presentation to the hospital.

Elderly patients have a higher risk for both mortality and morbidity following appendectomy than younger patients.[50] There is a growing body of literature about the nonoperative management of appendicitis. Given the operative risks, it is hoped that the geriatric population would be an appropriate group for further study on a change in practice to demonstrate outcomes similar to those undergoing surgery.[55]

Extra-Abdominal Causes of Abdominal Pain

The elderly, like the pediatric population, can manifest extra-abdominal abnormality as abdominal pain because of referred pain and inability to localize, or perhaps to communicate specific symptoms.

Congestive heart failure can often present as abdominal pain. The character of the pain is typically dull or described as a fullness, which will not be relieved until the heart failure is addressed. Importantly, acute myocardial infarction must always be on the differential with a complaint of nausea and epigastric discomfort. In one study, 45% of women over the age of 75 with an ST segment elevation myocardial infarction presented without chest pain, but simply with GI symptoms.[56]

Pneumonias have been reported as a frequent cause of referred abdominal pain, epically lower lobe infections.[57] Other pulmonary causes can include pulmonary embolus, heart failure, pneumothorax, and empyema. A low threshold for chest radiographs in recommended.

Genitourinary complaints are often difficult to tease out, because dysuria is not always present in the geriatric patient, and if there is a component of altered mental status, occult infections become very important to consider. One must be careful, however, when attributing the abdominal pain to a urinary tract infection. There is a high incidence of asymptomatic bacteria in the elderly, up to 18%, and this increases with age.[58] Prostatitis can also be a very difficult diagnosis to make, given its often vague symptoms.[59] A rectal examination is pivotal in the workup of abdominal pain, and especially with genitourinary complaints.

Urinary retention is also a very common cause of nonspecific abdominal pain and can be caused by several different abnormalities. Medications, especially the antihistamines and anticholinergics, can cause retention (**Fig. 2**). There can be physical outlet obstruction, or bladder dysfunction from a neurologic catastrophe, such as stroke, intracranial bleed, or spinal cord injury. Pyelonephritis can be a difficult diagnosis to make as well, because many elderly patients do not have the traditional costovertebral angle tenderness on examination.[60]

Other systems such as dermatologic are often missed. Herpes zoster should be considered. An attack of herpes zoster involving the thoracic dermatomes can sometimes cause severe right upper quadrant pain, which can be confused with other disease states such as acute cholecystitis.[61] Rashes can be a manifestation of other

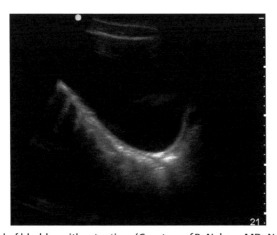

Fig. 2. Ultrasound of bladder with retention. (*Courtesy of* B. Nelson, MD, New York City, NY.)

abnormality, or they themselves a cause of abdominal pain in the elderly, so it is crucially important to fully undress patients for the physical examination.

Rectus sheath hematomas (RSH) must always be considered, especially in patients who are on anticoagulation, such as low-molecular-weight heparin or warfarin. There is a high mortality in this group, and imaging should be pursued on patients with an otherwise unexplained abdominal pain. The mortality risk from RSH is 4% overall, but may be as high as 25% in patients on anticoagulation.[62]

Depression or somatization in the elderly may present as abdominal pain, and practitioners should maintain a low threshold for performing a depression screening on patients. In one study, about 24% of elderly patients presenting to the ED with abdominal pain had negative workups in terms of an intra-abdominal diagnosis.[17] Although it is not clear whether those patients had a diagnosis of depression, the clinician should have a low threshold for performing a depression screen on patients presenting with abdominal pain that has no clear diagnosis.

Constipation

Constipation is a common condition in the elderly, with prevalence ranging from 24% to 50%.[63] It is defined as unsatisfactory defecation, infrequent stools, or difficulty with stool passage. In older adults, constipation may be associated with fecal impaction and fecal incontinence. Fecal impaction can cause mucosal ulceration, bleeding, and anemia. Laxatives are used daily by 10% to 18% of community-dwelling older adults and 74% of nursing home residents.[64]

There are important differences between constipation in the elderly and in the young. In young people, the condition is often caused by poor dietary choices, including lack of fiber. In the geriatric patient, medications, comorbidities, inactivity, and decreased gastric-emptying time as well as GI malignancies are important to consider.[23] In one study, a low-calorie diet, low fluid intake, high protein diet, and psychological distress were linked to constipation. Distress was defined as depression, anxiety, obsessive-compulsive disorder, and somatization disorder.[65]

A digital rectal examination should be performed on all patients with constipation to rule out mechanical obstruction of stool, or other pelvic floor abnormality, such as rectal or uterine prolapse. Blood in the stool, a change in the caliber of the stool, acute onset of constipation, or a strong family history of malignancy should trigger a more extensive workup.

In the elderly, given the risk of medication side effects, it is best to treat chronic constipation with dietary and activity changes. If that has already been tried, then a bulk laxative, like psyllium, would be safest. If an enema is indicated, then a warm water enema would be the safest to administer, as opposed to a medication-containing preparation.

Malignancy

About 10% of elderly patients that present to the ED with a nonsurgical abdominal pain will be found to have a malignancy.[66] Malignancies can present as different types of abdominal pain, but a history of unintentional weight loss, night sweats, and fatigue should raise suspicion for a malignancy. It may also present as peritonitis, ascites, perforation, or abdominal mass. Unfortunately, many cases of malignancy are discovered once they are already metastatic.[67] Different types of malignancies may have different presentations. For example, renal cell carcinomas may have flank pain and hematuria, but often are asymptomatic and diagnosed on imaging.[68] Colonic and rectal malignancies often present as constipation, or with dark or bloody stools.

Pharmacology

The elderly often have a long list of medications that can be the cause of clinical conditions and complicate the making of some diagnosis. They are more susceptible to different types of medication errors than in the younger population. PIM have been studied many times. A range of 12% to 20% of geriatric ED patients received PIM.[69,70] PIM include narcotics, NSAIDs, anti-inflammatories, sedative-hypnotics, muscle relaxants, and antihistamines. These medications can lead to such varied abnormality as altered mental status, renal failure, GI bleeding, and constipation. Unfortunately, they are often administered to the elderly inappropriately.

ED -dedicated pharmacist involvement can predict and prevent medication side effects and interactions. The geriatric population would logically have a high potential from benefit from clinic pharmacists in the ED.[71]

When treating patients over the age of 65, it is essential that the Beers list be consulted, before ordering any medications.[13] This list provides invaluable information and guidelines as to which medications may not be safe in older adults.

Disposition/Special Considerations

There are a growing number of specially designed Geriatric EDs that are being constructed in the United States. Traditional physical plants and layouts of EDs are not safe for older adults that may have hearing or visual impairment, or suffer from cognitive decline. Falls can occur, epically during times of crowding and inadequate staffing. Specially designed Geriatric EDs have more protocolized interventions of ancillary services like physical and occupational therapy, volunteers, and staff to arrange from home services, to help reduce the rate of hospital admissions.[72]

If the decision is made to discharge a patient with a presenting complaint of abdominal pain, it is important to document a repeat physical examination, and that the patient is tolerating oral intake, and a follow-up appointment with a primary care provider is made.[73] The patient should have a responsible adult to monitor and assist them should their condition worsen. If a definite follow-up time is unable to be made, the patient should be told to return to the ED for a recheck.

Many of the above-described clinical conditions require the use of CT scanning, often with intravenous contrast. The provider should be aware of the risk of renal failure with contrast studies and should use the glomerular filtration rate (GFR), as opposed to serum creatinine, to decide whether contrast would be safe in the patient; this is important because as aging occurs, the GFR will decrease. Decreased muscle mass and protein intake, both very common in the elderly, can result in the serum creatinine to be falsely elevated.[74] Although ultrasound has become more common at the bedside, it does remain operator-dependent and cannot show other, unexpected abnormalities that commonly occur in the elderly.

SUMMARY

By 2030, 1 in 5 Americans will be over the age of 65, with many more living to be greater than 100. Clinicians need to be vigilant so as to not miss potentially serious conditions that may be difficult to diagnose in the geriatric population. Any acute abdominal pain is important in an elderly patient. There is no single test that can help the clinician to make a decision about admission versus discharge.[75] Therefore, one would advocate a liberal policy for at least a period of observation, if not admission, for repeat abdominal examinations. Unfortunately, about 60% of abnormality in the geriatric patient requires surgery,[4] and their mortality is 10 times higher than that of the young.[76]

There are more often than not atypical presentations of common diseases and uncommon diseases as well. Having a lower index of suspicion for abnormality and ordering tests will help make diagnoses, and getting ancillary services like pharmacy involved in the patients' care can be of innumerable benefit.

REFERENCES

1. de Dombal FT. Acute abdominal pain in the elderly. J Clin Gastroenterol 1994; 19(4):331–5.
2. Brewer BJ, Golden GT, Hitch DC, et al. Abdominal pain. An analysis of 1,000 consecutive cases in a University hospital emergency room. Am J Surg 1976; 131(2):219–23.
3. van Geloven AA, Biesheuvel TH, Luitse JS, et al. Hospital admissions of patients aged over 80 with acute abdominal complaints. Eur J Surg 2000;166(11):866–71.
4. Birnbaumer D. The elder patient. In: Marx J, editor. Rosen's emergency medicine—concepts and clinical practice. Elsevier; 2013. p. 2351–6.
5. Rothrock SG, Greenfield RH, Falk JL. Acute abdominal emergencies in the elderly: clues to identifying serious illness. Part I—clinical assessment and diagnostic studies. Emerg Med Rep 1992;13:177–84.
6. Paranjape C, Dalia S, Pan J, et al. Appendicitis in the elderly: a change in the laparoscopic era. Surg Endosc 2007;21(5):777–81.
7. Wroblewski M, Mikulowski P. Peritonitis in geriatric inpatients. Age Ageing 1991; 20(2):90–4.
8. Clinch D, Banerjee AK, Ostick G. Absence of abdominal pain in elderly patients with peptic ulcer. Age Ageing 1984;13(2):120–3.
9. Potts FE, Vukov LF. Utility of fever and leukocytosis in acute surgical abdomens in octogenarians and beyond. J Gerontol A Biol Sci Med Sci 1999;54(2):M55–8.
10. Esses D, Birnbaum A, Bijur P, et al. Ability of CT to alter decision making in elderly patients with acute abdominal pain. Am J Emerg Med 2004;22(4):270–2.
11. McNamara RM, Rousseau E, Sanders AB. Geriatric emergency medicine: a survey of practicing emergency physicians. Ann Emerg Med 1992;21(7):796–801.
12. Hwang U, Platts-Mills TF. Acute pain management in older adults in the emergency department. Clin Geriatr Med 2013;29(1):151–64.
13. American Geriatrics Society 2012 Beers Criteria Update Expert Panel. American Geriatrics Society Updated Beers Criteria for potentially inappropriate medication use in older adults. J Am Geriatr Soc 2012;60(4):616–31.
14. Keller SM, Markovitz LJ, Wilder JR, et al. Emergency and elective surgery in patients over age 70. Am Surg 1987;53(11):636–40.
15. Davis P, Hayden J, Springer J, et al. Prognostic factors for morbidity and mortality in elderly patients undergoing acute gastrointestinal surgery: a systematic review. Can J Surg 2014;57(2):E44–52.
16. Aminzadeh F, Dalziel WB. Older adults in the emergency department: a systematic review of patterns of use, adverse outcomes, and effectiveness of interventions. Ann Emerg Med 2002;39(3):238–47.
17. Bugliosi TF, Meloy TD, Vukov LF. Acute abdominal pain in the elderly. Ann Emerg Med 1990;19(12):1383–6.
18. Schwab DP, Blackhurst DW, Sticca RP. Operative acute small bowel obstruction: admitting service impacts outcome. Am Surg 2001;67(11):1034–8 [discussion: 1038–40].
19. Kauvar DR. The geriatric acute abdomen. Clin Geriatr Med 1993;9(3):547–58.

20. Greenlee HB, Pienkos EJ, Vanderbilt PC, et al. Proceedings: acute large bowel obstruction. Comparison of county, Veterans Administration, and community hospital populations. Arch Surg 1974;108(4):470–6.
21. Bak MP, Boley SJ. Sigmoid volvulus in elderly patients. Am J Surg 1986;151(1): 71–5.
22. Hendrickson M, Naparst TR. Abdominal surgical emergencies in the elderly. Emerg Med Clin North Am 2003;21(4):937–69.
23. Ragsdale L, Southerland L. Acute abdominal pain in the older adult. Emerg Med Clin North Am 2011;29(2):429–48, x.
24. Fox-Orenstein A. Ileus and pseudo-obstruction. In: Friedman L, Feldman M, Brandt LJ, editors. Sleisenger and Fordtran's gastrointestinal and liver disease: pathophysiology/diagnosis/management. philadelphia: WB Saunders; 2010. p. 2121–43.
25. Batke M, Cappell MS. Adynamic ileus and acute colonic pseudo-obstruction. Med Clin North Am 2008;92(3):649–70, ix.
26. Kayani B, Spalding DR, Jiao LR, et al. Does neostigmine improve time to resolution of symptoms in acute colonic pseudo-obstruction? Int J Surg 2012;10(9): 453–7.
27. McSherry CK, Ferstenberg H, Calhoun WF, et al. The natural history of diagnosed gallstone disease in symptomatic and asymptomatic patients. Ann Surg 1985; 202(1):59–63.
28. Bedirli A, Sakrak O, Sözüer EM, et al. Factors effecting the complications in the natural history of acute cholecystitis. Hepatogastroenterology 2001;48(41): 1275–8.
29. Rosenthal RA, Andersen DK. Surgery in the elderly: observations on the pathophysiology and treatment of cholelithiasis. Exp Gerontol 1993;28(4–5):459–72.
30. Morrow DJ, Thompson J, Wilson SE. Acute cholecystitis in the elderly: a surgical emergency. Arch Surg 1978;113(10):1149–52.
31. Gruber PJ, Silverman RA, Gottesfeld S, et al. Presence of fever and leukocytosis in acute cholecystitis. Ann Emerg Med 1996;28(3):273–7.
32. Elwood DR. Cholecystitis. Surg Clin North Am 2008;88(6):1241–52, viii.
33. Martin SP, Ulrich CD. Pancreatic disease in the elderly. Clin Geriatr Med 1999;15: 579–605.
34. Hoffman E, Perez E, Somera V. Acute pancreatitis in the upper age groups. Gastroenterology 1959;36:675–85.
35. Kiriyama S, Gabata T, Takada T, et al. New diagnostic criteria of acute pancreatitis. J Hepatobiliary Pancreat Sci 2010;17(1):24–36.
36. Paajanen H, Jaakkola M, Oksanen H, et al. Acute pancreatitis in patients over 80 years. Eur J Surg 1996;162(6):471–5.
37. Lin KJ, García Rodríguez LA, Hernández-Díaz S. Systematic review of peptic ulcer disease incidence rates: do studies without validation provide reliable estimates? Pharmacoepidemiol Drug Saf 2011;20(7):718–28.
38. Hirschowitz BI, Lanas A. Atypical and aggressive upper gastrointestinal ulceration associated with aspirin abuse. J Clin Gastroenterol 2002;34(5):523.
39. Pilotto A, Salles N. Role of Helicobacter pylori infection in geriatrics. Helicobacter 2002;7:56–62.
40. Borum M. Peptic ulcer disease in the elderly. Clin Geriatr Med 1999;15(3):457–71.
41. Chang CC, Wang SS. Acute abdominal pain in the elderly: a review article. Int J Gerontol 2007;1:279–85.
42. Parks TG. Natural history of diverticula of the colon. Clin Gastroenterol 1974;4: 53–69.

43. Jun S. Epidemiology of diverticular disease. Best Pract Res Clin Gastroenterol 2002;16(4):529–42.
44. Adedipe A, Lowenstein R. Infectious emergencies in the elderly. Emerg Med Clin North Am 2006;24:443–8.
45. Place RJ, Simmang CL. Diverticular disease. Best Pract Res Clin Gastroenterol 2002;16:135–48.
46. Boley SJ, DiBiase A, Brandt LJ, et al. Lower intestinal bleeding in the elderly. Am J Surg 1979;137:57–63.
47. Berman PM. Diverticular disease of the colon in the elderly. Geriatrics 1972;27: 70–5.
48. Stollman N, Raskin JB. Hospitalizations for diverticular disease: effect of age on presentation. Am J Gastroenterol 1999;11:3110–21.
49. Peura DA, Lanza FL, Gostout CJ, et al. The American College of Gastroenterology Registry of bleeding. Am J Gastroenterol 1997;92:419–24.
50. Storm-Dickerson TL, Horattas MC. What we have learned over the past 20 years about appendicitis in the elderly? Am J Surg 2003;185:198–201.
51. Pooler BD, Lawrence EM, Pickhardt PJ. MDCT for suspected appendicitis in the elderly: diagnostic performance and patient outcome. Emerg Radiol 2012;19: 27–33.
52. Rosen MP, Ding A, Blake MA, et al. ACR Appropriateness Criteria® right lower quadrant pain–suspected appendicitis. J Am Coll Radiol 2011;8(11):749–55.
53. Hlibczuk V, Dattaro JA, Jin Z, et al. Diagnostic accuracy of noncontrast computed tomography for appendicitis in adults: a systematic review. Ann Emerg Med 2010;55:51–9.
54. Lunca S, Bouras G, Romedea NS. Acute appendicitis in the elderly patient: diagnostic problems, prognostic factors and outcomes. Rom J Gastroenterol 2004;13: 299–303.
55. Wray CJ, Kao LS, Millas SG, et al. Acute appendicitis: controversies in diagnosis and management. Curr Probl Surg 2013;50:54–86.
56. Milner KA, Vaccarino V, Arnold AL, et al. Gender and age differences in chief complaints of acute myocardial infarction (Worcester Heart Attack Study). Am J Cardiol 2004;93:606–8.
57. Lyon C, Clark D. Diagnosis of acute abdominal pain in older patients. Am Fam Physician 2006;74(9):1537–44.
58. Nicolle L. Asymptomatic bacteriuria in older adults. Geriatr Aging 2003;6(9):24–8.
59. Haughey M. Genitourinary and gynecologic emergencies in the elderly. Geriatric emergency medicine; principles and practice. Cambridge University Press; 2014. p. 219–36.
60. Gleckman RR. Acute pyelonephritis in the elderly. South Med J 1982;75(5):551.
61. Purcell T. Nonsurgical and extraperitoneal causes of abdominal pain. Emerg Med Clin North Am 1989;7(3):721.
62. Osinbowale O, Bartholomew J. Rectus sheath hematoma. Vasc Med 2008;13: 275–9.
63. Talley NJ, O'Keefe EA, Zinsmeister AR, et al. Prevalence of gastrointestinal symptoms in the elderly: a population-based study. Gastroenterol 1992;102(3):895.
64. Wald A, Scarpignato C, Mueller-Lissner S, et al. A multinational survey of prevalence and patterns of laxative use among adults with self-defined constipation. Aliment Pharmacol Ther 2008;28(7):917.
65. Towers A, Burgio K, Locher J, et al. Constipation in the elderly: influence of dietary, psychological, and physiological factors. J Am Geriatr Soc 1994;42(7):701.

66. Mehta S. Cancer in the elderly. API India; Chapter 33. Mumbai (India): Journal of the Association of Physicians; 1985. p. 242.
67. Hunter CP. Cancer in the elderly. New York: CRC Press; 2000. p. 339.
68. Sountoulides P, Metaxa L, Cindolo L. Atypical presentations and rare metastatic sites of renal cell carcinoma: a review of case reports. J Med Case Rep 2011;5:429.
69. Chin MH, Wang LC, Jin L, et al. Appropriateness of medication selection for older persons in an urban academic emergency department. Acad Emerg Med 1999; 6(12):1232–42.
70. Chen YC, Hwang SJ, Lai HY, et al. Potentially inappropriate medication for emergency department visits by elderly patients in Taiwan. Pharmacoepidemiol Drug Saf 2009;18(1):53–61.
71. Jacknin G, Nakamura T, Smally A, et al. Using pharmacists to optimize patient outcomes and costs in the ED. Am J Emerg Med 2014;32:673–7.
72. Hwang U. The geriatric emergency department. J Am Geriatr Soc 2007;55: 1873–6.
73. Martinez J, Mattu A. Abdominal pain in the elderly. Emerg Med Clin North Am 2006;24:371–88.
74. Dowling T, Wang E, Ferrucci L. Glomerular filtration rate equations overestimate creatinine clearance in older individuals enrolled in the Baltimore Longitudinal Study on Aging: impact on renal drug dosing. Pharmacotherapy 2013;33(9): 912–21.
75. O'Brien M. Acute abdominal pain. In: Tintinalli J, editor. Tintinalli's emergency medicine: a comprehensive study guide. Chapter 74. 7th edition. New York: McGraw-Hill; 2010.
76. Lewis LM, Banet GA, Blanda M, et al. Etiology and clinical course of abdominal pain in senior patients: a prospective, multicenter study. J Gerontol A Biol Sci Med Sci 2005;60:1071.

Abdominal Pain in the Immunocompromised Patient—Human Immunodeficiency Virus, Transplant, Cancer

Jonathan McKean, MD, Sarah Ronan-Bentle, MD, MS*

KEYWORDS

- Immunocompromised • Immunosuppressed • Human immunodeficiency virus
- Cytomegalovirus • Necrotizing enterocolitis

KEY POINTS

- Immunocompromised patients include those with human immunodeficiency virus, malignancy, and organ transplant and present frequently to emergency departments with abdominal pain.
- Opportunistic infections are a common cause of abdominal pain in the immunocompromised patient and include cytomegaolovirus, mycobacterium avium complex, and abdominal tuberculosis.
- Abdominal pain can also be caused by complications from surgery in transplant patients such as nosocomial infections, including pneumonia or urinary tract infection.
- Maintaining a broad differential diagnosis is required in immunocompromised patient evaluation.
- Emergency department evaluation of immunocompromised patients includes assessment of electrolytes and cross-sectional abdominal imaging.
- Emergency department disposition is most often admission.

INTRODUCTION

Immunocompromised patients include those with chronic illnesses being treated with immunomodulatory medications and those with the more severe form caused by impairment of a patient's own immune responses. **Box 1** lists examples of immunosuppressed states. In immunocompromised patients, abdominal pain is a nonspecific

---

Disclosures: The authors have nothing to disclose.
Department of Emergency Medicine, University of Cincinnati College of Medicine, 231 Albert Sabin Way, ML0769, Cincinnati, OH 45267-0769, USA
* Corresponding author.
E-mail address: ronanse@uc.edu

Emerg Med Clin N Am 34 (2016) 377–386
http://dx.doi.org/10.1016/j.emc.2015.12.002
emed.theclinics.com

Box 1
Classification of immunocompromised patients

Conditions

Mild-to-moderate immunosuppression
  Elderly
  Diabetes
  Uremia
  SLE
  RA
  Sarcoidosis
  Inflammatory bowel disease
  HIV with CD4 count >200
  Malignancy
  Posttransplant on maintenance immunosuppressive therapy

Severe immunosuppression
  HIV/AIDS with CD4 <200
  Neutropenia
  Posttransplant <60 d

Medications
  Steroids
  Anti-TNFα medications
  Methotrexate
  Cyclosporin
  Tacrolimus

Adapted from Spencer SP, Power N. The acute abdomen in the immune compromised host. Cancer Imag 2008;8:93.

---

symptom arising from extra-abdominal or retroperitoneal pathologic conditions, including genitourinary or pulmonary etiologies. Diagnosis of peritonitis in immunosuppressed patients is delayed because of delayed presentation and lack of definitive physical examination findings.[1] This is all secondary to the inability to mount an immune response. It is important to maintain vigilance and a broad approach in these patients.

HUMAN IMMUNODEFICIENCY VIRUS/AIDS

Patients with chronic immunosuppression secondary to human immunodeficiency virus (HIV)/AIDS who have abdominal pain warrant significant consideration when being evaluated in the emergency department. Although the advent of highly active antiretroviral therapy (HAART) has greatly diminished the incidence of opportunistic infections in this population, the emergency provider must still have a high index of suspicion owing to potential poor adherence to medication regimens and unknown HIV/AIDS status. Furthermore, because HAART has resulted in increased survival in those with this disease, further diagnostic challenge is presented in an aging and elderly HIV population.

Diagnostic Considerations

This article focuses on patients with known HIV as provided in the patient's history, but it is important to consider the possibility of an undiagnosed HIV infection with the appropriate clinical picture or historical risk factors. In the acute infectious setting, primary HIV may preferentially deplete CD4 cells in the gastrointestinal tract, with up to 60% of T lymphocytes being found in that distribution.[2,3] Abdominal pain, nausea, vomiting, and diarrhea may ensue. Unknown, untreated HIV infection may also result in significantly depleted CD4 count and subsequent opportunistic infection. If HIV status is known, the degree of immunosuppression is helpful in developing a comprehensive differential diagnosis, including the risk of opportunistic infections and neoplastic processes. Chart review for the patient's latest CD4 count and a current complete blood count with differential is helpful.

Opportunistic Infections

Intra-abdominal infection is always a consideration a cause of abdominal pain or other symptoms including nausea, vomiting, and diarrhea in the immunosuppressed patient. Positive HIV status in a patient with such symptoms should result in further risk stratification for opportunistic infections. However, because HIV-positive individuals are certainly susceptible to flora responsible for infections in immunocompetent individuals, it is important to include appropriate antibiotic coverage of enteric gram-negative rods and anaerobes.

CYTOMEGALOVIRUS

Cytomegalovirus (CMV) is a common infection found in the gastrointestinal tract of HIV-positive patients, and the colon is the most common site of involvement (47%).[4] Common presenting symptoms include abdominal pain, anorexia, fever, diarrhea, and weight loss. CMV has also been linked to appendicitis. CD4 count is an important consideration in this infection, as patients with a count less than 50 cells per international unit are at higher risk for life-threatening complications, namely, perforation of the colon and rarely the small bowel. CMV ileocolitis with subsequent bowel perforation or other surgical complications is reported to be responsible for most emergency laparotomies in AIDS patients and directly responsible for the deaths in 54% to 87% of all such patients.[4–6] Initial presentation may be insidious with isolated hematochezia as the only symptom. Thus, a high index of suspicion is recommended in these patients owing to the potentially devastating outcomes. Diagnostics in the emergency department rely on computed tomography (CT) imaging for evaluation of colitis or ulceration, with further inpatient diagnostics as needed. CT imaging in CMV often shows transmural colonic wall thickening, spanning from isolated involvement in recto-sigmoid or cecal regions to pan-colitis, with small bowel involvement typically presenting in terminal ileum.[7] A 3- to 6-week course of ganciclovir or foscarnet is recommended treatment[4,8]; however, because histopathology confirmation is often required, patients suspected of this disease will benefit from admission to the hospital for further studies and monitoring regardless of CT findings in the emergency department.

MYCOBACTERIUM AVIUM COMPLEX

Mycobacterium avium complex (MAC) is an opportunistic infection that involves the gastrointestinal tract. MAC is seen in patients with a CD4 count of less than100 cells per international unit.[8] In the context of a low CD4 count, CT imaging shows significant involvement of lymphoid tissue and mesenteric lymph nodes, splenomegaly, and small bowel thickening predominantly involving the jejunum.[9] In contrast, CMV involves mesenteric lymphadenopathy only 16% of the time.[10] Secondary to antibiotic resistance, in treatment of MAC, it is recommended to initiate antibiotic therapy with double antibiotic coverage of clarithromycin and ethambutol.[8]

ABDOMINAL TUBERCULOSIS

Increasing in frequency in developed countries, abdominal tuberculosis (ATB) should be considered in the HIV population with less severe immunosuppression (200–500 CD4 cells per international unit). Elucidating historical risk factors for contraction of this infection may raise suspicion. Although the abdomen is a less common anatomic location for this infection, it is disproportionately found to be present in immunosuppressed patients. Eighty percent to 85% of HIV patients with ATB will have no signs of pulmonary involvement. Up to 90% of cases favor the ileocecal region as the site of infection with presenting symptoms of right lower quadrant pain or mass.[7] Classically, ATB presents in a wet form with ascites or a dry form with adhesions and possible obstruction. Current recommendations suggest a minimum of a 6-month multidrug therapy for treatment, consisting of ethambutol, rifampin, isoniazid, and pyrazinamide for 2 months followed by 4 months of isoniazid and rifampin.[8]

AMEBIC COLITIS

Parasitic infections with ameba may be considered in the HIV-positive patient with a travel history or recent immigration from geographic regions with high incidences, including India, Africa, and parts of South and Central America. Those at risk for obtaining this infection include HIV-positive people, those younger than 50 years, men who have sex with men, and commercial sex workers.[7,11] Amebic colitis secondary to this infection bears mentioning, as it is difficult to differentiate from other infectious colitis sources both through clinical examination and CT imaging. However, it is treatable with metronidazole.[12] Intestinal collections of this infection may be misinterpreted as a nonspecific mass or cancer on CT.

OTHERS

- Hepatitis C has a high co-infection rate with HIV transmission (10%–40%) and is more likely to be acutely symptomatic compared with HIV-negative patients.[13,14]
- Gastrointestinal infections with *Salmonella* and *Campylobacter* are more likely in HIV-positive patients. Notably, these patients are more likely to have a systemic infection (20%–40%) from *Salmonella* compared with immunocompetent patients.[9]
- Acalculous cholecystitis is a more prevalent cause of abdominal pain in immunosuppressed patients than in immunocompetent patients. In HIV patients, acalculous cholecystitis is most often caused by infection from *Listeria*, CMV, *Cryptosporidium*, and microsporidia.[15]
- Hepatitis causing right upper quadrant pain can be caused by multiple opportunistic infectious agents including CMV and MAC.[15]

Treatment Regimen Complications

Protease inhibitors cause side effects of abdominal pain, nausea, vomiting, and diarrhea, which are often self-limited. In a patient who has more significant abdominal pain, particularly epigastric/right upper quadrant pain, pancreatitis should be considered. Pancreatitis has been implicated in HAART, although newer-generation medications are less likely to cause it.[16] It is thought that protease inhibitors may contribute to pancreatitis secondary to hyperlipidemia; however, pathophysiology of pancreatitis in HIV likely has multiple contributing factors.

Nucleoside reverse transcriptase inhibitors, including zidovudine, lamivudine, stavudine, and didanosine adversely affect mitochondrial DNA polymerase owing to structural similarity to reverse transcriptase. Because oxidative phosphorylation and fatty acid chain transport across mitochondrial membrane may be affected, increasing anaerobic metabolism and lactic acidosis can result. Unfortunately, there is no established timeline for onset of symptoms, with cases being reported between months 1 to 20 of therapy.[17] Management of mitochondrial toxicity and lactic acidosis is supportive; with discontinuation of offending agents, one may also consider the addition of metabolic precursors for reactions affected by inhibition of mitochondrial enzymes including thiamine, carnitine, and riboflavin.

Other Complications

In addition to infectious precipitants and medication regimen complications, one must consider gross physical intra-abdominal abnormalities as cause of abdominal pain in the HIV-positive patient presenting to the emergency department. Bowel perforation may be present secondary to infectious or inflammatory bowel disease. Small bowel obstruction may be present secondary to adhesions from these infections or from masses secondary to B-cell lymphoma, Kaposi sarcoma, or tuberculosis.[18] With potential for such serious complications, a high index of suspicion is required in the evaluation of these patients.

SOLID ORGAN TRANSPLANT

Solid organ transplantation presents a dynamic diagnostic challenge with regard to abdominal pain in the emergency department. These patients are exposed to risks that may change based on chronologic time from surgery or immunosuppressive course. Complications from these risks may manifest as acute or chronic abdominal pain; one clinical center's experience has found abdominal pain, in addition to fever, was the most frequent presenting complaint to the emergency department among their patients after liver transplant.[19] In patients with a primary intra-abdominal transplant site, including pancreas, liver, and kidney, it behooves the emergency provider to thoroughly evaluate even mild abdominal pain for potentially serious conditions.

Diagnostic Considerations

As with other classes of immunosuppression, the transplant patient on immunosuppressive therapy certainly raises concern for infection as a cause of abdominal pain. Furthermore, inhibition of appropriate inflammatory response threatens to blunt symptoms and physical examination findings that would normally be much more striking, which leads to more frequent perforation of appendicitis in liver transplant patients compared with an immunocompetent cohort.[20] There should be a low threshold for CT imaging in the emergency department for these patients.

Infections

For the solid organ transplant patient presenting to the emergency department with abdominal pain, infection should be high on the differential diagnosis. Although much discussion focuses on rare and atypical infectious processes, it is important to remember that often it is the same offending agent as in immunocompetent patients. Evaluation for diverticulitis, cholangitis, and other conditions and prompt administration of antibiotics for the usual pathogens is recommended. The timeline from the patient's surgical procedure and initiation of immunosuppressive therapy may help narrow differential diagnosis.[21]

First month

In the first month after surgery, suspicion should be highest for nosocomial infections related to the hospital stay and surgery. Incision cellulitis, intra-abdominal abscess, fungal infection, urinary tract infection, hospital acquired/ventilator-associated pneumonia, *Clostridium difficile*, or bacteremia secondary to central line placement should be explored.[21]

Months 1 to 6

Generally, within this timeframe the patient undergoes the greatest immunosuppression and is at the highest risk for opportunistic infections. Acute viral, such as CMV, and bacterial infections similar to those discussed previously for HIV-related abdominal pain may all be present in posttransplant patients during this time.

Months 6 to 12

Variability in immune response is seen in this group of patients. For those whose graft has taken well and require less pharmacotherapy to prevent rejection, this period represents a risk of infection similar to those in immunocompetent patients, such as community-acquired pneumonia and urinary tract infections, which present as abdominal pain. Other patients requiring a more intensive antirejection regimen continue to have a higher risk for opportunistic infections.

Seropositivity for certain viral strains including CMV, hepatitis C, and Epstein Barr virus have also been associated with a greater propensity for concomitant infections secondary to immunomodulation.[21,22]

Other Postoperative Complications

In addition to infection, other posttransplant diseases result in new-onset abdominal pain. Aside from known risks after abdominal surgery, such as adhesions and small bowel obstruction, the solid organ transplant patient may present with rare or unique causes of abdominal pain. The following list is by no means comprehensive, but rather a representation of the possible complications that may ensue.

Pancreatitis

After transplant of the pancreas, there is an expected early phase of pancreatitis known as physiologic acute graft pancreatitis related to reperfusion of the organ that occurs between 30 minutes and 72 hours after the procedure. With such an early onset, this response is managed during postoperative inpatient course. However, graft pancreatitis may have more delayed presentations. Generally, within the first 3 months after transplant, patients are at risk for early acute graft pancreatitis, presenting with abdominal pain and systemic inflammatory response. Most of these cases (60%–70%) result from vascular thrombosis to the graft or other causes including infection or immunologic response.[23] Clues to this diagnosis include laboratory markers for pancreatic inflammation and dysfunction (elevated amylase/lipase levels and hyperglycemia) with confirmatory CT imaging.

Pancreatitis is also found with disproportionate frequency in renal transplant patients compared with the general population and a significant increase in associated mortality.[24] Multiple suggested contributors to the development of pancreatitis among renal transplant patients include immunosuppression, hyperlipidemia, and viral infections. As with other causes of abdominal pain in the immunosuppressed patient, pancreatitis in transplant may present with subdued symptoms and examination findings in the setting of advanced disease, perhaps contributing to the increased mortality in this cohort.

Graft-versus-host disease

Graft-versus-host disease is a rare disease with a mortality rate greater than 85% in liver transplant patients.[25] More commonly associated with hematopoietic stem cell transplants, this disease develops in solid organ transplants because of the presence of lymphoid tissue in the donor organ.[26] Not only is the disease itself rare in this population, abdominal pain as the presenting symptom is also atypical. The skin and gastrointestinal tract are the most commonly affected areas; skin rash with diarrhea or abdominal pain in the posttransplant patient, particularly within 2 to 6 weeks after the procedure, should raise suspicion.[25,26]

Abdominal compartment syndrome

After large solid organ transplant, such as liver transplant, bowel edema, ascites, and organ donor/recipient size mismatch can lead to increased intra-abdominal pressure. Although more likely to be managed in the inpatient setting after initial surgery, worsening ascites or other causes of increased abdominal pressure as an outpatient may result in an emergency department visit for abdominal compartment syndrome. Bladder pressure may be measured as a barometer for this condition. With pressures greater than 25 mm Hg, insertion of a Foley catheter and nasogastric tube for bladder and stomach evacuation can start treatment. Pressures greater than 35 mm Hg require more definitive management with decompressive laparotomy.[27]

Many other cases are reported of postsurgical complications in the solid organ transplant patient population, ranging from diaphragmatic hernia to renal transplant torsion to aortoenteric fistula presenting with hematochezia. These are rare but potentially serious causes of abdominal pain and other gastrointestinal complaints that the emergency provider may encounter.[28–30]

CHEMOTHERAPY/NEUTROPENIA
Diagnostic Considerations

Patients with various malignancies have increased frequency of visits to the emergency department, and the frequency of emergency department visits increases near the end of life.[31,32] Of patients presenting with oncologic-related complaints, the most common presenting symptoms were gastrointestinal followed by pain.[31] Gastrointestinal manifestations can be directly related to the disease burden of the cancer or to complications of cancer treatment.

Opportunistic Infections

Those infections common to other immunocompromised patients including those with HIV/AIDs and posttransplant patients are also common in patients undergoing chemotherapy for treatment of malignancy. These include C difficile pseudomembranous colitis, CMV, and herpes simplex virus.

Neutropenic enterocolitis (NEC) or typhlitis is a disease that is increasingly recognized as the most common intestinal pathologic condition in patients presenting with the triad of neutropenia, fever, and abdominal pain after receiving antineoplastic chemotherapy. The incidence of NEC is not known, as it is likely underdiagnosed.[33] In hospitalized patients with hematologic malignancies and solid organ malignancies, the pooled incidence was reported at 5.2%. However, the true incidence is likely 50% in this population.[33] In addition, mortality rates are more than 50% because of complications such as colonic perforation and overwhelming sepsis.

The pathophysiology is not well understood. Some years ago, NEC was thought to remain within the ileocecal region because of the decreased vascularity of this portion of the colon. In published reports incorporating cross-sectional imaging studies with histopathology, NEC was found to be widely distributed throughout the colon, with only 28% of cases isolated to the cecum.[34]

Similar to posttransplant patients, patients who have undergone bone marrow transplant or have lymphoma are at risk of graft-versus-host disease, which affects the gastrointestinal tract.

In addition to the opportunistic infections and entities related to neutropenia specifically, patients undergoing chemotherapy have abdominal pain, vomiting, and diarrhea related to direct cytotoxic effects of the chemotherapy.

Other specific intra-abdominal conditions that occur more commonly in patients with colorectal cancer than in emergency department patients without cancer include bowel perforation and obstruction.

Other Immunocompromised Patients

In addition to the above-described conditions, it is important to be mindful of patients who present to the emergency department who are mildly or moderately immunocompromised because of other comorbidities or medications. See Table 1 for a description of conditions and medications that contribute to a relative state of immunocompromise. Recognizing that these medications contribute to a relative state of immunosuppression should alert the care provider to the unreliability of the abdominal examination and the need for additional laboratory evaluation and cross-sectional imaging. Early treatment should include volume replacement in addition to symptom control.

The evaluation of abdominal pain in the immunocompromised patient remains challenging. Many patients, whether they have a history of HIV or malignancy or transplant will require cross-sectional imaging of the abdomen and pelvis in the emergency department. Administration of broad-spectrum antibiotics should be considered early. Admission for continued resuscitation and subspecialty consultation or intervention is the usual course.

PEARLS AND PITFALLS

- Immunocompromised patients include those with with HIV, malignancy, and organ transplant and present frequently to emergency departments with abdominal pain.
- Opportunistic infections are a common cause of abdominal pain in the immunocompromised patient and include CMV, MAC, and abdominal tuberculosis.
- Abdominal pain can also be caused by complications from surgery in transplant patients such as nosocomial infections including pneumonia or urinary tract infection.
- Maintaining a broad differential diagnosis is required in immunocompromised patient evaluation.
- Emergency department evaluation of immunocompromised patients includes assessment of electrolytes and cross-sectional abdominal imaging.
- Emergency department disposition is most often admission.

REFERENCES

1. Golda T, Kreisler E, Mercader C, et al. Emergency surgery for perforated diverticulitis in the immunosuppressed patient. Colorectal Dis 2014;16(9):723–31.

2. Huppmann AR, Orenstein JM. Opportunistic disorders of the gastrointestinal tract in the age of highly active antiretroviral therapy. Hum Pathol 2010;41(12):1777–87.

3. Hill A, Balkin A. Risk factors for gastrointestinal adverse events in HIV treated and untreated patients. AIDS Rev 2009;11(1):30–8.
4. Michalopoulos N, Triantafillopoulou K, Beretouli E, et al. Small bowel perforation due to CMV enteritis infection in an HIV-positive patient. BMC Res Notes 2013;6:45.
5. Kram HB, Shoemaker WC. Intestinal perforation due to cytomegalovirus infection in patients with AIDS. Dis Colon Rectum 1990;33(12):1037–40.
6. Wexner SD, Smithy WB, Trillo C, et al. Emergency colectomy for cytomegalovirus ileocolitis in patients with the acquired immune deficiency syndrome. Dis Colon Rectum 1988;31(10):755–61.
7. Tonolini M, Bianco R. Acute HIV-related gastrointestinal disorders and complications in the antiretroviral era: spectrum of cross-sectional imaging findings. Abdom Imaging 2013;38(5):994–1004.
8. Cello JP, Day LW. Idiopathic AIDS enteropathy and treatment of gastrointestinal opportunistic pathogens. Gastroenterology 2009;136(6):1952–65.
9. Gazzard B. AIDS and the gastrointestinal tract. Medicine 2005;33(6):24–6.
10. Murray JGJ. Cytomegalovirus colitis in AIDS: CT features. Am J Roentgenol 1995; 165(1):67.
11. Nagata N, Shimbo T, Akiyama J, et al. Risk factors for intestinal invasive amebiasis in Japan, 2003-2009. Emerging Infect Dis 2012;18(5):717–24.
12. Ohnishi K, Murata M. Treatment of symptomatic amebic colitis in human immunodeficiency virus-infected persons. Int J Antimicrob Agents 1996;7(4):231–3.
13. Driver TH, Terrault N, Saxena V. Acute hepatitis C in an HIV-infected patient: a case report and review of literature. J Gen Intern Med 2013;28(5):734–8.
14. Anderson KB, Guest JL, Rimland D. Hepatitis C virus coinfection increases mortality in HIV-infected patients in the highly active antiretroviral therapy era: data from the HIV Atlanta VA Cohort Study. Clin Infect Dis 2004;39(10):1507–13.
15. Scott-Conner CE, Fabrega AJ. Gastrointestinal problems in the immunocompromised host. A review for surgeons. Surg Endosc 1996;10(10):959–64.
16. Oliveira NM, Ferreira FA, Yonamine RY, et al. Antiretroviral drugs and acute pancreatitis in HIV/AIDS patients: is there any association? A literature review. Einstein (Sao Paulo) 2014;12(1):112–9.
17. Margolis AM, Heverling H, Pham PA, et al. A review of the toxicity of HIV medications. J Med Toxicol 2014;10(1):26–39.
18. Gao GJ, Yang D, Lin KK, et al. Clinical analysis of 10 AIDS patients with malignant lymphoma. Cancer Biol Med 2012;9(2):115–9.
19. Turtay MG, Oguzturk H, Aydin C, et al. A descriptive analysis of 188 liver transplant patient visits to an emergency department. Eur Rev Med Pharmacol Sci 2012;16(Suppl 1):3–7.
20. Abt PL, Abdullah I, Korenda K, et al. Appendicitis among liver transplant recipients. Liver Transpl 2005;11(10):1282–4.
21. Fishman JA. Infections in immunocompromised hosts and organ transplant recipients: essentials. Liver Transpl 2011;17(Suppl 3):S34–7.
22. Hryniewiecka E, Soldacki D, Paczek L. Cytomegaloviral infection in solid organ transplant recipients: preliminary report of one transplant center experience. Transpl Proc 2014;46(8):2572–5.
23. Nadalin S, Girotti P, Konigsrainer A. Risk factors for and management of graft pancreatitis. Curr Opin Organ Transpl 2013;18(1):89–96.
24. Taylor K, Sinha S, Cowie A, et al. Challenges in diagnosing acute pancreatitis in renal transplant patients. Clin Transpl 2009;23(6):985–9.
25. Sun B, Zhao C, Xia Y, et al. Late onset of severe graft-versus-host disease following liver transplantation. Transpl Immunol 2006;16(3–4):250–3.

26. Rossi AP, Bone BA, Edwards AR, et al. Graft-versus-host disease after simultaneous pancreas-kidney transplantation: a case report and review of the literature. Am J Transpl 2014;14(11):2651–6.
27. Zhang W, Wang K, Qian X, et al. Abdominal compartment syndrome associated with capillary leak syndrome after liver transplantation. Transpl Proc. 2009;41(9):3927–30.
28. Lam HD, Mejia J, Soltys KA, et al. Right diaphragmatic hernia after liver transplant in pediatrics: a case report and review of the literature. Pediatr Transpl 2013;17(3):E77–80.
29. Lucewicz A, Isaacs A, Allen RD, et al. Torsion of intraperitoneal kidney transplant. ANZ J Surg 2012;82(5):299–302.
30. Higgins PD, Umar RK, Parker JR, et al. Massive lower gastrointestinal bleeding after rejection of pancreatic transplants. Nat Clin Pract Gastroenterol Hepatol 2005;2(5):240–4.
31. Swenson KK, Rose MA, Ritz L, et al. Recognition and evaluation of oncology-related symptoms in the emergency department. Ann Emerg Med 1995;26(1):12–7.
32. Barbera L, Taylor C, Dudgeon D. Why do patients with cancer visit the emergency department near the end of life? Cmaj 2010;182(6):563–8.
33. Nesher L, Rolston KV. Neutropenic enterocolitis, a growing concern in the era of widespread use of aggressive chemotherapy. Clin Infect Dis 2013;56(5):711–7.
34. Kirkpatrick ID, Greenberg HM. Gastrointestinal complications in the neutropenic patient: characterization and differentiation with abdominal CT. Radiology 2003;226(3):668–74.

Acute Abdominal Pain in the Bariatric Surgery Patient

Kyle D. Lewis, MD*, Katrin Y. Takenaka, MD, MEd,
Samuel D. Luber, MD, MPH

KEYWORDS

- Anastomotic leak • Anastomotic stenosis • Stomal ulcer • Hernia • Dilatation
- Band erosion • Band slippage • Gastric prolapse

KEY POINTS

- In general, bariatric procedures achieve weight loss by altering gastrointestinal absorption, restricting gastric size, or a combination of both.
- In bariatric patients, abdominal pain may be caused by complications specific to their particular surgical procedure or by nonspecific complications, such as surgical site infection, cholelithiasis, bleeding, and small bowel obstruction.
- The differential diagnosis of abdominal pain in the patient who has had a Roux-en-Y gastric bypass or a biliary pancreatic diversion includes anastomotic leak or stenosis, dumping syndrome, gastric remnant dilatation, stomal ulcer, and internal or incisional hernia.
- Following laparoscopic adjustable gastric banding, abdominal pain may be caused by esophagitis, hiatal hernia, gastroesophageal dilatation, band erosion, band slippage, gastric prolapse, stomal obstruction, or port infection.
- Patients who have had a sleeve gastrectomy may suffer from gastric leak, gastric stenosis, or gastroesophageal reflux.

INTRODUCTION

Obesity is present in epidemic proportions in the United States. Obese individuals are at increased risk of morbidity and mortality compared with those with normal body mass indices (BMIs).[1] Several studies have demonstrated the superiority of bariatric surgery over conventional therapy.[2–4] As a result, bariatric surgery has become more commonplace, and emergency physicians will undoubtedly encounter many

Disclosures: None.
Department of Emergency Medicine, University of Texas Medical School at Houston, 6431 Fannin, 4th Floor, Houston, TX 77030, USA
* Corresponding author.
E-mail address: kyle.d.lewis@uth.tmc.edu

patients who have undergone one of these procedures. This article reviews common bariatric surgery procedures, their complications, and the approach to acute abdominal pain in these patients.

OBESITY

Obesity is a widespread disease and essentially an evolving international epidemic even though it is not infectious in nature. In a study that examined data from the 2011 to 2012 National Health and Nutrition Examination Survey, more than one-third (34.9% or 78.6 million) of adults in the United States are obese. The age-adjusted prevalences of obesity by race are astounding: 47.8% of non-Hispanic blacks, 42.5% of Hispanics, 32.6% of non-Hispanic whites, and 10.8% of Asians.[5] The cost of obesity-related medical care is substantial, resulting in a 41.5% increase in per capita medical spending compared with adults of normal weight. In their article, Finkelstein and colleagues[6] estimate that these costs could amount to $147 billion per year.[6] Among the concomitant health care risks associated with obesity are heart disease, stroke, type II diabetes (DM), hypertension (HTN), hyperlipidemia (HLD), gallbladder disease, musculoskeletal disorders, and obstructive sleep apnea. Obese individuals also have an increased risk of mortality, dying 6 to 7 years earlier than those with a normal weight. Compounding the issue, obese smokers die 13 to 14 years earlier than non smokers with normal BMIs.[1]

CONVENTIONAL THERAPY

Diet and exercise are routinely promoted as integral parts of weight loss regimens by prominent laypeople and health care professionals. For example, healthier lifestyles have been advocated by First Lady Michelle Obama (the Let's Move campaign) and the National Football League (the Play 60 initiative). Unfortunately, lifestyle modifications may not be adequate for obese people trying to attain a healthier BMI. Several studies have shown that bariatric surgery results in greater improvements in BMI and higher rates of resolution of comorbidities, such as type II DM, HTN, and HLD, when compared with conventional therapy (including medication, lifestyle modifications, and education).[2–4]

BARIATRIC SURGERY ON THE RISE

Across the globe, the number of bariatric surgeries more than doubled between 2003 and 2011. In 2011, the United States and Canada combined, performed the greatest number of bariatric surgical procedures (101,645 cases or 29.8%) when compared with other countries worldwide. In the United States and Canada, the three most common procedures were Roux-en-Y gastric bypass (RYGB; 47,791 cases or 47.0%), adjustable gastric band (27,630 cases or 27.2%), and sleeve gastrectomy (SG; 19,486 cases or 19.2%). Of these, SG was the only one increasing in percentage of cases. Also of note, 18.6% of the 6705 bariatric surgeons worldwide reside in the United States and Canada alone.[7]

INCLUSION CRITERIA FOR BARIATRIC SURGERY

The formula to calculate BMI is weight (in kilograms) divided by height (in meters) squared. The National Institutes of Health and World Health Organization use BMI to classify degree of obesity and to aid in risk stratification. A normal BMI is 18.5 to 24.9 kg/m^2. A person with a BMI of 25 to 29.9 kg/m^2 is considered overweight. Obesity is defined as a BMI greater than or equal to 30 kg/m^2 (class 1, 30–34.9 kg/m^2; class 2, 35–39.9 kg/m^2; class 3, $\geq$40 kg/m^2).

These classifications have been defined based largely on data from white populations; however, evidence exists that supports using ethnic-specific definitions. For example, a study by He and colleagues[8] supports using lower BMI cutoffs in Chinese because of higher prevalences of obesity-related comorbidities for a given BMI. This is thought to be at least in part caused by ethnic differences in abdominal and hepatic fat distribution.[9]

The National Institutes of Health has established evidence-based guidelines for surgical management of obesity. To qualify for bariatric surgery, a candidate must demonstrate a BMI greater than or equal to 40 kg/m^2 without comorbidity or a BMI of 35 to 39.9 kg/m^2 with at least one serious comorbidity, including but not limited to type II DM, HTN, HLD, obstructive sleep apnea, gastroesophageal reflux disease, asthma, or obesity-hypoventilation syndrome. In addition, the person must have failed other nonsurgical methods of weight loss.[10] Most major insurance carriers and bariatric programs in the United States also require that patients undergo psychological assessment before surgery.[11] Weight loss outcomes have been shown to be related to patients' preoperative psychological preparation and their ability to make lifelong changes in their dietary habits and physical activity.[12]

BARIATRIC SURGERY PROCEDURES

To evaluate acute abdominal pain in the bariatric surgery patient, the clinician needs to understand the most common bariatric procedures. In general terms, these procedures achieve weight loss by altering gastrointestinal (GI) absorption, restricting gastric size, or a combination of the two. Malabsorptive procedures bypass the distal stomach and some degree of small bowel, reducing the absorption of food. Gastric restriction is attained by gastroplasty or gastric banding, resulting in a functionally smaller stomach, delayed gastric emptying, and early satiety. Additionally these procedures may impact hormones that control appetite and satiety (eg, ghrelin, glucagon-like peptide 1 [GLP-1], peptide YY [PYY], and cholecystokinin).[13,14] Common types of malabsorptive and restrictive procedures are discussed in more detail next.

MIXED MALABSORPTIVE/RESTRICTIVE PROCEDURES
Roux-en-Y Gastric Bypass

In the 1960s, the first gastric bypass was performed by Mason and Ito.[15] Since then, the surgery has undergone several modifications (**Fig. 1**). Currently the most common weight reduction procedure worldwide is the RYGB (47% of all bariatric surgeries).[7] Although multiple variations of the RYGB exist, the general concept includes the creation of a small proximal gastric pouch (usually 15–50 mL) connected to a Roux or connecting limb of small bowel (typically 75–150 cm in length and found 30–50 cm distal to the ligament of Treitz). The distal stomach is stapled, and the proximal jejunum is anastomosed to the Roux limb as a jejunojejunostomy. The gastric pouch provides a restrictive element, causing early satiety and thus reducing a patient's total intake. The Roux limb promotes the malabsorptive process by bypassing the distal stomach and proximal jejunum.[13] RYGB may affect secretion of ghrelin (causing appetite suppression) and GLP-1 and PYY (resulting in satiety).[13,14] Various studies have demonstrated an approximately 70% excess weight loss at 2-year follow-up and 54% at 10 years and beyond.[14,16] In addition, RYGB has been shown to have a more appreciable benefit on DM and other metabolic derangements.[14]

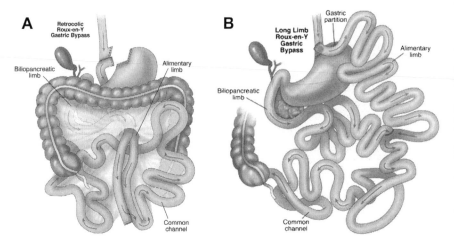

Fig. 1. (*A, B*) Examples of Roux-en-Y gastric bypass. (*From* Elder KA, Wolfe BM. Bariatric surgery: a review of procedures and outcomes. Gastroenterology 2007;132(6):2253; with permission.)

Biliary Pancreatic Diversion without and with Duodenal Switch

Biliary pancreatic diversion (BPD) is completed by performing a 50% to 80% gastrectomy removing the pylorus and dividing the ileum (**Fig. 2**). The distal ileum is attached to the proximal stomach, forming an alimentary limb. The proximal ileum is detached

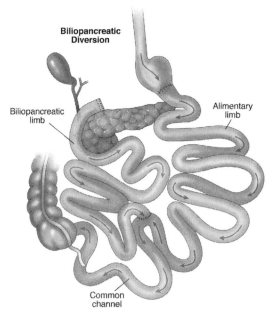

Fig. 2. Biliary pancreatic diversion. (*From* Elder KA, Wolfe BM. Bariatric surgery: a review of procedures and outcomes. Gastroenterology 2007;132(6):2253; with permission.)

becoming the biliopancreatic limb, which is then anastomosed to the alimentary limb about 50 cm PROXIMAL to the ileocecal valve.[13,17] In short, this results in restriction of the stomach and diversion of food, bile, and pancreatic secretions (malabsorptive component). BPD only comprises about 0.7% of bariatric procedures worldwide.[7] Excess weight loss was reported to be 68% and 71% at 2 and 4 years, respectively, after surgery.[16,18] BPD may be decreasing in favor because it is associated with higher rates of diarrhea, malnutrition, and stomal ulceration, and lower excess weight loss when compared with BPD with duodenal switch (BPD-DS).[19,20]

BPD-DS consists of an SG and an ileoduodenostomy distal to the pylorus. Thus, both the pylorus and proximal duodenum are preserved (**Fig. 3**).[13,17] This is performed as a single-stage procedure or with a staged approach (SG followed by BPD-DS). Controversy exists as to which is the preferred method.[21,22] BPD-DS accounts for 1.5% of bariatric procedures worldwide.[7] At 2 years after surgery, 85% excess BMI was lost.[16] The mean percentage weight loss for BPD $\pm$ DS (70.1%) was superior to that of RYGB (61.6%).[23] Furthermore this superior excess weight loss was maintained at 10 years and beyond.[14] In addition to RYGB, BPD-DS is the main surgical option for patients with BMI greater than 50 kg/m^2.[24]

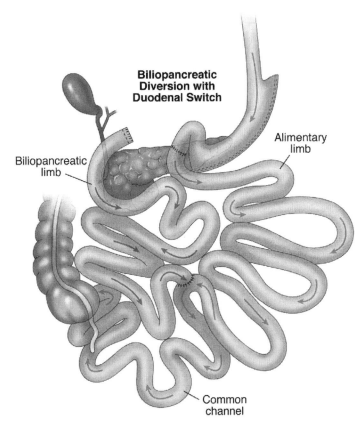

Fig. 3. Biliary pancreatic diversion with duodenal switch. (*From* Elder KA, Wolfe BM. Bariatric surgery: a review of procedures and outcomes. Gastroenterology 2007;132(6):2253; with permission.)

RESTRICTIVE PROCEDURES
Laparoscopic Adjustable Gastric Banding

About 18% of bariatric surgeries worldwide are laparoscopic adjustable gastric band-ing (LAGBs).[7] During LAGB (**Fig. 4**), an adjustable band is placed around the proximal stomach, creating a small gastric pouch. The band is filled with saline and is con-nected to a subcutaneous port located in the anterior abdominal wall, which can be accessed via a needle to adjust the amount of gastric restriction.[13,17] Besides its restrictive effects, LAGB also impacts appetite and satiety, possibly through vagal stimulation.[14] Of all bariatric surgeries, it has the lowest mortality rate (0.05%), one-tenth that of RYGB.[25] Even though excess weight loss is approximately only 47.5% at 2 years, longer term weight loss (≥10 years) is comparable with that of RYGB (47%–54.2%).[14,25,26]

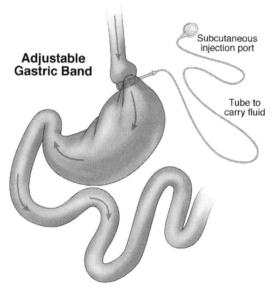

Fig. 4. Laparoscopic adjustable gastric banding. (*From* Elder KA, Wolfe BM. Bariatric sur-gery: a review of procedures and outcomes. Gastroenterology 2007;132(6):2253; with permission.)

Sleeve Gastrectomy

SG was initially reserved for high-risk patients with BMI greater than 60 kg/m² as an initial surgical intervention with subsequent RYGB (**Fig. 5**).[27] However, it is now considered a potential primary bariatric procedure. In 2011, it was the second most common type of bariatric surgery performed worldwide, constituting almost one-third of these cases.[7] During this procedure, the greater curvature of the stomach is resected, leaving a residual tubular structure behind.[13] As a result, the stomach cannot easily expand. SG also seems to affect ghrelin, GLP-1, and PYY levels and in-fluences satiety.[14,28] At 2 years follow-up, excess weight loss is 67.4%.[29] A study is currently underway evaluating the long-term outcome of SG, including maintenance of weight loss.[30]

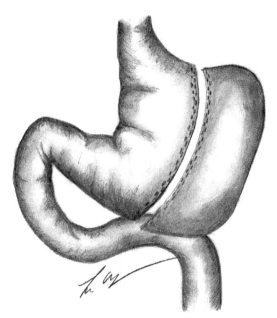

Fig. 5. Sleeve gastrectomy. (*Courtesy of* L. Aznaurova-Anderson, MD, Houston, TX.)

INTRAGASTRIC DUAL-BALLOON

In July 2015, the US Food and Drug Administration approved an intragastric dual-balloon device (ReShape Medical Inc, San Clemente, CA) for patients with BMI of 30 to 40 kg/m², who have failed to lose weight through diet and exercise, and who have one or more obesity-related comorbidities, such as DM or HTN.[31] The device is thought to induce satiety by occupying space in the stomach.[32] It is placed endoscopically and removed after 6 months. In a prospective, randomized controlled multicenter trial, patients with the dual-balloon device lost 25.1% excess weight, whereas those who relied on diet and exercise alone lost 11.3%.[33] The intragastric dual balloon offers a minimally invasive and reversible alternative to bariatric surgery (**Fig. 6**).

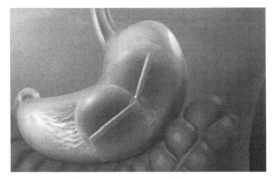

Fig. 6. Intragastric dual-balloon. (*From* Ponce J, Quebbemann BB, Patterson EJ. Prospective, randomized, multicenter study evaluating safety and efficacy of intragastric dual-balloon in obesity. Surg Obes Relat Dis 2013;9(2):291; with permission.)

APPROACH TO THE BARIATRIC PATIENT WITH ABDOMINAL PAIN IN THE EMERGENCY DEPARTMENT

As with any patient in the emergency department, initial evaluation and stabilization of the ABCs (airway, breathing, circulation, and so forth) is paramount. However, there may also be concerns specific to bariatric patients as described next.

Airway

In obese patients, airway management may be complicated by short necks and redundant soft tissues. Should the airway need to be secured, planning for a difficult intubation is crucial. If the initial approach for airway management fails, multiple backup plans may be needed (eg, direct and video-assisted laryngoscopy, supraglottic device, surgical cricothyroidotomy). Positioning the patient in a "ramped position" with elevation of the head and upper body to align the ear and sternum can help increase the chances of successful intubation and improve ventilation.[34]

Breathing

Once the patient's airway is secure, assessment of breathing ensues. Tachypnea may indicate a primary respiratory disorder (eg, pneumonia, pulmonary embolus, congestive heart failure) or a compensatory mechanism for metabolic acidosis (eg, caused by lactic acidosis or sepsis).[17] Obese patients have decreased functional residual capacity because of decreased chest wall compliance and increased intra-abdominal pressure.[34] As a result, they have a limited oxygen reserve.[34] Obesity hypoventilation syndrome may cause hypoxia, hypercapnea, and subsequent altered mental status. Bilevel positive airway pressure may be useful in this case along with supplemental oxygen. Oxygen saturation should be maintained between 88% and 92% to avoid overoxygenation and a resultant decrease in respiratory drive and hypercapnic narcosis.[35]

Circulation

Assessing the patient's circulation (ie, heart rate, blood pressure, distal pulses) can provide clues about illness. In several papers, a persistently elevated heart rate greater than 120 beats per minute may indicate a gastric leak (GL) and possible sepsis.[36,37] Due to the fact bariatric patients may not always present with typical signs (eg, fever, peritoneal signs) even in the face of serious illness, clinical indicators, such as persistent tachycardia, may be especially useful. If available, bedside ultrasound may help assess cardiac function, volume status (ie, collapsibility of the inferior vena cava), and the presence or absence of free fluid in the abdomen.

Other General Considerations

Once the patient is stabilized, a focused history and physical examination can help narrow the differential diagnosis. The provider should inquire about the presence of fever, vomiting, diarrhea, symptoms of dehydration (eg, lightheadedness, syncope, urine output), and GI bleeding (ie, hematemesis, hematochezia, melena). Additional information should include food intake, timing of last bowel movement, and adherence to the postbariatric surgery diet. Knowing what type of procedure was performed and when can also affect the provider's diagnostic considerations. The physical examination should focus on assessment of vital signs and volume status and searching for evidence of infection, sepsis, GI bleeding, and obstruction.

While the provider is evaluating the patient, intravenous (IV) access should be obtained and diagnostics ordered. Depending on the specific patient, the following testing may be useful: basic versus complete metabolic profile, complete blood count, lipase, blood gas (arterial or venous), lactic acid level, urinalysis, pregnancy test, stool hemoccult, and electrocardiogram. Imaging studies, such as plain radiographs, ultrasound, and computer tomography (CT) may be necessary for diagnosis as well. However, it is important to remember the potential limitations of imaging in the severely obese patient. General therapeutic options include IV fluids, pain control, and antiemetics. Blood products and antibiotics may be needed in patients with bleeding complications or sepsis respectively.

NONEXCLUSIVE COMPLICATIONS

In bariatric patients, abdominal pain may be caused by complications specific to a particular surgical procedure or by nonspecific complications.[36] General postsurgical complications include surgical site infection (SSI), cholelithiasis, bleeding, and small bowel obstruction. In addition, the clinician should consider other diagnoses, such as pneumonia and myocardial infarction.

Surgical Site Infection

SSIs may involve the skin, subcutaneous tissues, deeper soft tissues, and/or the abdominal cavity. These infections occur in up to about 15% of patients following bariatric surgery, although the incidence is lower after laparoscopic procedures (vs open surgeries).[36,38] Most SSIs occur within 2 to 3 weeks following surgery.[39] SSIs may be polymicrobial; however, the most commonly identified organisms are staphylococcal species.[38] Early recognition of an SSI is important as is source control (eg, opening the wound, abscess drainage, further operative intervention). Antibiotics are indicated in cases of cellulitis, deeper tissue infections, intra-abdominal abscess, or sepsis.

Cholelithiasis

Cholelithiasis is common after bariatric surgery because of rapid weight loss leading to increased mucin in the gallbladder, increased cholesterol in the bile, biliary stasis, and bile sludging.[40,41] The incidence of gallstones following bariatric procedures ranges from 30% to 53%.[40,42] However, only a minority of these patients (7%–15%) require cholecystectomy.[42] RYGB is associated with a higher rate of subsequent cholecystectomy than LABG or SG.[42] Due to this significant rate of cholelithiasis, some surgeons may opt to perform a cholecystectomy at the time of the bariatric procedure. Others may choose to prescribe prophylactic ursodeoxycholic acid and/or re-evaluate if biliary symptoms arise.[13,40]

If gallbladder disease is suspected in a bariatric surgery patient, the diagnostic and therapeutic approach is usually similar to that for all patients. Ultrasound can be used to detect gallstones, biliary sludge, and evidence of cholecystitis and choledocholithiasis. In patients with an RYGB, endoscopy may be complicated by postsurgical anatomic alterations.[40]

Postoperative Bleeding

Postoperative bleeding may have extraluminal or intraluminal causes. Extraluminal causes may include iatrogenic injury to the mesentery, liver, or spleen or bleeding from a trocar site. Patients with this type of bleeding may present with tachycardia, hypotension, fatigue, lightheadedness, or peritoneal signs from hemoperitoneum. Intraluminal bleeding may present as upper GI bleeding (UGIB) (ie, hematemesis, melena, hematochezia, or hypotension).[17] Between 0.6% and 4% of bariatric surgeries are complicated by UGIB within 2 weeks of the procedure. Laparoscopic RYGB is associated with a higher incidence than open RYGB and other bariatric procedures.[43] Although bleeding may arise from any anastomosis or staple line, the gastrojejunal anastomosis is the most common site of early UGIB following RYGB.[17,43] Late UGIB may occur years later because of gastric or duodenal ulcerations, stomal ulcers, or bleeding from the gastric pouch.[13,17]

In patients with postoperative bleeding, initial resuscitation potentially includes management of the ABCs, fluid resuscitation, blood product administration, correction of coagulopathy, and dosing of IV proton pump inhibitors. This supportive care suffices in many cases.[13,43] However, endoscopy and/or surgical intervention may be necessary if the patient is hemodynamically unstable, does not adequately respond to medical management, or has recurrent bleeding.[13,36,43] Depending on the patient's postprocedure anatomy, endoscopy may not be able to reach the site of bleeding (eg, if the bleeding arises from a bypassed part of the GI tract).[13]

Small Bowel Obstruction

Bowel obstructions are more commonly seen months after surgery (rather than in the early days to weeks following the procedure). They may be caused by hernias (incisional, internal, umbilical), adhesions, and kinking of the Roux limb. In addition, patients with anastomotic leaks may present in a similar fashion.[36] Because upper GI radiographs can be insensitive (especially in the case of internal hernias), CT may be more useful.[13] However, negative imaging may not obviate diagnostic laparoscopy if there is a strong clinical suspicion of obstruction.

Patients with an ileus or partial obstruction may be managed conservatively with bowel rest, IV fluids, and repletion of electrolytes.[36] Those with a complete obstruction are more likely to require diagnostic and/or therapeutic laparoscopy.[44]

SURGICAL COMPLICATIONS BY PROCEDURE

The 30-day morbidity following any bariatric procedure ranges from 3% to 20%.[45,46] Restrictive surgeries are associated with lower complication rates than the mixed malabsorptive/restrictive procedures.[47] During this same time period, the mortality rate is 0.1% to 1.2%.[23,45,47,48] Early mortality is most commonly caused by pulmonary emboli, sepsis, and anastomotic leaks.[47,49] Complications specific to certain procedures are discussed next (**Table 1**).

ROUX-EN-Y GASTRIC BYPASS
Anastomotic or Staple Line Leak

The incidence of anastomotic leaks ranges from 0.1% to 5.8%.[17,36,38,50] Several studies have shown the leak-associated mortality to be 14% to 17%.[51] These leaks most commonly occur at the gastrojejunal anastomosis but can also occur at the gastric pouch, gastric remnant, jejunojejunostomy site, or secondary to another GI injury.[13,17,36,51] This is typically an early complication of RYGB (most commonly within 1 week after surgery).[17] Patients may present with any combination of abdominal pain, persistent tachycardia, shortness of breath, fever, hypotension, and unexplained sepsis.[17,38,51] However, it is important to remember that the absence of abdominal pain does not exclude this diagnosis.[36]

Controversy exists as to the use of imaging studies, such as upper GI radiographs with water-soluble contrast and CT. Although these studies may help diagnose a leak, they may also delay definitive care of the patient.[36,38,50,51] Conservative management (bowel rest, IV fluid resuscitation, broad-spectrum antibiotics) may suffice in hemodynamically stable patients with mild symptoms.[51] Other management options in stable

Table 1
Complications associated with procedures

Procedure	Complication	Timing	Diagnostic Tests	Treatment
Roux-en-Y gastric bypass (30%)	Anastomotic leak	Weeks to months	Gastrograffin UGI or CT abdomen	Antibiotics, surgical exploration
	GI obstruction	Weeks to months	Abdominal radiographs	NGT decompression
	Stomal stenosis	6 mo	Endoscopy or UGI contrast study	Endoscopy and dilatation
	Internal hernia	Months	CT abdomen	Surgical
	Ventral incisional hernia	Months to years	Clinical, CT abdomen	Surgical
	Stomal ulcer	Months	Endoscopy	PPI, *Helicobacter pylori* treatment, smoking/NSAID cessation
	Dumping syndrome	Months to years	Clinical	Nutritional education
	GERD	Months to years	Clinical	PPI, nutritional education
Laparoscopic adjustable gastric banding (27%)	Esophageal/gastric pouch dilatation	Days to weeks	UGI series	PPI, nutritional education
	Port infection	Days to weeks	Clinical	Antibiotics, port removal
	Hiatal hernia	Weeks to months	UGI series, endoscopy	PPI, nutritional education, surgery if severe
	Gastric slippage	Days to months	UGI contrast study, abdominal radiographs	Surgery
	Esophagitis	Months to years	Clinical	PPI, nutritional education
	GERD	Months to years	Clinical	PPI, nutritional education
Sleeve gastrectomy (19%)	Anastomotic leak	Weeks to months	Gastrograffin UGI or CT abdomen	Antibiotics, surgical exploration
	Gastric stenosis	Days to weeks	UGI series, endoscopy	Endoscopy and dilatation, conversion to RYGB
	GERD	Months to years	Clinical	PPI, nutritional education
Biliopancreatic diversion with duodenal switch (1.5%)	Anastomotic leak	Weeks to months	Gastrograffin UGI or CT abdomen	Antibiotics, surgical exploration
	GI obstruction	Weeks to months	Abdominal radiographs	NGT decompression
	Stomal stenosis	6 mo	Endoscopy or UGI contrast study	Endoscopy and dilatation
	Internal hernia	Months	CT abdomen	Surgical
	Ventral incisional hernia	Months to years	Clinical, CT abdomen	Surgical
	Stomal ulcer	Months	Endoscopy	PPI, *H pylori* treatment, smoking/NSAID cessation
	Dumping syndrome	Months to years	Clinical	Nutritional education
	GERD	Months to years	Clinical	PPI, nutritional education

Abbreviations: GERD, gastroesophageal reflux disease; NGT, nasogastric tube; NSAID, nonsteroidal anti-inflammatory drug; PPI, proton pump inhibitor; UGI, upper gastrointestinal.

patients include percutaneous drainage or endoluminal stenting.[50] Patients with more severe symptoms or sepsis require operative intervention.[36,38,50,51]

Anastomotic Stenosis

Anastomotic stenosis occurs in 3% to 20% of RYGBs.[17,51,52] Although it may occur at any anastomosis, the gastrojejunostomy site is the most common.[36,51] Additionally, it is more common following laparoscopic RYGB than the open technique.[13,36] Stenosis formation may be related to anastomotic leaks, tension at the anastomosis, tissue ischemia, or marginal ulceration.[13,36] This complication most commonly develops 3 to 6 months postoperatively, and patients typically present with nausea, vomiting, abdominal pain, and/or progressive dysphagia.[17,36,51]

Endoscopy seems to be more useful than upper GI radiographs, being more sensitive diagnostically and potentially therapeutic.[13,17] Most of these stenoses can be treated with endoscopic dilatation, although operative revision is needed in some cases.[17,51]

Dumping Syndrome

Dumping syndrome occurs in about 40% of patients up to 12 to 18 months after RYGB.[17,53] Incidentally it has also been reported following partial or complete gastrectomy (including SG).[53] Symptoms of dumping syndrome begin following meals, particularly after ingestion of simple carbohydrates.

Early symptoms are caused by rapid gastric emptying and passage of stomach contents into the small bowel. The hyperosmolar intestinal contents may result in fluid shifts into the intestinal lumen. These patients may present with GI (nausea, diarrhea, abdominal pain) or vasomotor symptomatology (palpitations, diaphoresis, flushing, hypotension, syncope). Late symptoms occur 1 to 3 hour after meals as a result of hypoglycemia. Rapid gastric emptying transiently elevates glucose concentrations in the gut, which in turn triggers insulin secretion. After the intestinal contents are absorbed, hypoglycemia occurs, causing typical manifestations (ie, palpitations, diaphoresis, weakness, tremor, altered mental status, and/or syncope).[53]

Treatment in the emergency department is supportive (eg, IV fluids, antiemetics, electrolyte repletion). Patients should be counseled to eat smaller, more frequent meals that are high in fiber, complex carbohydrates, and protein. They should avoid eating sugars and lactose, and drinking during or after meals for at least 2 hours. Patients who are refractory to these interventions may be placed on a somatostatin analog by their surgeon.[53]

Gastric Remnant Dilatation

Gastric remnant dilatation is a rare complication of RYGB, occurring in up to 0.8% of patients following laparoscopic RYGB.[54,55] If this diagnosis is not discovered in a timely manner, gastric perforation, peritonitis, and sepsis may ensue. Potential causes include gastroparesis, gastrojejunostomy leak, jejunojejunostomy obstruction, hemorrhage, and gastric remnant ulceration.[54,55] Patients with gastric remnant distention may present with left upper quadrant or epigastric pain, nausea, vomiting, hiccups, tachycardia, or left upper quadrant tympany. Treatment options include prokinetics, gastrostomy tube for decompression, and surgical intervention.[54]

Marginal or Stomal Ulcers

Marginal ulcers occur in up to 20% of patients following RYGB.[13,51] Although these ulcers are probably multifactorial, various etiologic factors include increased gastric acid secretion, tissue ischemia, staple line dehiscence, nonsteroidal anti-inflammatory drug

(NSAID) use, *Helicobacter pylori* infection, smoking, and increased tissue tension.[13,17,36,56] Patients usually present 2 to 4 months postoperatively with nausea, vomiting, retrosternal or epigastric pain, dyspepsia, or UGIB.[17,51] The diagnosis is established by endoscopy. Treatment includes proton pump inhibitors, sucralfate, smoking cessation, *H pylori* therapy, and discontinuation of NSAIDs. Surgical intervention (ie, resection, reanastomosis) may be indicated for recurrent bleeding or refractory pain.[13,17,36,57]

Internal Hernia

Internals hernias are more common after laparoscopic RYGBs than open procedures with an incidence of up to 16%.[13,58,59] They are thought to occur because of abdominal-wall defects created during surgery.[58] Patients with internal hernias may present with nausea, vomiting, abdominal pain, and/or obstructive symptoms. Although CT is more sensitive than upper GI radiographs, a negative CT does not definitively rule out this diagnosis because herniation may be intermittent. Because delayed diagnosis is associated with a significant mortality if strangulation occurs, diagnostic laparoscopy should be considered for patients with persistent symptoms even if imaging is negative (**Figs. 7** and **8**).[13,58,59]

Ventral Incisional Hernia

The incidence of incisional hernias is low with the laparoscopic approach but much higher when conducted in an open fashion (ranging from 8% to 25%).[60,61] Clinical presentation, diagnosis, and management are similar to those of incisional hernias following other operations.

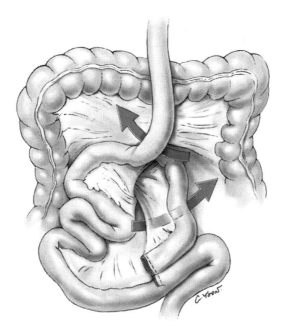

Fig. 7. Potential sites of internal hernia after antecolic RYGB. (*From* Carmody B, DeMaria EJ, Jamal M, et al. Internal hernia after laparoscopic Roux-en-Y gastric bypass. Surg Obes Relat Dis 2005;1(6):544; with permission.)

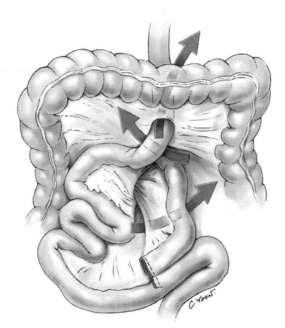

Fig. 8. Potential sites of internal hernia after retrocolic RYGB. (*From* Carmody B, DeMaria EJ, Jamal M, et al. Internal hernia after laparoscopic Roux-en-Y gastric bypass. Surg Obes Relat Dis 2005;1(6):545; with permission.)

BILIARY PANCREATIC DIVERSION WITHOUT AND WITH DUODENAL SWITCH

BPD and BPD-DS are associated with complications similar to RYGB: infection, bleeding, cholelithiasis, small bowel obstruction, anastomotic leaks and stenoses, marginal ulcers, and internal hernias.[62,63] The clinical presentation, diagnosis, and management of these conditions are as described previously. Other adverse symptoms include abdominal bloating and loose stools. Furthermore, postprandial vomiting and epigastric pain may occur because of rapid ileal distention.[17]

LAPAROSCOPIC ADJUSTABLE GASTRIC BANDING
Esophagitis

Esophagitis may occur in up to 30% of patients following LAGB.[64] These patients may present with reflux-like symptoms, such as dysphagia, chest pain, and dyspepsia. This may be related to such conditions as gastroesophageal reflux, hiatal hernia (HH) formation, gastric prolapse, and overly tight gastric bands.[65,66] Treatment is usually initiated based on a clinical presentation and includes acid-suppression therapy and nutritional counseling (ie, consumption of smaller, more frequent meals).

Hiatal Hernia

Because HHs occur in about 53% of severely obese people, they may be present preoperatively.[67] They have also been found postoperatively in association with band slippage, pouch and esophageal dilation, and gastric prolapse.[67,68] One hypothesis is that a "backpressure syndrome" of chronic overpressurization on the proximal pouch contributes to the worsening of a pre-existing or formation of a new HH.[67] Patients with HHs may present with reflux-like symptoms and may be diagnosed using upper GI radiography or endoscopy. Although initial management is similar to that for esophagitis, surgical revision of the LABG or HH repair may be necessary.

Gastroesophageal Dilatation

Gastric pouch and esophageal dilatation may occur in about 15% and 13% to 14% of patients, respectively, following LAGB.[64,69] Possible etiologies include an overly restrictive or improperly placed band, excessive vomiting, and dietary noncompliance.[17,36,63] Symptoms may include dysphagia, epigastric pain, and inability to tolerate oral intake. Upper GI imaging can establish the diagnosis. Pouch dilatation is usually relieved by deflation of the band. However, esophageal dilatation can cause irreversible damage if not diagnosed and treated in a timely manner. Should complete deflation of the band not resolve the esophageal dilatation, revision or removal of the band or conversion to RYGB may be necessary.[36,63]

Band Erosion

In a review of 25 studies about band erosion (BE) following LAGB (that included more than 15,000 patients), the incidence was 1.46%.[70] Various causes have been postulated including intraoperative injury to the gastric wall, chronic infection, overly tightened band, tissue ischemia, excessive food intake, smoking, NSAID use, and alcohol consumption.[36,63,70,71] Although BE can present between 5 and 51 months after surgery, the mean time of presentation in one study was 22 months.[72] Clinical presentations vary depending on whether the BE results in free leakage of gastric contents or containment by inflammation and scar tissue. The three most common presentations were (1) lack of satiety and failed weight loss, (2) port site infection, and (3) abdominal pain.[70] However, patients may also present with frank peritonitis.[36]

Although upper GI radiography may demonstrate leakage of contrast from the BE site, endoscopy is the preferred diagnostic tool.[17,36,70] Treatment involves surgical removal of the band and repair of any identifiable gastric injury.[17,36]

Band Slippage and Gastric Prolapse

Gastric pouch enlargement can result from downward band slippage or upward herniation/prolapse of the stomach through the band.[63] Reported incidences range from 2.3% to 15%.[66] Clinical presentations mimic those of overly restrictive bands and gastric pouch dilatation: dysphagia, reflux, vomiting, epigastric pain, and food intolerance.[17,36,63] However, unlike gastric pouch dilatation, symptoms of band slippage/gastric prolapse are not improved by deflation of the band.[36,63]

The diagnosis should be evident on an upper GI series. Emergency department management includes repletion of electrolytes and IV fluids. However, timely surgical intervention is needed to avoid complications, such as gastric ischemia, tissue necrosis, and perforation.[17,36,63]

Stomal Obstruction

Stomal obstruction blocks the passage of food from the gastric pouch into the distal stomach. It may occur as either an early or late complication of LAGB. Early stomal obstruction may be caused by postoperative edema, hematoma, an overly restrictive band, incorporation of excess tissue in the band, insufficiently chewed food, or pills.[17,63,73] Late obstructions can result from iatrogenic band adjustment, gastric pouch dilatation, band slippage/gastric prolapse, or BE.[17,63] Patients often present with obstructive symptomatology, such as reflux, vomiting, dysphagia, and epigastric pain. The obstruction is typically evident on upper GI imaging. Conservative treatment is usually first line: IV hydration and band deflation. Endoscopy may be needed if pills or a food bolus is causing the obstruction. Surgery may be required if there is complete obstruction, lack of improvement with conservative management, or evidence of tissue ischemia or perforation.[17,36,63]

Port Infection

Port infections have an incidence ranging from 0.3% to 9% and may occur during the immediate postoperative period, following port access/band adjustment, or at any point while the port is in place.[38,74] Patients commonly present with local tenderness, erythema, warmth, and swelling over the port site. It is imperative to consider BE if a port infection occurs outside of the immediate postoperative period.[36]

This is usually a clinical diagnosis, although endoscopy and/or CT may be needed to rule out other pathology, such as BE or intra-abdominal abscess.[38,74] Treatment of an isolated port infection involves systemic antibiotics (to cover skin flora) and possibly port removal.[36,74]

SLEEVE GASTRECTOMY
Gastric Leak

The incidence of GLs ranges in the literature from 0% to 7%.[75–77] They most commonly arise from the staple line in the proximal stomach near the gastroesophageal junction probably caused by a combination of mechanical stress and tissue ischemia.[63,76–78] Clinical presentations may be subtle but most commonly include fever, tachycardia, and abdominal pain.[76]

Early identification and treatment of GLs are vital to decrease the associated morbidity and mortality. Unfortunately upper GI radiography is notoriously insensitive for this diagnosis.[75,76] In the stable patient, CT may be more useful (83%–93% sensitivity, 75%–100% specificity).[76] However, re-exploration definitively diagnoses a GL. This procedure should be considered if there is a strong clinical suspicion for GL or if the patient is unstable. Nonoperative management is often the initial approach in stable patients. This includes IV fluids, parenteral antibiotics, and nutrition. Other possibilities include endoscopic or percutaneous drainage and endoluminal stenting.[63,76] Surgical intervention is usually necessary in unstable patients and those with early postoperative leaks. Chronic fistulae are generally managed nonoperatively and may require an average of 44 weeks to close.[76]

Gastric Stenosis

Gastric stenosis is an uncommon complication with a reported incidence ranging from 0.1% to 3.9%.[79] In this condition, delayed gastric emptying or true obstruction results from twisting of the gastric tube or an anatomic stricture. Patients commonly present with dysphagia, nausea, vomiting, or oral intolerance.[79,80]

Although gastric stenosis can be diagnosed with an upper GI series or endoscopy, the latter also has the potential to be of use therapeutically.[80] Patients who present during the immediate postoperative period may be managed conservatively with IV hydration and bowel rest. If there is no improvement, then endoscopic dilation is the next step. For patients with more chronic strictures, treatment options include endoscopy (ie, dilation or stent placement) or surgery (ie, conversion to RYGB).[63,79,80]

Gastroesophageal Reflux Disease

Although most studies have been inconclusive as to the effect of SG on gastroesophageal reflux disease, a recent meta-analysis demonstrated a trend toward an increased prevalence after SG.[81] Patients present with typical reflux-like symptoms including regurgitation and dyspepsia. Most respond to treatment with proton pump inhibitors, prokinetic agents, and nutritional/lifestyle modifications.[80]

SUMMARY

Obesity is present in epidemic proportions in the United States, and bariatric surgery has become more common. Thus, emergency physicians will undoubtedly encounter many patients who have undergone one of these procedures. Knowledge of the anatomic changes caused by these procedures aids the clinician in understanding potential complications and devising an organized differential diagnosis when evaluating the bariatric surgery patient with abdominal pain.

REFERENCES

1. Peeters A, Barendregt JJ, Willekens F, et al. Obesity in adulthood and its consequences for life expectancy: a life-table analysis. Ann Intern Med 2003;138(1): 24–32.
2. Heo YS, Park JM, Kim YJ, et al. Bariatric surgery versus conventional therapy in obese Korean patients: a multicenter retrospective cohort study. J Korean Surg Soc 2012;83(6):335–42.
3. Mingrone G, Panunzi S, De Gaetano A, et al. Bariatric surgery versus conventional medical therapy for type 2 diabetes. N Engl J Med 2012;366(17):1577–85.
4. Gloy VL, Briel M, Bhatt DL, et al. Bariatric surgery versus non-surgical treatment for obesity: a systematic review and meta-analysis of randomised controlled trials. BMJ 2013;347:f5934.
5. Ogden CL, Carroll MD, Kit BK, et al. Prevalence of childhood and adult obesity in the United States, 2011-2012. JAMA 2014;311(8):806–14.
6. Finkelstein EA, Trogdon JG, Cohen JW, et al. Annual medical spending attributable to obesity: payer-and service-specific estimates. Health Aff (Millwood) 2009;28(5):w822–31.
7. Buchwald H, Oien DM. Metabolic/bariatric surgery worldwide 2011. Obes Surg 2013;23(4):427–36.
8. He W, Li Q, Yang M, et al. Lower BMI cutoffs to define overweight and obesity in china. Obesity (Silver Spring) 2015;23(3):684–91.
9. Nazare JA, Smith JD, Borel AL, et al. Ethnic influences on the relations between abdominal subcutaneous and visceral adiposity, liver fat, and cardiometabolic risk profile: the international study of prediction of intra-abdominal adiposity and its relationship with cardiometabolic risk/intra-abdominal adiposity. Am J Clin Nutr 2012;96(4):714–26.
10. National Heart, Blood, and Lung Institute Obesity Education Initiative. The practical guide: identification, evaluation, and treatment of overweight and obesity in adults, vol. 80. Bethesda (MD): National Institutes of Health; 2000. Available at: https://www.nhlbi.nih.gov/files/docs/guidelines/prctgd_c.pdf. Accessed August, 2015.
11. Sheets CS, Peat CM, Berg KC, et al. Post-operative psychosocial predictors of outcome in bariatric surgery. Obes Surg 2015;25(2):330–45.
12. Sogg S, Friedman KE. Getting off on the right foot: the many roles of the psychosocial evaluation in the bariatric surgery practice. Eur Eat Disord Rev 2015;23(6): 451–6.
13. Elder KA, Wolfe BM. Bariatric surgery: a review of procedures and outcomes. Gastroenterology 2007;132(6):2253–71.
14. O'Brien PE. Controversies in bariatric surgery. Br J Surg 2015;102(6):611–8.

15. Mason EE, Ito C. Gastric bypass in obesity. Surg Clin North Am 1967;47(6): 1345–51.

16. Nelson DW, Blair KS, Martin MJ. Analysis of obesity-related outcomes and bariatric failure rates with the duodenal switch vs gastric bypass for morbid obesity. Arch Surg 2012;147(9):847–54.

17. Ellison SR, Ellison SD. Bariatric surgery: a review of the available procedures and complications for the emergency physician. J Emerg Med 2008;34(1):21–32.

18. Murr MM, Balsiger BM, Kennedy FP, et al. Malabsorptive procedures for severe obesity: comparison of pancreaticobiliary bypass and very very long limb Roux-en-Y gastric bypass. J Gastrointest Surg 1999;3(6):607–12.

19. Marceau P, Hould FS, Simard S, et al. Biliopancreatic diversion with duodenal switch. World J Surg 1998;22(9):947–54.

20. Marceau P, Biron S, Hould FS, et al. Duodenal switch improved standard biliopancreatic diversion: a retrospective study. Surg Obes Relat Dis 2009;5(1):43–7.

21. Iannelli A, Schneck AS, Topart P, et al. Laparoscopic sleeve gastrectomy followed by duodenal switch in selected patients versus single-stage duodenal switch for superobesity: case-control study. Surg Obes Relat Dis 2013;9(4):531–8.

22. Rezvani M, Sucandy I, Klar A, et al. Is laparoscopic single-stage biliopancreatic diversion with duodenal switch safe in super morbidly obese patients? Surg Obes Relat Dis 2014;10(3):427–30.

23. Buchwald H, Avidor Y, Braunwald E, et al. Bariatric surgery: a systematic review and meta-analysis. JAMA 2004;292(14):1724–37.

24. Laurenius A, Taha O, Maleckas A, et al. Laparoscopic biliopancreatic diversion/duodenal switch or laparoscopic Roux-en-Y gastric bypass for super-obesity-weight loss versus side effects. Surg Obes Relat Dis 2010;6(4):408–14.

25. O'Brien PE, Dixon JB. Lap-band: outcomes and results. J Laparoendosc Adv Surg Tech A 2003;13(4):265–70.

26. O'Brien PE, MacDonald L, Anderson M, et al. Long-term outcomes after bariatric surgery: fifteen-year follow-up of adjustable gastric banding and a systematic review of the bariatric surgical literature. Ann Surg 2013;257(1):87–94.

27. Cottam D, Qureshi FG, Mattar SG, et al. Laparoscopic sleeve gastrectomy as an initial weight-loss procedure for high-risk patients with morbid obesity. Surg Endosc 2006;20(6):859–63.

28. Ramon JM, Salvans S, Crous X, et al. Effect of Roux-en-Y gastric bypass vs sleeve gastrectomy on glucose and gut hormones: a prospective randomised trial. J Gastrointest Surg 2012;16(6):1116–22.

29. van Rutte PW, Smulders JF, de Zoete JP, et al. Outcome of sleeve gastrectomy as a primary bariatric procedure. Br J Surg 2014;101(6):661–8.

30. Biter LU, Gadiot RP, Grotenhuis BA, et al. The sleeve bypass trial: a multicentre randomized controlled trial comparing the long term outcome of laparoscopic sleeve gastrectomy and gastric bypass for morbid obesity in terms of excess BMI loss percentage and quality of life. BMC Obes 2015;2:30.

31. U.S. Food and Drug Administration. ReShape integrated dual balloon system - P140012. U.S. Food and Drug Administration Web site. Available at: http://www.fda.gov/MedicalDevices/ProductsandMedicalProcedures/DeviceApprovalsand Clearances/Recently-ApprovedDevices/ucm456293.htm. Accessed March 11, 2015.

32. Ponce J, Quebbemann BB, Patterson EJ. Prospective, randomized, multicenter study evaluating safety and efficacy of intragastric dual-balloon in obesity. Surg Obes Relat Dis 2013;9(2):290–5.

33. Ponce J, Woodman G, Swain J, et al. The REDUCE pivotal trial: a prospective, randomized controlled pivotal trial of a dual intragastric balloon for the treatment of obesity. Surg Obes Relat Dis 2015;11(4):874–81.
34. Aceto P, Perilli V, Modesti C, et al. Airway management in obese patients. Surg Obes Relat Dis 2013;9(5):809–15.
35. Price H. Effects of carbon dioxide on the caridovascular system. Anesthesiology 1960;21:652–63.
36. Tanner BD, Allen JW. Complications of bariatric surgery: implications for the covering physician. Am Surg 2009;75(2):103–12.
37. Agarwala A, Kellum JM. Prevention, detection, and management of leaks following gastric bypass for obesity. Adv Surg 2010;44:59–72.
38. Chopra T, Zhao JJ, Alangaden G, et al. Preventing surgical site infections after bariatric surgery: value of perioperative antibiotic regimens. Expert Rev Pharmacoecon Outcomes Res 2010;10(3):317–28.
39. Christou NV, Jarand J, Sylvestre JL, et al. Analysis of the incidence and risk factors for wound infections in open bariatric surgery. Obes Surg 2004;14(1):16–22.
40. Melmer A, Sturm W, Kuhnert B, et al. Incidence of gallstone formation and cholecystectomy 10 years after bariatric surgery. Obes Surg 2015;25(7):1171–6.
41. Coupaye M, Castel B, Sami O, et al. Comparison of the incidence of cholelithiasis after sleeve gastrectomy and Roux-en-Y gastric bypass in obese patients: a prospective study. Surg Obes Relat Dis 2015;11(4):779–84.
42. Tsirline VB, Keilani ZM, El Djouzi S, et al. How frequently and when do patients undergo cholecystectomy after bariatric surgery? Surg Obes Relat Dis 2014; 10(2):313–21.
43. Garcia-Garcia ML, Martin-Lorenzo JG, Torralba-Martinez JA, et al. Emergency endoscopy for gastrointestinal bleeding after bariatric surgery. Therapeutic algorithm. Cir Esp 2015;93(2):97–104.
44. Bradley JF 3rd, Ross SW, Christmas AB, et al. Complications of bariatric surgery: the acute care surgeon's experience. Am J Surg 2015;210(3):456–61.
45. Stenberg E, Szabo E, Agren G, et al. Early complications after laparoscopic gastric bypass surgery: results from the Scandinavian obesity surgery registry. Ann Surg 2014;260(6):1040–7.
46. Topart P, Becouarn G, Ritz P. Comparative early outcomes of three laparoscopic bariatric procedures: sleeve gastrectomy, Roux-en-Y gastric bypass, and biliopancreatic diversion with duodenal switch. Surg Obes Relat Dis 2012;8(3):250–4.
47. Piche ME, Auclair A, Harvey J, et al. How to choose and use bariatric surgery in 2015. Can J Cardiol 2015;31(2):153–66.
48. Maggard MA, Shugarman LR, Suttorp M, et al. Meta-analysis: surgical treatment of obesity. Ann Intern Med 2005;142(7):547–59.
49. Mason EE, Renquist KE, Huang YH, et al. Causes of 30-day bariatric surgery mortality: with emphasis on bypass obstruction. Obes Surg 2007;17(1):9–14.
50. Jacobsen HJ, Nergard BJ, Leifsson BG, et al. Management of suspected anastomotic leak after bariatric laparoscopic Roux-en-y gastric bypass. Br J Surg 2014;101(4):417–23.
51. Walsh C, Karmali S. Endoscopic management of bariatric complications: a review and update. World J Gastrointest Endosc 2015;7(5):518–23.
52. Go MR, Muscarella P 2nd, Needleman BJ, et al. Endoscopic management of stomal stenosis after Roux-en-Y gastric bypass. Surg Endosc 2004;18(1):56–9.
53. Tack J, Deloose E. Complications of bariatric surgery: dumping syndrome, reflux and vitamin deficiencies. Best Pract Res Clin Gastroenterol 2014;28(4):741–9.

54. Han SH, White S, Patel K, et al. Acute gastric remnant dilation after laparoscopic Roux-en-Y gastric bypass operation in long-standing type I diabetic patient: case report and literature review. Surg Obes Relat Dis 2006;2(6):664–6.
55. Chan E, Ramirez I, Szomstein S, et al. Incidence, etiology, and management of gastric remnant dilation following laparoscopic Roux-en-Y gastric bypass for morbid obesity: analysis of 1963 consecutive cases. Poster presentation at: 2008 Society of American Gastrointestinal and Endoscopic Surgeons. Philadelphia, April 9-12, 2008.
56. Rasmussen JJ, Fuller W, Ali MR. Marginal ulceration after laparoscopic gastric bypass: an analysis of predisposing factors in 260 patients. Surg Endosc 2007;21(7):1090–4.
57. Sanyal AJ, Sugerman HJ, Kellum JM, et al. Stomal complications of gastric bypass: incidence and outcome of therapy. Am J Gastroenterol 1992;87(9): 1165–9.
58. Altieri MS, Pryor AD, Telem DA, et al. Algorithmic approach to utilization of CT scans for detection of internal hernia in the gastric bypass patient. Surg Obes Relat Dis 2015;11(6):1207–11.
59. Higa KD, Ho T, Boone KB. Internal hernias after laparoscopic Roux-en-Y gastric bypass: incidence, treatment and prevention. Obes Surg 2003;13(3):350–4.
60. Iljin A, Szymanski D, Kruk-Jeromin J, et al. The repair of incisional hernia following Roux-en-Y gastric bypass-with or without concomitant abdominoplasty? Obes Surg 2008;18(11):1387–91.
61. Nguyen NT, Goldman C, Rosenquist CJ, et al. Laparoscopic versus open gastric bypass: a randomized study of outcomes, quality of life, and costs. Ann Surg 2001;234(3):279–89 [discussion: 289–91].
62. Michielson D, Van Hee R, Hendrickx L. Complications of biliopancreatic diversion surgery as proposed by scopinaro in the treatment of morbid obesity. Obes Surg 1996;6(5):416–20.
63. Mathus-Vliegen EM. The cooperation between endoscopists and surgeons in treating complications of bariatric surgery. Best Pract Res Clin Gastroenterol 2014;28(4):703–25.
64. Mittermair RP, Obermuller S, Perathoner A, et al. Results and complications after Swedish adjustable gastric banding-10 years experience. Obes Surg 2009; 19(12):1636–41.
65. Skomorowski M, Cappell MS. Endoscopic findings with severely symptomatic esophagitis from an overly restrictive laparoscopic adjustable gastric band. Surg Obes Relat Dis 2014;10(1):e9–10.
66. Kia L, Kahrilas PJ. An unusual complication after laparoscopic gastric lap band placement. Gastroenterology 2014;147(6):e9–10.
67. Azagury DE, Varban O, Tavakkolizadeh A, et al. Does laparoscopic gastric banding create hiatal hernias? Surg Obes Relat Dis 2013;9(1):48–52.
68. Parikh MS, Fielding GA, Ren CJ. U.S. experience with 749 laparoscopic adjustable gastric bands: intermediate outcomes. Surg Endosc 2005;19(12):1631–5.
69. Milone L, Daud A, Durak E, et al. Esophageal dilation after laparoscopic adjustable gastric banding. Surg Endosc 2008;22(6):1482–6.
70. Brown WA, Egberts KJ, Franke-Richard D, et al. Erosions after laparoscopic adjustable gastric banding: diagnosis and management. Ann Surg 2013; 257(6):1047–52.
71. Abu-Abeid S, Keidar A, Gavert N, et al. The clinical spectrum of band erosion following laparoscopic adjustable silicone gastric banding for morbid obesity. Surg Endosc 2003;17(6):861–3.

72. Suter M, Giusti V, Heraief E, et al. Band erosion after laparoscopic gastric banding: occurrence and results after conversion to Roux-en-Y gastric bypass. Obes Surg 2004;14(3):381–6.
73. Louri N, Darwish B, Alkhalifa K. Stoma obstruction after laparoscopic adjustable gastric banding for morbid obesity: report of two cases and treatment options. Obes Rev 2008;9(6):518–21.
74. Freeman L, Brown WA, Korin A, et al. An approach to the assessment and management of the laparoscopic adjustable gastric band patient in the emergency department. Emerg Med Australas 2011;23(2):186–94.
75. Gagner M, Deitel M, Kalberer TL, et al. The second international consensus summit for sleeve gastrectomy, March 19-21, 2009. Surg Obes Relat Dis 2009;5(4): 476–85.
76. Kim J, Azagury D, Eisenberg D, et al, American Society for Metabolic and Bariatric Surgery Clinical Issues Committee. ASMBS position statement on prevention, detection, and treatment of gastrointestinal leak after gastric bypass and sleeve gastrectomy, including the roles of imaging, surgical exploration, and nonoperative management. Surg Obes Relat Dis 2015;11(4):739–48.
77. Galloro G, Ruggiero S, Russo T, et al. Staple-line leak after sleve gastrectomy in obese patients: a hot topic in bariatric surgery. World J Gastrointest Endosc 2015;7(9):843–6.
78. Lalor PF, Tucker ON, Szomstein S, et al. Complications after laparoscopic sleeve gastrectomy. Surg Obes Relat Dis 2008;4(1):33–8.
79. Burgos AM, Csendes A, Braghetto I. Gastric stenosis after laparoscopic sleeve gastrectomy in morbidly obese patients. Obes Surg 2013;23(9):1481–6.
80. Sarkhosh K, Birch DW, Sharma A, et al. Complications associated with laparoscopic sleeve gastrectomy for morbid obesity: a surgeon's guide. Can J Surg 2013;56(5):347–52.
81. Oor JE, Roks DJ, Unlu C, et al. Laparoscopic sleeve gastrectomy and gastroesophageal reflux disease: a systematic review and meta-analysis. Am J Surg 2016;211(1):250–67.

Abdominal Pain Mimics

Jessica Palmer, MD[a], Elizabeth Pontius, MD, RDMS[a,b],*

KEYWORDS

- Abdominal pain • Mimics • Diagnoses

KEY POINTS

- Emergency department providers have become skilled at triaging patients with abdominal pain requiring surgical interventions.
- Abdominal pain mimics, medical conditions that cause the sensation of abdominal pain without abdominal abnormality, continue to puzzle the best physicians.

As any emergency physician can attest, abdominal pain makes up a significant portion of chief complaints. Eleven percent of emergency department (ED) visits are attributed to abdominal pain each year.[1] Fortunately, with improvements in technology and advancements in imaging, ED providers have become skilled at triaging patients with abdominal pain requiring surgical interventions. However, abdominal pain mimics, medical conditions that cause the sensation of abdominal pain without abdominal abnormality, continue to puzzle the best physicians. In this article, abdominal pain mimics, which includes diagnoses that cannot be missed, conditions that require urgent evaluation, and additional conditions to consider when broadening a differential diagnosis, are discussed (**Box 1**).

Box 1
Abdominal pain mimics

Metabolic

Diabetic ketoacidosis

Alcoholic ketoacidosis

Calcium abnormalities

Thyrotoxicosis

Uremia

Disclosure: The authors have no financial disclosures.
[a] Department of Emergency Medicine, MedStar Washington Hospital Center, 110 Irving Street Northwest NA 11-77, Washington, DC 20010, USA; [b] Department of Emergency Medicine, Georgetown University School of Medicine, Washington, DC, USA
* Correspondence author.
E-mail address: epontius@gmail.com

Emerg Med Clin N Am 34 (2016) 409–423
http://dx.doi.org/10.1016/j.emc.2015.12.007
0733-8627/16/$ – see front matter © 2016 Elsevier Inc. All rights reserved.

emed.theclinics.com

Porphyria

Pheochromocytoma

Adrenal crisis

Hematologic

Sickle cell disease

Neutropenic enterocolitis

Spontaneous splenic rupture

Immunologic

Angioedema

Henoch-Schonlein purpura

Systemic lupus erythematosus

Polyarteritis nodosa

Food allergy

Infectious

Pneumonia

Tuberculosis

Lyme disease

Pharyngitis (Lemierre syndrome)

Toxic

Mushroom intoxication

Alcohol intoxication

Metal poisoning

Envenomation

Opioid withdrawal

Cardiopulmonary

Atypical acute coronary syndrome

Pulmonary embolism

Pneumonia

Congestive heart failure

Functional

Abdominal migraine

Cyclic vomiting

Irritable bowel syndrome

Neurologic

Herpes zoster

Abdominal epilepsy

Environmental

Heat stroke

Adapted from Fields JM, Dean A. Systemic causes of abdominal pain. Emerg Med Clin North Am 2011;29:196–7; with permission.

CANNOT MISS DIAGNOSES

Atypical acute coronary artery syndrome, diabetic ketoacidosis, pulmonary embolism (PE), and congestive heart failure make up a group of diagnoses associated with significant morbidity and mortality if missed. These patients may present with abdominal pain as the sole complaint, and the practitioner must assess their cardiac, metabolic, and thromboembolic risk factors to ensure an accurate, timely diagnosis.

Acute Coronary Syndrome

Coronary artery disease is the number one cause of death in the United States.[2] Acute coronary syndrome (ACS), a clinical diagnosis that includes ST segment elevation myocardial infarction, non-ST segment myocardial infarction, and unstable angina, accounts for 3.5 million hospital admissions worldwide each year.[3] The typical presentation of ACS includes chest pain, shortness of breath, diaphoresis, and often pain in the left arm or jaw. ACS with an atypical presentation is an oft-missed diagnosis in the ED with grave consequences.[4] Symptoms are often dependent on a patient's age and gender. Younger patients (less than age 70) with ACS tend to present with typical symptoms such as chest pain and present earlier in the progression of symptoms.[5] On the other hand, the older patient population, greater than 70, who tend to be female and diabetic, often present only with gastrointestinal symptoms: abdominal pain, nausea, and vomiting. The pathophysiology behind this atypical presentation stems from autonomic neuropathy that occurs with longstanding diabetes mellitus. Researchers are still unsure why women tend to experience atypical symptoms more commonly than men. To avoid diagnostic delays, an early cardiac evaluation should be considered in high-risk patients (elderly female patients with history of diabetes, hypertension, and congestive heart failure) with nonfocal abdominal pain. An electrocardiogram with cardiac enzymes should be considered in addition to electrolytes, a liver function panel, and lipase. With a normal cardiac workup, the practitioner should pursue other abdominal pain causes. Keeping atypical ACS in the differential will prevent late treatment and reduce morbidity and mortality.

Diabetic Ketoacidosis

Hyperglycemic crises are becoming increasingly common as the incidence of diabetes mellitus continues to increase. Abdominal pain occurs in a significant proportion of patients with diabetic ketoacidosis. Patients are often unable to delineate between abdominal pain as a cause for their hyperglycemia (ie, a viral gastroenteritis with increasing insulin requirements or reduced insulin administration) or abdominal discomfort caused by worsening hyperglycemia and ketoacidosis. Umpierrez and Freire,[6] in a prospective 2003 study, found a direct correlation between abdominal pain and metabolic acidosis in patients with diabetic ketoacidosis. Patients with abdominal pain, nausea, and vomiting had significantly lower bicarbonate levels and a lower pH. Interestingly, there was no association between abdominal pain and severity of hyperglycemia or dehydration. Very rarely did these patients have intra-abdominal abnormality, and the researchers recommended hydration and insulin therapy to close the anion gap before performing an aggressive abdominal pain workup or exploratory laparotomy, because often symptoms resolved with resolution of the metabolic acidosis. Patients with hyperglycemic hyperosmolar nonketotic state were significantly less likely to have abdominal pain. Gastroparesis from poorly controlled blood glucose, ileus from the metabolic derangements associated with diabetic ketoacidosis, and pancreatitis may also contribute to abdominal pain in patients with diabetic ketoacidosis. Clinicians should aim to manage electrolyte derangements and pain, in addition to performing gastric emptying studies, if applicable.

Pulmonary Embolism

Clinicians consider PE when patients present with cardiopulmonary symptoms, such as pleuritic chest pain, shortness of breath, or even simply anxiety. However, abdominal pain can also be the presenting symptom of this diagnosis associated with tremendous morbidity and mortality. Nearly 7% of PEs have associated gastrointestinal complaints that range from vague discomfort to an acute abdomen.[7] Although the mechanism still remains unclear, pain may be due to hepatic congestion (due to right heart strain), distention of Glisson capsule, or even diaphragmatic irritation from pulmonary infarction.[8,9] It is crucial to maintain a high index of suspicion for PE in high-risk patients: those with active malignancy, known hypercoagulable states, patients on exogenous estrogens, or patients who present with concerning histories such as shortness of breath, chest pain, or lower extremity edema following injuries, recent surgeries, or prolonged sedentary periods. Clinical decision-making rules such as the Geneva, Wells, or PERC (pulmonary embolism rule-out criteria) criteria should not be used in patients with abdominal pain, for which the provider has a high index of suspicion, because this may result in significant morbidity and mortality from a missed diagnosis. Clinicians should consider a computed tomographic (CT) angiogram of the chest to rule out a PE in high-risk patients. If positive, patients should receive therapeutic dosing of anticoagulation before admission for further monitoring.

Congestive Heart Failure

Congestive heart failure is an increasingly common end-stage cardiac disease caused by a functional or structural cardiac defect impairing the heart's ability to fill and pump the ventricles.[10] Patients typically present with cardiopulmonary complaints such as chest pain, palpitations, or worsening shortness of breath. Interestingly, many patients experience abdominal pain: both localized and general. Patients may present with right upper quadrant pain that mimics that of hepatitis or cholecystitis. Similar to patients with abdominal pain and PE, patients in decompensated congestive heart failure can have hepatic congestion from right heart strain causing pain over the right upper quadrant on abdominal examination. In patients with new onset congestive heart failure, increasing distention of the splanchnic circulation can lead to bowel edema and a resultant adynamic ileus. These patients typically present with abdominal distention and nonfocal abdominal pain on examination, similar to a bowel obstruction. It is important to assess for cardiac risk factors, in addition to ruling out intra-abdominal abnormality before attributing abdominal pain to decompensated heart failure. In the pediatric population, children and adolescents with a new presentation of heart failure from dilated cardiomyopathies tend to present with abdominal complaints such as pain, anorexia, nausea, and vomiting.[11] Practitioners should have a higher index of suspicion in this younger patient population and incorporate cardiac laboratory tests, a chest radiograph, and even a bedside echocardiogram, into their initial workup.

CONDITIONS REQUIRING URGENT EVALUATION

Several conditions requiring urgent but noncritical evaluation may also present with abdominal pain. Diseases such as community-acquired pneumonia, sickle cell disease, hereditary angioedema, mushroom intoxication, black widow spider envenomation, adrenal crisis, and hematologic malignancies require urgent evaluation by a practitioner.

Community-Acquired Pneumonia

Community-acquired pneumonia has been associated with abdominal pain in select patient populations. Although adult patients with community-acquired pneumonia tend to present with productive cough, fever, and malaise, pediatric patients often complain solely of abdominal pain. The pathophysiology behind abdominal pain in patients with pneumonia is multifaceted. In patients with lower lobar pneumonias, diaphragmatic irritation from infiltrates can cause upper abdominal pain and occasionally mimic cholecystitis, particularly in adults.[12] Authors of case reports in the pediatric population of acute abdomens from lower lobar and retrocardiac pneumonias attributed the abdominal complaint to innervation by the lowest intercostal nerves of both the lower costal pleura and the anterior abdominal wall.[13] In addition, there are case reports of reactive mesenteric adenitis from lobar or segmental pneumonias, often mimicking acute appendicitis in the pediatric population.[14] It is important to consider chest radiographs in patients who present with fevers and productive cough, despite their complaint of abdominal pain, given the possibility of referred pain from an extra-abdominal cause.

Sickle Cell Disease

Sickle cell disease, a hemoglobinopathy characterized by a genetic variation in the β-globin chain of hemoglobin, is a common hematologic condition. During periods of illness, dehydration, or hypoxia, sickle red blood cells tend to become inflexible, occluding small venules and leading to microinfarcts. Patients experience severe pain, often localized to the abdomen. Abdominal pain in the sickle cell population should be approached similarly to abdominal pain in other patient populations. In the sickle cell population, a complete blood count with differential and reticulocyte count should also be drawn in addition to traditional abdominal pain laboratory tests.

Sickle cell hemoglobin C and hemoglobin SC-thalassemia patients tend to be prone to splenic infarction due to high viscosity blood from normal hemoglobin counts. These patients present with left upper quadrant pain, nausea, and vomiting and may have a friction rub on cardiac examination.[15] Splenic sequestration occurs when high volumes of red blood cells pool in the spleen due to an unclear cause. Patients tend to be young and have splenomegaly, hypotension, anemia, and very high reticulocyte counts.[16] Definitive treatment is splenectomy.

Hepatic sequestration can also occur. Patients complain of right upper quadrant pain due to microinfarction of the liver. Patients tend to have a mild transaminitis that improves over 1 to 2 weeks without intervention. Patients can have mesenteric microthrombi precluding them to bowel necrosis, particularly during pain crises. These patients tend to present similarly to patients with mesenteric ischemia. Abdominal pain is nonfocal, often out of proportion to examination. In patients who appear toxic, resuscitation is key, as is early surgical intervention. In patients with less clear-cut symptoms, a thorough evaluation including complete blood counts with differentials and reticulocyte counts, in addition to abdominal laboratory tests: complete metabolic profile, liver function panel, and lipase, must be considered. Hydration is crucial, as is pain control. The practitioner should consider advanced imaging such as CT scans of the abdomen and pelvis with intravenous (IV) contrast to evaluate for evidence of bowel necrosis.

Patients with sickle cell disease are also susceptible to pneumonias from encapsulated organisms; therefore, as mentioned above, a chest radiograph, especially in patients with upper respiratory complaints, is reasonable. Only when intra-abdominal abnormality is ruled out should the practitioner attribute a sickle cell patient's pain to a pain crisis.

Hereditary Angioedema

Hereditary angioedema (HAE) is a condition characterized by either a defect or a deficiency in the C1 receptor resulting in excess bradykinin production. Angioedema attacks may be precipitated by stress, trauma, infection, or hormonal fluctuations. As a result, patients have vasodilation and edema, particularly affecting the skin, upper airways, and gastrointestinal system. These patients present with vague abdominal pain, nausea, and vomiting, as well as airway complaints. Because of excessive vasodilation, patients tend to feel light-headed. They will not have pruritus or hives, because HAE does not affect the histamine pathway or mast cells; these symptoms separate HAE from allergic reaction or anaphylaxis. Providers should initially ensure a patient's airway is intact without evidence of oral edema. Patients with airway concerns should be intubated early.

Abdominal pain initially begins as mild discomfort. With worsening edema, patients experience abdominal distention and even ascites. Nausea and vomiting follow thereafter, with progression of intestinal edema leading to obstruction. Patients may have dilated loops of bowel on radiography.[17] Eventually the nausea begins to subside, but patients experience an exponential increase in the severity of their pain. Patients may appear to have an acute abdomen and often undergo multiple unnecessary surgical procedures in their lifetime. Symptoms peak around 1 to 3 days and resolve spontaneously thereafter. In addition to monitoring electrolytes, providers should acquire imaging to rule out any surgical cause. ED care is primarily supportive with hydration, antiemetics, and pain control. Several treatment options currently exist, including C1 and kallikrein inhibitors. These treatment options are very expensive and, if used, should be administered early and with the assistance of a pharmacist. Traditionally, fresh frozen plasma (FFP) was used, because it contains C1 esterase inhibitor to replenish low supplies. FFP, similar to all blood products, carries a risk of blood-borne pathogens, and there is anecdotal evidence that angioedema can be worsened by the kinin, which is also found in FFP. Regardless, FFP should be used when C1 and kallikrein inhibitors are not available, because it is effective during HAE attacks.[18] There is no role for antihistamines or steroids in these patients.

Amanita Intoxication

Several toxic ingestions may present with abdominal pain. There are at least 50 species of mushrooms that are poisonous to humans. *Amanita* mushrooms account for more than 90% of fatal mushroom poisonings in the world, but are rare in the United States[19] and limited to the coastal Pacific Northwest, Pennsylvania, New Jersey, and Ohio. Amatoxins are found in several mushrooms, including *Amanita*, *Lepiota*, and *Galerina* species. Amatoxins primarily include α-, β-, and γ-amanitins, with the α-amanitin being most dangerous. This toxin is absorbed intestinally before being excreted into bile and shunted into the enterohepatic circulation for clearance. The toxin has a lengthy enterohepatic clearance, absorption by hepatocytes, and hepatocellular necrosis that places patients at risk for fulminant hepatic failure. Of the *Amanita* species, *Amanita phalloides* is associated with the highest morbidity and mortality.

A phalloides poisoning occurs in 3 stages. The initial stage, or incubation stage, is an asymptomatic stage that occurs within 6 to 12 hours of mushroom consumption. The second stage, typically 6 to 16 hours after consumption, is known as the gastrointestinal stage. In this stage, phalloidin, another enterotoxin, causes gastroenteritis-like symptoms due to alteration in the cell membrane of enterocytes.[20] These patients will present with nonspecific gastrointestinal symptoms such as non-focal abdominal pain, nausea, vomiting, and diarrhea. Symptoms last approximately 24 hours. The final stage, known as the cytotoxic stage, is associated with highest morbidities and mortalities. This stage is α-amanitin-mediated, and patients present in hepatic failure with jaundice, coagulopathy, and encephalopathy. To worsen the clinical picture, the enterotoxin continues to cycle between the intestinal and entero-hepatic circulation, perpetuating hepatocyte necrosis. Practitioners should have a high index of suspicion in patients with known mushroom consumption or new onset hepatic failure. It is important to check electrolytes, liver function tests, a coagulation profile, and ammonia in patients with suspected amanita poisoning.

Treatment includes repeated activated charcoal (as often as every 2–4 hours), because this may prevent intestinal absorption of the toxin. Because of the latency phase, patients tend to present later in their course, and most sources still advise giving activated charcoal even if a significant amount of time has passed since inges-tion.[21] Additional treatment regimens center on agents that compete with the ama-toxin for binding sites. Penicillin G competes with amatoxin for binding sites on serum proteins and prevents uptake by hepatocytes. IV dosing is 1,000,000 IU/kg for the first day, followed by 500,000 IU/kg for 2 days. Silibinin, a silymarin derivative, acts similarly to penicillin G by competing with amatoxin for binding sites on trans-membrane transporters, preventing the amatoxin from penetrating hepatocytes. Silibinin may also reduce enterohepatic recirculation. It must be used within 48 hours of ingestion to be effective. IV dosing is 20 to 50 mg/kg/d for 48 to 96 hours. Studies have not shown a benefit to combining silibinin with penicillin G. N-acetylcysteine, known for its hepatic free radical scavenging effects, may be beneficial, despite the lack of confirmatory data. The IV dose is 150 mg/kg over 15 minutes, followed by 50 mg/kg over 4 hours, followed by 100 mg/kg over 16 hours. In patients with wors-ening liver failure despite the aggressive use of antidotes, liver transplantation may be the only solution.

Black Widow Spider Envenomation

Black widow spider bites, another rare toxidrome, may present with abdominal pain. Black widow spiders (*Latrodectus mactans*) are the most toxic of the *Latrodectus* genus. The female black widow spiders are approximately 2 cm long with a red-orange hourglass on their abdomen. Bites tend to be small and often go unnoticed by patients. α-Latrotoxin, the toxin released with black widow envenomations, opens cation channels in presynaptic neurons, resulting in a massive release of various neurotransmitters (primarily norepinephrine and acetylcholine), leading to neurologic and autonomic symptoms. Symptoms typically begin within 1 hour of envenomation and include pain, anxiety, agitation, and autonomic dysfunction, including hyperten-sion, tachycardia, and diaphoresis.[22] Patients experience muscle cramping of large muscle groups, including extremities, back, and abdomen. Often patients can have abdominal rigidity that mimics that of an acute abdomen. Initial laboratory tests aim to rule out other causes of a patient's symptoms, and any pertinent imaging should be used in a similar fashion. Care is primarily supportive. Antivenin (*L mactans*) is immunoglobulin G derived from horses inoculated with black widow venom. Relief is typically experienced after a single (2.5 mL) vial, but no prospective trials have confirmed an outcome benefit of the administration of antivenin.[23] Opioids are frequently needed for pain control. Calcium gluconate and benzodiazepines were historically used but few studies support their usage. Deaths from *L mactans* envenomations are quite rare, and patients tend to require hospital admission solely for pain control.

Adrenal Crisis

Adrenal crisis is primarily a state of mineralocorticoid deficiency.[24] It is precipitated by stress or infection, particularly in patients who have chronic undiagnosed adrenal insufficiency or patients who are unable to take their stress doses of glucocorticoids during illness due to protracted nausea and vomiting. Patients on chronic oral or inhaled steroids who abruptly stop their steroid regimens may also experience a crisis.

There are case reports of patients in adrenal crisis who present with acute abdomens; the mechanism is unclear. Similarly to other abdominal pain mimics, clinicians who encounter patients with known adrenal insufficiency and abdominal pain should rule out other pathologic causes of abdominal pain. Assessing electrolytes, a liver function panel, and lipase, in addition to performing a thorough abdominal examination and acquiring imaging, as the data and examination suggest, is imperative to ensuring that an intra-abdominal cause for a patient's abdominal pain is not missed. Untreated adrenal crises end in significant morbidity and mortality. These patients are very ill and necessitate admission for further evaluation, including hypothalamic-pituitary axis testing, and treatment.

As a result, patients present most commonly with hypovolemia and hypotension. Resuscitation, in these patients, is the priority. Patients should receive 1 to 3 L of normal saline, unless they require dextrose solutions (5% dextrose) for hypoglycemia, within the first 12 to 24 hours of presentation. Steroids also play a major role in resuscitation. In patients with known adrenal insufficiency in crisis, the clinician should administer 100 mg IV hydrocortisone promptly. The patient should receive 50 mg IV hydrocortisone every 8 hours thereafter. Hydrocortisone has mineralocorticoid properties, which eliminate the need for additional mineralocorticoid administration. In patients with undiagnosed adrenal insufficiency, the provider should consider giving 4 mg IV dexamethasone instead of hydrocortisone because it does not alter serum cortisol levels. Electrolyte monitoring also is crucial in the patient presenting with adrenal crisis. These patients have hyponatremia and hyperkalemia from aldosterone deficiency. With normal saline boluses and mineralocorticoid properties of hydrocortisone, patients tend to improve their electrolyte abnormalities within a few days.

Hematologic Malignancies

Patients with hematologic malignancies including leukemia and lymphoma can experience abdominal pain related to their underlying cancer. Neutropenic entercolitis (NEC) and spontaneous splenic rupture are 2 conditions associated with hematologic malignancies that may present to the ED with abdominal pain. NEC, also known as typhlitis, is a condition caused by breakdown of the gut membrane due to chemotherapy. The condition was first identified in the pediatric population undergoing chemotherapy for leukemia, but has been seen in neutropenic patients of all ages, particularly those with underlying hematologic malignancies. The pathophysiology of NEC is multifactorial. Cytotoxic medications lead to compromise of the bowel wall integrity. Neutropenia (absolute neutrophil count <500 cells/μL) causes patients to have a poor immune response to injury and promotes the spread of microorganisms, both bacterial and fungal. As a result, they have a polymicrobial intestinal infection, typically of the cecum (thought to be due to its distensible nature and poor vascularity), that frequently leads to bowel necrosis. Patients present classically with right lower quadrant pain (although theoretically both the small and the large bowels can be affected) and a prolonged fever (tends to occur 2–3 weeks after chemotherapy) and are often bacteremic. Providers should consider NEC in febrile patients with abdominal pain on active chemotherapy, especially patients who recently received induction chemotherapy, severely neutropenic individuals, or patients on immunosuppressants. NEC is diagnosed radiographically. A CT scan with both oral and IV contrast should be performed, as a patient's renal function allows. Practitioners should avoid the use of barium enemas and colonoscopy in this population, because patients are prone to bowel perforation and subsequent bacteremia. CT scans will show evidence of bowel wall thickening, pneumatosis, or free air.[25] In patients with thrombocytopenia, intramural hemorrhage is also possible. Patients should have blood and urine cultures performed and started on an antibiotic regimen that covers *Pseudomonas aeruginosa*, *Escherichia coli*, other enteric gram-negative species, including anaerobes.[26] In patients without evidence of perforation, peritonitis, or severe bleeding, treatment should be conservative with bowel rest, IV hydration, pain control, and nasogastric tube insertion. Although neutropenic and immunocompromised populations are considered poor surgical candidates, if a patient has free air, uncontrolled hemorrhage from underlying coagulopathy, or clinical deterioration attributed to bowel necrosis, surgical intervention is indicated.

Spontaneous splenic rupture is a rare condition associated with hematologic malignancies that presents with abdominal pain. Occasionally, splenic rupture precedes a patient's cancer diagnosis. The pathophysiology of spontaneous splenic rupture is unclear but thought to be due to 3 mechanisms. First, the spleen is infiltrated by malignant lymphoproliferative and myeloproliferative cells. Because the splenic capsule is not distensible, it becomes prone to capsular rupture and subsequent splenic hemorrhage. Second, thrombocytopenia, common with myelodysplastic, predisposes these patients to hemorrhage. Finally, patients with hematologic malignancies are prone to splenic infarctions, which alter the vasculature of the spleen, increasing the likelihood of rupture.[27] Patients present with severe left upper quadrant pain and are often in hemorrhagic shock. Clinicians should have a high index of suspicion for spontaneous splenic rupture in patients with known hematologic malignancies who recently received induction chemotherapy who present with left upper quadrant pain and hypotension. These patients may decompensate quickly. Bedside ultrasound can assess for hemoperitoneum, but providers may consider CT scans to assess hemodynamically stable patients. Clinicians should check a complete blood count with differential, in addition to basic abdominal laboratory tests: electrolytes, a liver function panel, and lipase. Providers should use blood products to transfuse hypotensive patients and involve surgery early, as splenectomy is frequently necessary.

UNUSUAL CAUSES TO CONSIDER

Beyond the life-threatening and urgent causes, there are a wide variety of unusual causes of abdominal pain. These causes include acute intermittent porphyria, rheumatologic diseases, infectious causes, neurologic causes, and functional causes.

Acute Intermittent Porphyria

Porphyrias encompass 8 metabolic disorders of heme biosynthesis. They lead to skin lesions, neurologic symptoms, and visceral symptoms. Porphyrias are separated into acute porphyrias, chronic cutaneous porphyrias, and rare recessive porphyrias. A subset of acute porphyrias, the acute intermittent porphyrias, present with intermittent attacks of severe abdominal pain.[28,29] Other signs and symptoms include nausea, vomiting, dark reddish urine, constipation or diarrhea, sweating, tachycardia, and hypertension.[29–31] Patients often become dehydrated and develop electrolyte abnormalities, particularly hyponatremia, which is seen in 40% of cases.[29] Neurologic complications may also occur, including seizures, neuropathy, paresis, and alterations of consciousness ranging from apathy to agitation.[29,32] Testing a 24-hour urine sample for porphyrins makes the diagnosis. Attacks can be triggered by hormonal changes during menstruation, fasting, smoking, alcohol abuse, sun overexposure, infections, and certain medications.[28–30,32] Management includes discontinuing any contributing medications and supportive care. Electrolyte abnormalities should be corrected.[28] Acute intermittent porphyrias are rare autosomal-dominant disorders, although they have low penetrance, with only 10% to 20% of carriers exhibiting symptoms.[30–32] The chronic cutaneous porphyrias and rare recessive porphyrias typically do not cause abdominal pain.[29,32]

Systemic Lupus Erythematosus

Up to 40% of patients with systemic lupus erythematosus may develop abdominal pain secondary to intestinal vasculitis, otherwise known as lupus enteritis.[33,34] The pain typically presents insidiously, developing pain over hours to days and without peritoneal signs, with associated nausea, vomiting, diarrhea, fever, and tachycardia.[33,35] Occasionally, bowel ischemia can result, leading to perforation and hemorrhage.[35,36] Diagnosis can be made with CT scanning, which shows bowel wall thickening, a "target sign" of increased bowel wall enhancement, intestinal segment dilation, enlarged mesenteric vessels, and increased attenuation of mesenteric fat.[34] Treatment consists of high-dose corticosteroids or cyclophosphamide.[33–35] Patients with an acute abdomen, and patients who do not respond to treatment, should have evaluation to look for other causes of abdominal pain, such as peptic ulcer disease, pancreatitis, pelvic inflammatory disease, appendicitis, and cholecystitis.[33,36]

Henoch-Schönlein Purpura

Henoch-Schönlein purpura is the most common vasculitis in children and is associated with gastrointestinal complaints in 50% to 75% of patients. The most common manifestation is colicky abdominal pain, which is thought to be due to bowel ischemia, although patients may have bleeding, ulcers, intussusception, or pneumatosis intestinalis.[37,38] Abdominal pain may precede or follow the classic rash of palpable purpura on the abdomen, buttocks, and lower extremities.[38] After exclusion of significant abdominal abnormality, treatment consists of corticosteroids.[37,39]

Polyarteritis Nodosa

Polyarteritis nodosa is a necrotizing vasculitis, which affects medium-sized vessels.[40] It commonly involves the renal arteries, resulting in hypertension, but may affect multiple organ systems.[41] When the gastrointestinal tract is involved, patients may exhibit abdominal pain and gastrointestinal bleeding.[40] Diagnosis can be difficult in the ED because patients have nonspecific symptoms and laboratory findings, usually requiring testing for specific antibodies.[41] Treatment with corticosteroids and cyclophosphamide is effective.[40,41]

Lemierres Syndrome

Lemierre syndrome (LS) is a rare complication of tonsillopharyngitis, which was more common in the preantibiotic era.[42] LS is caused by *Fusobacterium necrophorum* in 70% to 80% of cases, but *Streptococcus*, *Bacteroides*, *Peptostreptococcus*, and *Eikenella* species may also lead to its development. In LS, the bacteria penetrate the parapharyngeal space to the posterior lateral compartment of the neck, seeding the internal jugular vein. The resulting thrombophlebitis of the vein then leads to septic emboli to the lungs, liver, and spleen.[42–44] Abdominal pain may come from primary abdominal abnormality as well as from referred pain from pleural complications. Patients present with signs of severe sepsis, and symptoms of a throat infection may have resolved by the time of presentation, which may lead to a delay in diagnosis.[42] In patients in whom LS is suspected, the internal jugular vein should be examined by ultrasound for evidence of thrombophlebitis, although CT and MRI may also be used.[42,44] Although LS was fatal in the preantibiotic era, recovery is good with appropriate antibiotic treatment, with a 6% mortality rate.[42,44,45] The use of anticoagulants is controversial.[44,45]

Tuberculosis

Abdominal tuberculosis is a rare manifestation of extrapulmonary tuberculosis, affecting 3% to 5% of patients.[46] It can affect any part of the gastrointestinal system, including the bowel, peritoneum, and hepatobiliary system.[47] Patients have nonspecific symptoms, but most commonly present with abdominal pain, ascites, abdominal distension, fever, and weight loss.[46,47] Complications include bowel perforation, bowel obstruction from strictures, and abscess formation.[47,48] Ascitic fluid, if present, can be sent for mycobacterial cultures, although the results may not be available for 6 weeks.[46]

Lyme Disease

Lyme disease is caused by *Borrelia burgdorferi*, transmitted by an Ixodid tick bite. Patients present with a variety of musculoskeletal, neurologic, and cardiovascular symptoms. Neurologic symptoms typically cause pain, which can include abdominal pain. The diagnosis is supported when the history includes a tick bite and the classic rash of erythema migrans; however, 50% of patients do not recall a tick bite and cutaneous findings are absent in 20%.[49] Lyme disease typically resolves with antibiotic treatment using doxycycline, amoxicillin, or cefuroxime.[50]

Varicella Zoster

Varicella zoster, or shingles, is an acute reactivation of the latent varicella zoster virus, which resides in dorsal root ganglia, cranial nerve, and enteric ganglia cells after chickenpox.[51,52] Patients typically report onset of pain before onset of the pathognomonic rash. If the dermatome affected overlies the abdomen, patients may present to the ED complaining of abdominal pain.[51] In addition, although rare, patients may develop visceral zoster, which may mimic an acute abdomen or lead to complications such as colonic pseudo-obstruction.[51–53] Treatment with antivirals is effective.[52,53]

Abdominal Epilepsy

Abdominal epilepsy is an unusual cause of chronic, recurrent abdominal pain. Diagnosis is made by 4 criteria: paroxysmal gastrointestinal complaints that are unexplained by other testing (pain, nausea, vomiting, bloating, diarrhea), central nervous system complaints (headache, confusion, fatigue, dizziness), electroencephalogram with findings specific for seizure disorder (temporal lobe seizures, generalized spike and wave discharges, and frontal lobe seizures), and improvement with anticonvulsant medications.[54–56] Treatment can be initiated with carbamazepine, phenytoin, and valproic acid.[56]

Abdominal Migraine

Abdominal migraines are a variant of migraine headaches, which typically appear during childhood and adolescence.[57,58] Diagnostic criteria include the following:

a. At least 5 attacks meeting criteria B–D
b. Attacks of abdominal pain lasting 1 to 72 hours
c. Pain which is midline, periumbilical, or poorly localized, dull or sore in nature, and of moderate to severe intensity
d. At least 2 associated symptoms of anorexia, nausea, vomiting, or pallor
e. Symptoms are not attributable to another cause.

Patients should avoid triggers, such as alcohol, stress, and certain foods, and may be treated with abortive migraine medications.[58]

PEARLS AND PITFALLS

- Abdominal pain mimics are medical conditions that cause the sensation of abdominal pain without abdominal abnormality.
- Clinicians should initially rule out all intra-abdominal causes of abdominal pain.
- Cannot miss diagnoses, which may present with abdominal pain, include
  o Atypical ACS
  o Diabetic ketoacidosis
  o PE
  o Congestive heart failure
- Some abdominal pain mimics require urgent intervention, including
  o Lower lobe pneumonia
  o Sickle cell disease
  o HAE
  o Amantia poisoning
  o Black widow spider envenomation
  o Adrenal crisis
  o Hematologic malignancies
- Once the life-threatening abdominal pain mimics have been ruled out, the ED practitioner may want to consider some unusual causes of abdominal pain, including porphyrias, lupus enteritis, Henoch-Schonlein purpura, polyarteritis nodosa, Lemierre syndrome, tuberculosis, Lyme disease, herpes zoster, abdominal epilepsy, and abdominal migraine.

REFERENCES

1. Bhuiya F, Pitts SR, McCaig LF. Emergency department visits for chest pain and abdominal pain: United States, 1999–2008. Hyattsville (MD): National Center for Health Statistics; 2010. NCHS data brief, no 43.
2. US National Center for Health Statistics. National Vital Statistics Reports. Deaths: preliminary data for 2010. 2012. Available at: http://www.cdc.gov/nchs/data/nvsr/nvsr60/nvsr60_04.pdf. Accessed August 28, 2015.
3. Grech ED, Ramsdale DR. Acute coronary syndrome: unstable angina and non-ST segment elevation myocardial infarction. BMJ 2003;326:1259–61.
4. Brieger D, Eagle KA, Goodman SG, et al, GRACE Investigators. Acute coronary syndromes without chest pain, an underdiagnosed and undertreated high-risk group: insights from the Global Registry of Acute Coronary Events. Chest 2004;126:461–9.

5. Hwang SY, Park EH, Shin ES, et al. Comparison of factors associated with atypical symptoms in younger and older patients with acute coronary syndrome. J Korean Med Sci 2009;24(5):789–94.
6. Umpierrez G, Freire AX. Abdominal pain in patients with hyperglycemic crises. J Crit Care 2002;17(1):63–7.
7. Israel HL, Goldstein F. The varied clinical manifestations of pulmonary embolism. Ann Intern Med 1957;47:202–26.
8. Gantner J, Keffeler JE, Derr C. Pulmonary embolism: an abdominal pain masquerader. J Emerg Trauma Shock 2013;6:280–2.
9. Potts DE, Sahn SA. Abdominal manifestations of pulmonary embolism. JAMA 1976;235(26):2835–7.
10. Ho KK, Pinsky JL, Kannel WB, et al. The epidemiology of heart failure: the Framingham Study. J Am Coll Cardiol 1993;22:6A.
11. Hollander SA, Addonizio LJ, Chin C, et al. Abdominal complaints as a common first presentation of heart failure in adolescents with dilated cardiomyopathy. Am J Emerg Med 2013;31:684.
12. Armeni E, Mylona V, Karlis G, et al. Pneumonia presenting with lower right abdominal pain and migratory polyarthritis. Respir Med Case Rep 2012;5:29–30.
13. Pezone I, Iezzi ML, Leone S. Retrocardiac pneumonia mimicking acute abdomen: a diagnostic challenge. Pediatr Emerg Care 2012;28(11):1230–1.
14. Swischuk L. Acute abdomen: suspected appendicitis: computer topography: surprise. Pediatr Emerg Care 2010;26(7):536–7.
15. Ebert E, Nagar N, Hagspiel K. Gastrointestinal and hepatic complications of sickle cell disease. Clin Gastroenterol Hepatol 2010;8(6):483–9.
16. Dickerhoff R. Splenic sequestration in patients with sickle cell disease. Klin Padiatr 2002;214(2):70–3.
17. Longhurst H, Cicardi M. Hereditary angio-oedema. Lancet 2012;379(9814):474–81.
18. Buyantseva LV, Sardana N, Craig TJ. Update on treatment of hereditary angioedema. Asian Pac J Allergy Immunol 2012;30:89–98.
19. Chen W-C, Kassi M, Saeed U, et al. A rare case of amatoxin poisoning in the state of Texas. Case Rep Gastroenterol 2012;6(2):350–7.
20. Santi L, Maggioli C, Mastroroberto M, et al. Acute liver failure caused by Amanita phalloides poisoning. Int J Hepatol 2012;2012:487480.
21. Enjalbert F, Rapior S, Nouguier-Soulé J. Treatment of amatoxin poisoning: 20-year retrospective analysis. J Toxicol Clin Toxicol 2002;40:715–57.
22. Dart RC, Bogdan G, Heard K, et al. A randomized, double-blind, placebo-controlled trial of a highly purified equine F(ab) antibody black widow spider antivenom. Ann Emerg Med 2013;61:458–67.
23. Offerman SR, Daubert GP, Clark RF. The treatment of black widow spider envenomation with antivenin latrodectus mactans: a case series. Perm J 2011;15(3):76–81.
24. Cronin CC, Callaghan N, Kearney PJ, et al. Addison disease in patients treated with glucocorticoid therapy. Arch Intern Med 1997;157(4):456–8.
25. Kirkpatrick IDC, Greenberg HM. Gastrointestinal complications in the neutropenic patient: characterization and differentiation with abdominal CT. Radiology 2003;226(3):668–74.
26. Cloutier R. Neutropenic enterocolitis. Emerg Med Clin North Am 2009;27(3):415–22.
27. Goddard SL, Chesney AE, Reis MD. Pathological splenic rupture: a rare complication of chronic myelomonocytic leukemia. Am J Hematol 2007;82:405–8.

28. Besur S, Schmeltzer P, Bonkovsky HL. Acute porphyrias. J Emerg Med 2015; 49(3):305–12.
29. Puy H, Gouya L, Deybach JC. Porphyrias. Lancet 2010;375(9718):924–37.
30. Klobucić M, Sklebar D, Ivanac R, et al. Differential diagnosis of acute abdominal pain–acute intermittent porphyria. Med Glas (Zenica) 2011;8(2):298–300.
31. Mungan NÖ, Yilmaz BS, Nazoglu S, et al. A 17-year-old girl with chronic intermittent abdominal pain. Acute intermittent porphyria. Pediatr Ann 2015;44(4): 139–41.
32. Ventura P, Cappellini MD, Biolcati G, et al. A challenging diagnosis for potential fatal diseases: recommendations for diagnosing acute porphyrias. Eur J Intern Med 2014;25(6):497–505.
33. Buck AC, Serebro LH, Quinet RJ. Subacute abdominal pain requiring hospitalization in a systemic lupus erythematosus patient: a retrospective analysis and review of the literature. Lupus 2001;10(7):491–5.
34. Lee CK, Ahn MS, Lee EY, et al. Acute abdominal pain in systemic lupus erythematosus: focus on lupus enteritis (gastrointestinal vasculitis). Ann Rheum Dis 2002;61(6):547–50.
35. Lian TY, Edwards CJ, Chan SP, et al. Reversible acute gastrointestinal syndrome associated with active systemic lupus erythematosus in patients admitted to hospital. Lupus 2003;12(8):612–6.
36. Kwok SK, Seo SH, Ju JH, et al. Lupus enteritis: clinical characteristics, risk factor for relapse and association with anti-endothelial cell antibody. Lupus 2007; 16(10):803–9.
37. McCarthy HJ, Tizard EJ. Clinical practice: diagnosis and management of Henoch–Schönlein purpura. Eur J Pediatr 2010;169(6):643–50.
38. Fatima A, Gibson DP. Pneumatosis intestinalis associated with Henoch-Schönlein purpura. Pediatrics 2014;134(3):e880–3.
39. Toshihiko K, Tomonobu A. Henoch-Schonlein purpura with preceding abdominal pain. Clin Case Rep 2015;3(6):513–4.
40. Aruny JE 1, Perazella MA. An odd case of hypertension. Am J Med 2006; 119(9):748–50.
41. Goodman R, Dellaripa PF, Miller AL, et al. Clinical problem-solving. An unusual case of abdominal pain. N Engl J Med 2014;370(1):70–5.
42. Hoehn S, Dominguez TE. Lemierre's syndrome: an unusual cause of sepsis and abdominal pain. Crit Care Med 2002;30(7):1644–7.
43. Isaac A, Baker N, Wood MJ. A young man with sore throat, acute abdomen and respiratory failure. J Postgrad Med 2003;49:166.
44. David HA. 21-year-old male with fever and abdominal pain after recent peritonsillar abscess drainage. Am J Emerg Med 2009;27(4):515.e3–4.
45. Thoufeeq MH, Salloum W, Win SS, et al. Lemierre's syndrome secondary to Fusobacterium necrophorum infection, a rare cause of hepatic abscess. Acta Gastroenterol Belg 2009;72(4):444–6.
46. Kılıç Ö, Somer A, Hançerli Törün S, et al. Assessment of 35 children with abdominal tuberculosis. Turk J Gastroenterol 2015;26(2):128–32.
47. Awasthi S, Saxena M, Ahmad F, et al. Abdominal tuberculosis: a diagnostic dilemma. J Clin Diagn Res 2015;9(5):EC01–3.
48. Elgendy AY, Mahmoud A, Elgendy IY. Abdominal pain and swelling as an initial presentation of spinal tuberculosis. BMJ Case Rep 2014. http://dx.doi.org/10. 1136/bcr-2013-202550.
49. Chan J, Ahmed A, Stacey B. Acute abdominal pain: an unusual medical cause. Acute Med 2009;8(1):26–8.

50. Shapiro ED. Clinical practice: Lyme disease. N Engl J Med 2014;370:1724–31.
51. Olmez D, Boz A, Erkan N. Varicella zoster infection: a rare cause of abdominal pain mimicking acute abdomen. J Clin Med Res 2009;1(4):247–8.
52. Gershon AA, Chen J, Gershon MD. Use of saliva to identify varicella zoster virus infection of the gut. Clin Infect Dis 2015;61(4):536–44.
53. Edelman DA, Antaki F, Basson MD, et al. Ogilvie syndrome and herpes zoster: case report and review of the literature. J Emerg Med 2010;39(5):696–700.
54. Dutta SR, Hazarika I, Chakravarty BP. Abdominal epilepsy, an uncommon cause of recurrent abdominal pain: a brief report. Gut 2007;56(3):439–41.
55. Kshirsagar VY, Nagarsenkar S, Ahmed M, et al. Abdominal epilepsy chronic recurrent abdominal pain. J Pediatr Neurosci 2012;7(3):163–6.
56. Mondal R, Sarkar S, Bag T, et al. A pediatric case series of abdominal epilepsy. World J Pediatr 2014;10(1):80–2.
57. D'Onofrio F, Cologno D, Buzzi MG, et al. Adult abdominal migraine: a new syndrome or sporadic feature of migraine headache? a case report. Eur J Neurol 2006;13(1):85–8.
58. Evans RW, Whyte C. Cyclic vomiting syndrome and abdominal migraine in adults and children. Headache 2013;53(6):984–93.

Index

Note: Page numbers of article titles are in **boldface** type.

Emerg Med Clin N Am 34 (2016) 425–433
http://dx.doi.org/10.1016/S0733-8627(16)30011-6
0733-8627/16/$ – see front matter © 2016 Elsevier Inc. All rights reserved.

Printed and bound by CPI Group (UK) Ltd, Croydon, CR0 4YY

11/05/2025

01866604-0001